EMBRACING THE HEART OF CAREGIVING

A COMPASSIONATE GUIDE FOR DEMENTIA CARE

RAE A. STONEHOUSE

LIVE FOR EXCELLENCE PRODUCTIONS

INTRODUCTION

Welcome to a journey that delves deep into the essence of caregiving, specifically tailored for those caring for loved ones with dementia. This guide serves as a beacon for navigating the complexities and challenges that come with dementia care, offering solace, understanding, and practical advice to support you through this profoundly transformative experience. It celebrates the resilience of the human spirit and aims to provide a source of comfort and hope for the path that lies ahead.

Caring for someone with dementia goes beyond the provision of physical care; it's about connecting on a soulful level, finding ways to communicate beyond words, and fostering moments of joy in confusion. It involves embracing vulnerability, both in ourselves and in those we care for, and nurturing a connection that reaches the core of our being.

Within these pages, you'll find a compilation of insights, stories, and strategies designed to guide you through the facets of dementia care. From confronting the initial challenges and managing the emotional impact to finding meaning and fulfillment in your role, this guide is here to offer the tools and perspectives needed to navigate your caregiving journey with empathy and resilience.

We begin by addressing the unique aspects of stepping into a caregiving role for someone with dementia, acknowledging the emotions and responsibilities that go along with this journey. Understanding the emotional terrain and mastering the practicalities of dementia care lay the groundwork for a nurturing caregiving experience.

As the journey progresses, the significance of self-care and resilience comes to the forefront. Recognizing that caregiving is a marathon, not a sprint, especially in the context of dementia, we share strategies for maintaining your well-being, establishing boundaries, and cultivating a support network that empowers and sustains you.

At the heart of dementia caregiving is the profound connection formed between caregiver and care recipient. We explore the transformative power of sharing personal stories, the solace found in community, and the deep impact of empathy and understanding. These connections not only enrich the caregiving experience but also promote a sense of belonging and mutual support.

Ultimately, we reflect on the transformative power of the dementia caregiving journey. Despite its inherent challenges, caregiving for someone with dementia can be an immensely rewarding source of personal growth, fulfillment, and strengthened relationships. It offers an opportunity to rediscover the depth of love, compassion, and humanity.

As a retired registered nurse with over 40 years in psychiatry and mental health, I never imagined my post-retirement role would be a caregiver. My wife, Sandra, also a retired nurse, began showing signs of dementia a few years ago. After working the night shift for 20 years, we thought her disorganization, trouble expressing herself, and periodic confusion might be from stopping her sleep medication. But after seeing her doctor and doing some tests, we found out she has frontal lobe dementia.

Sandra's ability to do daily tasks has been slowly declining. As her caregiver, I help her with these tasks while trying to keep her as independent as possible. Sometimes, it's a real challenge. For instance, I might have to ask her to "take your top off" up to 20 times when getting her ready for bed. She often can't follow simple instructions.

It's tough when she tries to talk to me but forgets her main point. I ask questions to understand her better, but it usually doesn't help. She also tends to ruminate, getting stuck on thoughts where she misunderstands and feels hurt by something I said.

Writing these paragraphs took me months. Thinking about her losses and what lies ahead often made me feel down. My nursing background helps me understand the dementia process, but it's different when it's your own loved one. I worry about her not recognizing me one day and having to find alternative living arrangements.

When we were both working, she cared for the elderly. I used to tease her, saying, "Okay, dear… you'll be staying with us from now on." Little did I know how true that might be.

So, I'm on this caregiving journey with you. Our paths will differ, but we'll share many experiences. My philosophy is to take each day as it comes and make the best of it. I believe every day above ground is a good one, and I try to make it the best I can with what I have.

This guide is an invitation to embrace the dementia caregiving journey with an open heart and a spirit of resilience. It honors the dedication and love that caregivers provide daily, often without recognition. May you find in these pages the encouragement, insight, and support you need to navigate your caregiving journey with grace and strength. Welcome to "Embracing the Heart of Caregiving: A Compassionate Guide for Dementia Care."

I wish you the best on your caregiving journey. I hope this book eases some of the anxiety you may feel. This isn't the path we chose, but it's the one we're on.

Warm regards, Rae A. Stonehouse

COPYRIGHT

ISBN:

Ebook: 978-1-998813-69-8

Paperback: 978-1-998813-70-4

Audiobook: 978-1-998813-71-1

∿

PART ONE
DEMENTIA ESSENTIALS: A CONCISE GUIDE FOR CAREGIVERS

Defining Dementia:

Let's begin by establishing a solid foundation: understanding the condition you're facing is important.

Dementia is a broad term that encompasses a range of cognitive impairments, including difficulties with thinking, memory, and decision-making, which significantly interfere with daily life. Rather than being a single disease, dementia is a collection of symptoms caused by various brain disorders. Let's explore some of the primary types of dementia you may encounter:

Alzheimer's Disease: As the most common form of dementia, Alzheimer's accounts for about 60-80% of all cases. This progressive condition gradually erodes an individual's ability to remember, think lucidly, and regulate emotions. While researchers are still unraveling the precise causes, evidence suggests that a combination of genetic, lifestyle, and environmental factors contribute to its development. Early detection and intervention can substantially improve quality of life and potentially slow the progression of symptoms.

Vascular Dementia: The second most common type, vascular dementia, represents around 10% of cases. It occurs when the brain is deprived of adequate blood supply, often due to a stroke or cardiovascular issues. Symptoms can vary significantly depending on the specific brain regions affected, underlining the importance of accurate diagnosis and targeted treatment.

Frontotemporal Dementia: This group of dementias primarily affects the frontal and temporal lobes of the brain and is less common than Alzheimer's or vascular dementia. Frontotemporal dementia can profoundly change an individual's personality, behavior, and language abilities. It usually manifests in younger individuals, typically those under 65.

Other forms of dementia include Lewy body dementia, Parkinson's disease dementia, and mixed dementia, which involves a combination of Alzheimer's and vascular dementia. Each type presents unique symptoms and progression patterns, emphasizing the critical nature of accurate diagnosis and personalized care plans.

Gaining a comprehensive understanding of the types of dementia and their underlying causes is essential for providing effective support to those living with the condition. Early recognition and interventions can significantly enhance an individual's quality of life and potentially slow the advancement of symptoms, underscoring the importance of timely action and informed care.

Dementia Dynamics: Recognizing Signs and Understanding Progression

Dementia is a condition that gradually affects the brain, affecting memory, thought processes, behavior, and the ability to carry out daily tasks. Recognizing the signs and understanding the typical progression of the condition can help individuals and their families seek support and care.

Common Symptoms of Dementia:

Memory Loss: One of the earliest signs of dementia is forgetting recent events, appointments, or conversations. Individuals may struggle to remember names or misplace objects often.

Cognitive Decline: Dementia can present challenges in reasoning, problem-solving, and decision-making. Tasks that require planning or complex thought become increasingly difficult to navigate.

Confusion: People with dementia may feel disoriented even in familiar surroundings or have trouble recognizing well-known faces.

Mood Changes: Dementia can trigger shifts in personality, such as increased irritability, anxiety, or even depression.

Communication Difficulties: Finding the right words, following conversations, or expressing thoughts coherently can become challenging for those with dementia.

As Dementia Progresses, Additional Challenges May Arise:

Difficulty with Self-Care: As the condition advances, basic personal care tasks like dressing or bathing can become increasingly difficult to manage independently.

Agitation and Aggression: Feelings of frustration or being overwhelmed may cause individuals to show more agitated or aggressive behavior.

Hallucinations and Delusions: In later stages, some individuals with dementia may experience hallucinations or hold beliefs that are not grounded in reality.

Loss of Mobility: Coordination and physical ability may decline over time, affecting the person's capacity to walk or perform various tasks.

Severe Memory Loss: As dementia progresses, recognizing loved ones or recalling significant life events can become increasingly challenging.

The progression of dementia can vary significantly from person to person. Factors such as the specific type of dementia, overall health, and individual characteristics can influence the trajectory of the condition. Early detection and effective management strategies can contribute to enhancing the quality of life for those living with dementia and provide invaluable support to their caregivers.

If you or someone you care about is showing signs of dementia, it is important to consult with a healthcare provider for a comprehensive assessment and guidance. They can offer personalized recommendations and connect you with relevant resources to navigate this challenging journey with greater understanding and support.

~

UNDERSTANDING DEMENTIA: THE VALUE OF EARLY DETECTION AND DIAGNOSIS

DEMENTIA IS a condition that significantly affects an individual's thinking, memory, and behavior. Early detection plays an important role in managing the condition effectively, as it opens doors to treatments and planning that can make a substantial difference in the lives of those affected. By identifying dementia early, individuals and their families can access support, better manage symptoms, and prepare for the challenges that lie ahead.

Cognitive Assessments: The First Step

The diagnostic process often begins with cognitive assessments, which are designed to evaluate an individual's thinking abilities, including memory, attention, language, and problem-solving skills. These assessments provide a baseline measurement of cognitive function and can be used to track changes over time, helping to identify early signs of dementia. When cognitive assessments indicate potential concerns, further evaluations may be recommended to confirm the diagnosis.

Brain Imaging: Visualizing the Inner Workings

Advanced imaging techniques, such as magnetic resonance imaging (MRI) and positron emission tomography (PET) scans, provide valuable insights into the brain's structure and function. These scans can identify changes associated with specific types of dementia, such as Alzheimer's disease or vascular dementia. Additionally, brain imaging can help rule out other potential causes of memory problems, such as tumors or strokes, ensuring an accurate diagnosis.

Comprehensive Diagnostic Approach

Beyond brain scans and cognitive assessments, healthcare professionals use a range of diagnostic tools to evaluate individuals suspected of having dementia. Blood tests can detect markers of brain dysfunction or inflammation, while genetic testing can identify individuals at higher risk for certain forms of dementia. Neuropsychological testing provides a more in-depth assessment of cognitive functions, aiding in the differentiation between various types of dementia.

The Significance of Early Detection

Early detection of dementia is imperative, as it presents opportunities to slow disease progression, alleviate symptoms through medication, cognitive training, and lifestyle changes. An early diagnosis also lets individuals and their families plan for the future, explore care options, and participate in clinical trials for novel treatments. Early detection helps combat the stigma surrounding dementia, fostering a better understanding and support system for those affected by the condition.

Chapter Summary:

Early detection of dementia is important for providing the best care and support to individuals and their loved ones. Using tools such as cognitive assessments and brain imaging, healthcare professionals can identify dementia in its early stages, enabling timely interventions and support. By raising awareness about the importance of early detection, we can collectively work toward improving the quality of life for those living with dementia and their families.

NAVIGATING THE CHALLENGES OF DAILY LIFE WITH DEMENTIA

DEMENTIA PROFOUNDLY AFFECTS the lives of those experiencing the condition and their loved ones who provide care and support. Beyond memory loss, dementia affects communication, independence, and the ability to perform everyday tasks. Understanding these changes is important for everyone involved to adapt and support one another effectively.

Communication Challenges:

Individuals with dementia often encounter difficulties in engaging in conversations as they once did. They may struggle to find the right words, comprehend others, or feel disoriented in familiar surroundings. These challenges can transform simple interactions or following instructions into significant obstacles, leading to feelings of frustration and isolation.

Shifting Independence:

Dementia can erode an individual's ability to perform tasks they previously managed independently, such as dressing, preparing meals, or managing finances. This shift in independence can be emotionally challenging for both the person with dementia and their loved ones, evoking feelings of anxiety, sadness, and a sense of loss over the changes in their identity and capabilities.

Adapting Daily Activities:

Even routine activities like bathing, eating, and mobility can become increasingly difficult as dementia progresses. As the condition advances, the individual may require more assistance, placing more demands on caregivers. Managing behavioral changes, memory issues, and confusion adds another layer of complexity to maintaining a consistent routine and fostering a sense of normalcy.

Supporting Caregivers:

Caring for someone with dementia can be physically, emotionally, and mentally taxing. Caregivers often face unique challenges, such as managing their own well-being while providing round-the-clock support. Caregivers must have access to resources, respite services, and support networks to maintain their own health and resilience throughout the caregiving journey.

Chapter Summary:

Life with dementia is multifaceted and requires immense patience, understanding, and compassion. Ensuring those affected by dementia receive care and support is important in managing the daily challenges they face. Equally important is giving caregivers the resources and support to deliver the best care while maintaining their own well-being.

By deepening our understanding of how dementia impacts daily life, we can work toward enhancing the quality of life for individuals with dementia and their caregivers. This includes promoting awareness, developing innovative care strategies, and fostering a supportive community that recognizes and addresses the unique needs of those navigating the complex journey of dementia.

~

THE VITAL ROLE OF CAREGIVERS IN SUPPORTING INDIVIDUALS WITH DEMENTIA:

CAREGIVERS FORM the foundation of care for individuals living with dementia, providing the essential physical, emotional, and cognitive support crucial for their well-being. This role requires dedication, compassion, and resilience, as it directly affects the quality of life of those affected by dementia. Let's explore the various aspects of caregiving and emphasize the importance of supporting caregivers themselves.

Physical Support:

Caregivers help with daily living activities, such as bathing, dressing, eating, mobility, and medication management. These tasks require patience, clear communication, and a thorough understanding of the individual's abilities and needs. Ensuring the safety and physical well-being of someone with dementia is a significant responsibility that caregivers undertake.

Emotional Support:

Dementia can be an emotional roller coaster for those experiencing it, often leading to feelings of confusion, frustration, and anxiety. Caregivers provide comfort, reassurance, and a supportive presence, creating a nurturing environment that combats loneliness and helps the individual feel understood and connected to their loved ones. Maintaining social connections and engagement is a critical part of emotional support.

Cognitive Support:

Engaging in mentally stimulating activities is essential for individuals with dementia. Caregivers play an important role in helping with activities that promote cognitive stimulation, such as memory exercises, puzzles, or reminiscence therapy. Establishing a structured daily routine that supports cognitive health and overall well-being can significantly contribute to maintaining cognitive function and mental wellness.

Importance of Caregiver Self-Care:

While caregivers often focus on the needs of those they care for, it is crucial that they also attend to their own well-being. Caregiving can be emotionally and physically demanding, and without proper self-care, caregivers may experience burnout. Engaging in self-care activities, such as exercise, relaxation techniques, social support, and respite care, is essential for caregivers to maintain their own health and resilience.

Supportive Resources for Caregivers:

Caregivers should not feel alone in their journey. Many resources are available to provide support, education, and guidance. These may include caregiver support groups, educational programs, respite care services, and counseling. Accessing these resources can help caregivers navigate the challenges they face, learn effective strategies, and connect with others who understand their experiences.

Caregivers play an important role in supporting individuals living with dementia, significantly enhancing their quality of life. However, it is equally important to recognize and support the needs of caregivers themselves. By focusing on caregiver well-being and providing access to supportive resources, we can make sure caregivers are equipped to continue their invaluable work.

Supporting caregivers is not only beneficial for their own health and resilience but also directly affects the quality of care they provide to individuals with dementia. By fostering a supportive environment for caregivers, we can help maintain the dignity, independence, and overall well-being of those living with dementia.

~

NAVIGATING DEMENTIA CARE: EXPLORING TREATMENT APPROACHES

Dementia poses significant challenges to the mind, affecting memory, cognitive abilities, and daily functioning. Although there is no cure for dementia, various strategies can be used to manage symptoms and enhance the quality of life for those affected. Let's explore these approaches, which include medication, cognitive exercises, and lifestyle changes.

Medication:

Pharmacological interventions are available to help manage dementia symptoms, particularly in the early stages of the condition. These medications work by either increasing brain chemicals associated with memory and cognitive processes or regulating neurotransmitters to improve cognitive function. Commonly prescribed medications include cholinesterase inhibitors such as donepezil, rivastigmine galantamine and memantine. It is important to work closely with a healthcare professional to determine the most appropriate medication and dosage based on individual needs and medical history.

Cognitive Exercises:

Cognitive training involves engaging in specific activities and exercises designed to stimulate and improve brain functions like memory, attention, and problem-solving skills. These exercises can be performed individually or in a group setting and may include puzzles, memory games, and tasks that challenge cognitive abilities. Research suggests that regular participation in cognitive training activities can help slow down cognitive decline and promote brain health. Caregivers can work with healthcare professionals to develop a personalized cognitive training program tailored to the individual's abilities and interests.

Lifestyle Modifications:

Lifestyle changes are an essential part of managing dementia. This approach focuses on promoting brain health through regular physical exercise, a balanced and nutritious diet, adequate sleep, social engagement, and mentally stimulating activities. Exercise has been shown to have positive effects on cognitive function and may reduce the risk of developing dementia. Encouraging individuals with dementia to stay socially connected and engage in hobbies that challenge the brain can further support cognitive well-being and overall quality of life.

Importance of a Multidisciplinary Approach:

Effective dementia care often involves a multidisciplinary team of healthcare professionals, including doctors, nurses, occupational therapists, and social workers. This collaborative approach makes sure all parts of an individual's care are addressed, from medical management to support for daily living activities and emotional well-being. Caregivers should actively participate in the care planning process and communicate regularly with the healthcare team to make sure the individual's needs are met and any concerns are promptly addressed.

Navigating dementia care requires a comprehensive approach that combines medication, cognitive exercises, and lifestyle changes. These strategies aim to manage symptoms, slow down cognitive decline, and enhance the overall quality of life for individuals with dementia. Working closely with healthcare professionals to develop a personalized care plan that considers the individual's unique needs, preferences, and medical history is essential for effective dementia management.

By adopting a holistic and multidisciplinary approach to dementia care, caregivers can provide the best support to their loved ones, helping them maintain dignity, independence, and a sense of well-being throughout their journey with dementia.

∼

ENVISIONING THE FUTURE: ADVANCES IN DEMENTIA RESEARCH

DEMENTIA AFFECTS millions of individuals and families worldwide, presenting a complex and emotionally challenging journey. While there is currently no cure for dementia, ongoing research efforts are dedicated to unraveling its mysteries and developing innovative approaches to improve the lives of those affected. By highlighting the importance of compassion, awareness, and scientific progress, we can not only seek answers but also provide support and hope to individuals with dementia and their caregivers.

Current Research Landscape:

Contemporary dementia research encompasses a wide range of disciplines and approaches, including genetics, biomarker identification, drug development, lifestyle interventions, and novel treatment strategies. Genetic studies aim to identify specific genes that increase the risk of developing dementia, enabling the development of personalized therapies and precision medicine approaches.

Biomarker research focuses on identifying measurable indicators, such as blood proteins or brain imaging changes, that can provide insights into the underlying mechanisms and progression of dementia. These biomarkers can aid in early diagnosis, tracking disease progression, and evaluating the effectiveness of treatments.

Drug development efforts are exploring diverse pathways to target the complex nature of dementia. Researchers are investigating anti-inflammatory drugs, compounds that enhance the clearance of harmful proteins, and treatments that improve neuronal communication and function. These innovative approaches hold promise for slowing down or even halting the progression of dementia.

Lifestyle interventions are increasingly recognized as powerful tools in the prevention and management of dementia. Studies have highlighted the positive impact of regular physical activity, a nutritious diet, social engagement, and mentally stimulating activities on brain health and cognitive function. Encouraging individuals to adopt healthy lifestyle habits can play a significant role in reducing the risk of cognitive decline and improving overall well-being.

Future Directions:

As we look to the future of dementia research, several exciting avenues are emerging. Combination therapies that target multiple parts of the disease simultaneously are showing promise in addressing the complex nature of dementia. Early detection markers are being developed to enable timely interventions and maximize the effectiveness of treatments.

Stem cell therapies are another area of ongoing research, exploring the potential to regenerate damaged neurons and restore cognitive function. While still in the early stages, these regenerative approaches hold immense potential for the future of dementia treatment.

Equally important is the need for increased awareness and the reduction of stigma surrounding dementia. Educating communities about the condition and promoting a supportive and inclusive environment is important for improving the quality of life for individuals with dementia and their caregivers.

The journey of dementia research is one of hope, determination, and unwavering commitment to improving the lives of those affected by this condition.

As we continue to make scientific advancements, our ultimate goal remains clear: to develop effective treatments, provide support, and foster a society that embraces and empowers individuals with dementia.

By combining cutting-edge research, compassionate care, and widespread awareness, we can work toward a future where the impact of dementia is mitigated, and those navigating this challenging journey are supported every step of the way. Together, we can strive for a world where dementia is met with understanding, innovation, and unwavering support.

~

FREQUENTLY ASKED QUESTIONS:

1. What exactly is dementia? Think of dementia as an umbrella term for a bunch of symptoms that mess with a person's brain powers - like remembering stuff, thinking, and making decisions. It's not just one disease but a mix of several, where the brain starts to decline more than what we'd expect from just getting older. Alzheimer's is the most common type, but there are others like vascular dementia, frontotemporal dementia, and more.

2. How do I spot dementia in someone I care about? Keep an eye out for signs like forgetting recent events or conversations, trouble keeping up with personal care, getting confused in familiar places, mood swings, and having a hard time with daily tasks. These symptoms can start off mild but get worse over time. Catching them early can help in managing the situation better.

3. Why is it important to catch dementia early? Finding out about dementia early opens up the chance to slow down the disease with certain treatments, plan for the future, and adjust daily life to manage better. It can make a big difference in maintaining quality of life for the person affected and helps everyone involved to prepare and adapt.

4. How can we manage daily life with dementia? It's about staying patient, adapting to changes, and finding new ways to support independence and communication. Break tasks into simpler steps, maintain a calm and structured environment, and keep engaging with activities that stimulate the mind. And don't forget, taking care of yourself as a caregiver is super important too. You need to be your best to give your best.

5. What's being done to find a cure for dementia? There's a ton of research going into understanding dementia better, from looking into genetics to developing new drugs and exploring lifestyle changes that might lower the risk. While we don't have a cure yet, the progress is promising, focusing on treatments that could slow down symptoms or even prevent dementia from getting worse. Staying informed and supportive is key.

I hope these answers help clear up some of the fog around dementia care. Remember, you're not alone in this. There's a whole community out there ready to support you and your loved one through this journey.

$\sim$

CASE STUDY:

LET'S dive into a story that brings all these points to life. Imagine Sarah, a 58-year-old woman who's been noticing changes in her mom, Ellen, who is 82. Ellen, a retired schoolteacher, began forgetting conversations and appointments, which was unusual for someone who always prided herself on her sharp memory. Sarah saw this as the first red flag.

Defining the Challenge: Ellen's journey began with small moments of forgetfulness, but soon, she started struggling with daily tasks, like managing her finances and remembering to take her medication. Sarah realized these weren't just senior moments; they were signs of something deeper. After a visit to the doctor, Ellen was diagnosed with Alzheimer's disease, the most common dementia.

Recognizing Symptoms and Understanding Progression: Sarah saw firsthand how dementia affected her mom. Ellen would forget recent events and mix up names. She struggled with planning and became easily confused, even in familiar settings. These changes weren't just hard on Ellen; they were hard on Sarah too, as she had to watch her vibrant, independent mom face these challenges.

The Value of Early Detection and Diagnosis: Sarah learned the importance of catching dementia early. Through cognitive assessments and brain imaging, Ellen's healthcare team could outline a treatment plan. This early intervention let them manage Ellen's symptoms better and gave Sarah time to plan, including looking into care options and support networks.

Navigating Daily Life with Dementia: As Ellen's dementia progressed, daily life became more challenging. Sarah stepped in as a caregiver, helping with tasks Ellen once did on her own. They faced communication barriers and had to find new ways to connect. Sarah also introduced routines that helped Ellen feel more secure and less confused.

The Essential Role of Caregivers in Dementia Care: Sarah realized that being a caregiver was about providing physical, emotional, and mental support. She adapted her communication to meet Ellen where she was, found activities to keep her mom's mind engaged, and took care of herself too. She learned that self-care wasn't selfish; it was necessary to be the best caregiver she could be.

Navigating Dementia Care: Understanding Treatment Approaches: Together with Ellen's healthcare team, Sarah explored medications, cognitive training, and lifestyle changes to manage the symptoms. They found that a mix of treatments worked best for Ellen, slowing down the progression and improving her quality of life.

Exploring the Horizon: The Future of Dementia Research: Sarah also became an advocate for dementia research, hoping that future advancements could change the course of this disease. She stays updated on new studies and participates in awareness campaigns, hoping to make a difference not just for her mom but for others facing the same journey.

Lessons Learned:

- **Early detection is key**: It opens doors to treatments and planning that can significantly affect.

- **Caregiving is multifaceted**: It involves physical, emotional, and cognitive support.
- **Self-care for caregivers is important**: To provide the best care, caregivers need to look after their own well-being.
- **Treatment is individual**: What works for one person might not work for another, so it's important to tailor the approach.
- **Hope and advocacy**: Staying informed and supporting dementia research can lead to better outcomes.

Sarah's story with Ellen is a testament to the journey many face with dementia. It's about adapting, finding support, and holding onto hope as they navigate this challenging path together.

∿

PART ONE WRAP-UP:
ACTION ITEMS FOR THE CAREGIVER:

HERE'S a straightforward list of action items for caregivers, inspired by Sarah and Ellen's journey, to help manage the care of a loved one with dementia:

1. **Educate Yourself on Dementia**: Learn about the types of dementia, symptoms, progression, and management strategies to better understand what your loved one is going through.
2. **Seek an Early Diagnosis**: If you notice signs of cognitive decline in your loved one, encourage them to see a healthcare provider for a thorough assessment.
3. **Develop a Care Plan**: Work with healthcare professionals to create a tailored care plan that addresses medication, cognitive training, and lifestyle changes.
4. **Improve Communication**: Adapt your communication style to your loved one's needs, using simple, clear sentences and maintaining patience.
5. **Create a Safe Environment**: Make necessary changes to the living space to ensure it's safe and comfortable, reducing the risk of falls and confusion.

6. **Establish a Routine**: Routines can help reduce confusion and anxiety for people with dementia, providing a sense of stability.
7. **Engage in Cognitive Activities**: Include brain-stimulating activities like puzzles, memory games, or simple tasks they enjoy to help maintain cognitive function.
8. **Encourage Physical Activity**: Incorporate regular, gentle exercise into their routine to support overall health and well-being.
9. **Monitor Nutrition and Hydration**: Ensure they're eating a balanced diet and staying hydrated, which can affect cognitive health and energy levels.
10. **Manage Behavioral Changes**: Learn strategies to deal with agitation, aggression, or other behavioral changes calmly and effectively.
11. **Seek Support for Yourself**: Connect with caregiver support groups, consider respite care options, and make time for your own mental and physical health.
12. **Plan for the Future**: Discuss and arrange legal, financial, and long-term care planning to prepare for the progression of the disease.
13. **Stay Informed About Research**: Keep up with the latest in dementia research and treatment options and consider participating in studies or advocacy efforts.
14. **Spread Awareness and Reduce Stigma**: Help educate others about dementia to foster understanding and support within the community.
15. **Celebrate the Good Moments**: Focus on creating positive experiences and cherishing your quality time with your loved one.

By following these action items, caregivers can provide compassionate, effective care for their loved ones with dementia while also taking care of their own well-being.

～

IN OUR NEXT PART...

In our next Part, we dig into the deeply personal and often challenging journey of navigating dementia's progression, illuminated through the heartrending yet inspiring story of Mr. Johnson and his daughter Linda. This narrative serves as a guiding light, offering important insights into the gradual onset and advancement of dementia, while underscoring the critical importance of early detection, the power of informed and compassionate caregiving, and the profound impact of these conditions on both the individual and their loved ones. As we explore Mr. Johnson's path from the initial subtle signs to the need for comprehensive support, we'll uncover the layers of complexity involved in managing dementia and the emotional toll it exacts on families.

Through Linda's reflections and experiences, we aim to offer readers not just an understanding of dementia's clinical stages, but a glimpse into the emotional resilience, adaptive strategies, and unwavering love that caregiving entails.

The lessons Linda shares from her journey—ranging from the significance of patience and flexibility to the essential nature of self-care and the value of cherishing every moment—resonate as universal truths for many navigating similar paths.

As we piece together their story, we invite you to reflect on the broader implications of dementia on individuals and families, fostering a deeper empathy and connection among those touched by this condition.

This Part not only seeks to educate but also to inspire and support caregivers and families facing the realities of dementia, reminding us the strength found in shared experiences and the indomitable spirit of those who care for their loved ones through life's most challenging chapters.

∾

PART TWO
NAVIGATING THE JOURNEY: UNDERSTANDING DEMENTIA'S PROGRESSION

UNDERSTANDING THE STAGES OF DEMENTIA: A GUIDE FOR CAREGIVERS

DEMENTIA IS a condition that gradually affects a person's cognitive abilities, affecting memory, communication, reasoning, and decision-making skills. It is an umbrella term that encompasses various symptoms resulting from different underlying diseases, with Alzheimer's disease being the most common cause.

Understanding the stages of dementia provides a roadmap for caregivers and loved ones, offering insights into the challenges and adaptations that may lie ahead. While the progression of dementia can vary depending on the specific type and individual, a general pattern is often observed.

Early Stage: Subtle Changes and Mild Impairment

In the early stage of dementia, subtle changes in memory and cognitive function begin to emerge. The person may experience mild forgetfulness, such as difficulty recalling recent conversations or struggling to find the right words. The individual often maintains a significant level of independence, although assistance and support can help ease the transition.

Caregivers can offer gentle reminders, establish routines, and encourage the use of memory aids like calendars and notes. It is important to provide a supportive environment that promotes independence while ensuring safety and well-being.

Middle Stage: Increasing Challenges and Confusion

As dementia progresses to the middle stage, the challenges become more pronounced. Memory loss intensifies, and confusion becomes more frequent. Everyday tasks, such as dressing or preparing meals, may become increasingly difficult. Behavioral changes, including frustration, agitation, or restlessness, may also become more noticeable.

Caregivers play an important role in this stage, assisting with daily activities, offering reassurance, and creating a structured and familiar environment. Patience, compassion, and flexibility are essential qualities for caregivers during this phase.

Late Stage: Extensive Support and Care

In the late stage of dementia, cognitive abilities are severely impaired, and the individual requires comprehensive support and care. Communication may become very limited, and the person may struggle to recognize familiar faces or surroundings. Physical abilities also decline, making tasks like walking or eating challenging.

At this stage, caregivers must focus on the person's comfort, dignity, and quality of life. Providing a safe and nurturing environment, managing medical needs, and offering emotional support are key aspects of care. Seeking more support from healthcare professionals, support groups, or respite care services can help caregivers manage the demands of this stage.

Importance of Support and Resources

Navigating the stages of dementia can be emotionally and physically demanding for both the person with dementia and their caregivers. It is essential to access resources and support throughout the journey. This may include educational materials, support groups, counseling services, and respite care options.

Caregivers should also focus on their own well-being, as caring for a loved one with dementia can be mentally and physically exhausting. Taking breaks, seeking help when needed, and engaging in self-care activities are important for maintaining the caregiver's health and resilience.

Understanding the stages of dementia equips caregivers with the knowledge and insights needed to provide care and support at each phase of the journey. By recognizing the challenges and adapting to the changing needs of the person with dementia, caregivers can foster an environment of comfort, dignity, and compassion.

Accessing resources, seeking support, and prioritizing self-care are essential parts of effective dementia caregiving. By working with healthcare professionals and support networks, caregivers can navigate the complexities of dementia with grace, empathy, and resilience.

∾

RECOGNIZING THE EARLY WARNING SIGNS OF DEMENTIA

Dementia is a condition that gradually affects cognitive functions, including memory, reasoning, language, and the ability to perform everyday tasks. Identifying the early signs of dementia is important, as it allows for timely intervention, proper planning, and access to appropriate support. This guide will help you understand the subtle changes that may show the onset of dementia.

Memory Lapses:

One of the most common early signs of dementia is memory loss that goes beyond occasional forgetfulness. This may involve difficulty recalling recent events, forgetting important dates or appointments, or repeatedly asking the same questions. If memory lapses start to interfere with daily life, it's essential to take note.

Difficulty with Familiar Tasks:

Individuals in the early stages of dementia may struggle with tasks that were once second nature to them. This could include preparing a simple meal, managing finances, or operating household appliances. If a person finds themselves confused or unable to complete routine activities, it may be a cause for concern.

Disorientation and Confusion:

Dementia can cause disorientation, even in familiar surroundings. A person may have trouble remembering dates, navigating well-known routes, or recognizing faces of family members or friends. If someone often feels lost or confused, it's important to pay attention.

Changes in Mood and Behavior:

Dementia can affect a person's mood and behavior, leading to unexplained mood swings, increased irritability, or a loss of interest in previously enjoyed activities. If a typically outgoing person becomes withdrawn or a generally even-tempered individual becomes easily agitated, it may be a sign of underlying cognitive changes.

Language and Communication Difficulties:

Early-stage dementia can affect a person's ability to communicate effectively. They may struggle to find the right words, have difficulty following conversations, or experience problems with reading and writing. If you notice a significant change in someone's language skills, it's worth noting.

Impaired Judgment and Decision-Making:

Dementia can affect a person's judgment and decision-making abilities. They may make poor financial choices, such as overspending on unnecessary items or falling victim to scams. They may have difficulty assessing risks in everyday situations. If someone's judgment seems impaired, it's important to address the issue.

Decreased Attention and Focus:

Individuals with early-stage dementia may have trouble maintaining focus or concentration. They may struggle to follow storylines in books or television shows, or have difficulty completing tasks that require sustained attention. If a person's ability to stay focused noticeably declines, it's important to act.

Exhibiting one or more of these signs doesn't necessarily mean a person has dementia. These symptoms can overlap with other health conditions, so it's essential to consult with a healthcare professional for a proper evaluation and diagnosis.

Taking Action:

If you suspect you or a loved one may be experiencing the early signs of dementia, it's important to seek medical advice promptly. Early diagnosis allows for better management of the condition, planning for the future, and access to appropriate support services.

Additionally, engaging in mentally stimulating activities, maintaining social connections, and adopting a healthy lifestyle may help slow the progression of dementia. This includes regular exercise, a balanced diet, and staying socially and intellectually active.

Chapter Summary:

Recognizing the early warning signs of dementia is an important step in providing timely support and care for those affected. By understanding the subtle changes in memory, behavior, communication, and daily functioning, you can take proactive measures to address the situation.

If you have concerns about yourself or a loved one, trust your instincts and seek professional guidance. Early intervention can make a significant difference in managing dementia and ensuring the best quality of life for all involved.

~

NAVIGATING THE STAGES OF DEMENTIA: A COMPASSIONATE GUIDE

DEMENTIA IS a complex and progressive condition that affects a person's cognitive abilities, gradually changing their perception, memory, and interaction with the world around them. Understanding the stages of dementia can help caregivers and loved ones provide support and care throughout the journey. This guide aims to shed light on the different phases of dementia and offer insights into navigating each stage with compassion and understanding.

Stage 1 - Mild Cognitive Impairment (MCI):

The journey often begins with Mild Cognitive Impairment (MCI), characterized by subtle changes in memory or cognitive function. At this stage, individuals may experience occasional lapses in memory or have difficulty concentrating on tasks. These changes may be noticeable to the person or their close family members, but they typically do not significantly interfere with daily life. Not everyone with MCI will progress to dementia, but it can be an early warning sign.

Stage 2 - Early-Stage Dementia:

As the condition progresses, the challenges become more apparent. In the early stage of dementia, memory loss becomes more pronounced, and individuals may struggle with tasks that were once familiar, such as planning meals or managing finances. Mood changes, confusion, and disorientation may also become more frequent. At this stage, individuals can still maintain some independence, but they may require occasional assistance and support from caregivers.

Stage 3 - Moderate Stage Dementia:

In the moderate stage of dementia, the need for support and assistance goes up significantly. Individuals may have difficulty with basic daily activities, such as dressing, grooming, and maintaining personal hygiene. They may struggle to recognize familiar faces or remember recent events.

Communication becomes more challenging, with word-finding difficulties and confusion becoming clearer. Caregivers play an important role in providing a structured and supportive environment, offering guidance and assistance with daily tasks.

Stage 4 - Severe Stage Dementia:

As dementia progresses to the severe stage, individuals become increasingly dependent on others for care and support. Memory loss becomes more extensive, and the ability to recognize loved ones or recall cherished memories may go down. Communication becomes severely impaired, with limited verbal expression and understanding. Physical abilities also decline, requiring help with mobility and basic needs. Caregivers must focus on the individual's comfort, safety, and dignity, providing round-the-clock care and support.

Stage 5 - End Stage Dementia:

In the final stage of dementia, individuals become fully dependent on others for all parts of care. They may lose the ability to communicate verbally and have significantly reduced physical capabilities. This stage requires compassionate and attentive care to ensure the individual's comfort and well-being. Caregivers focus on providing a peaceful and nurturing environment, attending to the person's basic needs, and offering emotional support.

Understanding the Uniqueness of Each Journey:

Every person's journey through dementia is unique. The progression and duration of each stage may vary depending on the type of dementia, such as Alzheimer's disease, vascular dementia, or Lewy body dementia. Some individuals may progress through the stages more rapidly, while others may have a slower progression.

The Role of Early Detection and Support:

Early recognition of dementia symptoms is important for providing timely support and care. If you notice changes in a loved one's memory, behavior, or cognitive abilities, it's essential to consult with a healthcare professional for a proper evaluation. Early diagnosis allows for better planning, access to resources, and the implementation of care strategies.

Throughout the journey, it's important to surround the person with dementia with a strong support system. This includes family members, friends, healthcare professionals, and support groups. Patience, understanding, and a focus on maintaining the individual's dignity and quality of life are key aspects of providing compassionate care.

Chapter Summary:

Navigating the stages of dementia requires knowledge, compassion, and a willingness to adapt to the changing needs of the individual. By understanding the unique challenges and features of each stage, caregivers can provide the proper level of support and care, ensuring the best quality of life for their loved one.

Remember, no one must face this journey alone. Seeking support, resources, and guidance from healthcare professionals and support organizations can make a significant difference in managing the challenges of dementia. With love, patience, and understanding, moments of joy and connection can still be found along the way.

~

THE MIDDLE OF THE ROAD: NAVIGATING MIDDLE STAGE DEMENTIA

As DEMENTIA PROGRESSES to the middle stage, the challenges become more pronounced for both the person with dementia and their caregivers. This stage is often described as a journey through a thickening fog, where everyday tasks become increasingly difficult, and confusion becomes more frequent. Understanding the features of middle stage dementia and putting effective strategies into practice can help caregivers navigate this challenging phase with compassion and resilience.

The Challenges of Middle Stage Dementia:

Memory Decline: Memory loss becomes more significant in the middle stage of dementia. The person may have difficulty remembering recent events, familiar faces, or how to perform routine tasks. This can lead to confusion, frustration, and a sense of disorientation.

Communication Difficulties: Engaging in conversations becomes more challenging as the person struggles to find the right words or follow the flow of a discussion. They may have trouble expressing their thoughts or understanding complex sentences, leading to feelings of isolation and disconnection.

Behavioral Changes: Middle stage dementia can bring about changes in behavior and emotions. The person may experience restlessness, agitation, or a desire to wander. They may also exhibit mood swings, anxiety, or irritability, which can be difficult for caregivers to manage.

Increased Dependence: As dementia progresses, the person becomes more reliant on others for help with daily activities such as dressing, eating, and personal hygiene. This increased dependence can be emotionally and physically demanding for caregivers.

Strategies for Caregivers:

Simplify Communication: When communicating with a person in the middle stage of dementia, use clear and concise language. Give one instruction at a time and allow ample time for processing. Visual cues, such as pictures or gestures, can also help convey messages more effectively.

Establish a Routine: Creating a predictable daily routine can provide a sense of structure and familiarity for the person with dementia. Maintain consistent times for meals, activities, and bedtime. This can help reduce confusion and anxiety.

Prioritize Safety: As the risk of wandering increases, ensuring the person's safety becomes a top priority. Put safety measures into practice in the home, such as securing doors and installing locks. Consider using a GPS tracking device or an identification bracelet to help locate the person if they wander.

Practice Self-Care: Caregiving can be physically and emotionally exhausting. Caregivers must prioritize their own well-being. Engage in activities that bring joy and relaxation, such as hobbies or exercise. Seek support from family, friends, or support groups, and consider respite care options to allow for breaks and rest.

Focus on Connection: Despite the challenges, it's important to remember that the person with dementia is still the same individual at their core. Find moments of connection and joy through shared activities, laughter, or simply sitting together in peaceful companionship.

These moments can bring comfort and strengthen the bond between caregiver and care recipient.

Chapter Summary:

Navigating the middle stage of dementia requires patience, understanding, and a willingness to adapt to the changing needs of the person with dementia. By putting effective communication strategies into practice, establishing routines, focusing on safety, and practicing self-care, caregivers can provide the best support during this challenging phase.

The journey through dementia is unique for every individual and family. Seeking guidance from healthcare professionals, support groups, and local resources can provide valuable insights and assistance along the way.

Above all, approach this stage with compassion and love. While the road may be difficult, finding moments of connection and joy can bring light to the journey. With the right support and strategies, caregivers can navigate the fog of middle stage dementia and provide the care and comfort their loved ones need.

◦∼◦

THE LONG GOODBYE: NAVIGATING LATE-STAGE DEMENTIA

WHEN DEMENTIA ENTERS its late stage, it's like entering a different world —one where the mind and body start to walk separate paths. This stage is tough, not just for the person going through it, but also for those around them trying to help. Let's break down what this stage means and how to handle its challenges with care and compassion.

Cognitive Twilight

- **Memory's Fade**: Remembering faces, names, or even significant life events becomes a distant dream. The person you care for might not recognize you anymore, which is heart-wrenching but part of this stage's reality.
- **Lost in Time and Space**: The idea of time, places, and even the people around them becomes a jumble. Familiar settings may look alien, making the world a confusing place to be.
- **Words Slip Away**: Trying to chat can become a puzzle where the pieces don't fit. Words might be scarce, and understanding others can be just as tough. It's like being in a country where you don't speak the language.
- **Emotions on the Edge**: You might see more tears, anger, or

even laughter at odd times. These emotional roller coasters are part of the journey, as control over feelings slips away.

Physical Journey

- **Moving Mountains**: Simple movements become monumental tasks. Standing, walking, or even sitting up might need a helping hand. This makes the risk of falling a constant worry.
- **Swallowing Sand**: Eating and drinking aren't just about taste anymore; they're about safety. Swallowing can become a challenge, leading to risks of choking or not getting enough nutrition.
- **The Unspoken**: Control over when and where to go to the bathroom fades away. It's a delicate topic but handling it with dignity is important for their comfort and health.
- **Daily Living Dances**: The rhythm of daily life—eating, washing, dressing—changes. Each step needs more help, more patience, and more love.

Lighting the Path

Navigating this stage is about providing comfort, preserving dignity, and ensuring safety. Here are a few beacons to guide you:

- **Speak Without Words**: When words don't work, use touch, music, or being there to communicate. Sometimes, a hand held is worth a thousand words.
- **Create a Safe Haven**: Make the living space safe and comfortable. Think about easy-to-navigate areas, soft lighting, and removing trip hazards.
- **Nourish Gently**: Pay close attention to how they eat and drink. Soft foods, hydration, and patience during meals can help avoid complications.
- **Respect and Dignity**: Keep routines for personal care that respect their dignity. It's about making sure they feel cared for in every action.

The Heart of Care

Late-stage dementia asks us to redefine what it means to connect, to care, and to love. It's about finding peace in moments of presence, comfort in the calm, and joy in the simple act of being together. Remember, you're not alone on this journey. Contact communities, professionals, and resources that can help light the way. Together, we can navigate the twilight with grace and love.

Navigating the Challenges of Late-Stage Dementia:

Late-stage dementia marks a profound shift in the journey, where the person's cognitive and physical abilities significantly decline. This stage can be emotionally challenging for both the person with dementia and their caregivers, as it requires a deep level of understanding, patience, and compassion. This guide aims to shed light on the complexities of late-stage dementia and provide insights on how to navigate this phase with love and dignity.

The Cognitive Decline:

Memory Fade: In late-stage dementia, the person's ability to recognize faces, names, and even cherished memories may diminish. They may struggle to identify loved ones, which can be heartbreaking for caregivers. It's important to remember that this is a part of the disease and not a reflection of the person's feelings or the strength of your relationship.

Disorientation: The concept of time, place, and familiar surroundings becomes increasingly confusing for the person with dementia. They may feel lost or disoriented, even in their own home. Providing a safe, comforting, and familiar environment can help alleviate some of this confusion.

Communication Challenges: Verbal communication becomes severely impaired in late-stage dementia. The person may struggle to find the right words, express their thoughts, or understand others. This can lead to frustration and isolation. Finding alternative ways to communicate, such as through gentle touch, music, or simply being present, can help maintain a sense of connection.

Emotional Fluctuations: As the person loses control over their cognitive functions, they may experience intense emotional upheavals. Tears, anger, or unexpected laughter may occur at seemingly inappropriate times. It's important to approach these emotional outbursts with patience, understanding, and a calming presence.

The Physical Journey:

Mobility Challenges: As dementia progresses, the person's physical abilities decline. They may have difficulty standing, walking, or even sitting up without help. This increased risk of falls requires close supervision and support. Adapting the living space to ensure safety and ease of navigation becomes a priority.

Eating and Swallowing Difficulties: Swallowing disorders (dysphagia) are common in late-stage dementia, making eating and drinking a challenge. Choking risks and inadequate nutrition become concerns. Caregivers must pay close attention to the person's eating habits, offer soft, easily swallowable foods, and ensure proper hydration.

Incontinence: Loss of bladder and bowel control is a sensitive issue that arises in late-stage dementia. Handling these situations with dignity and respect is paramount. Establishing a toileting routine, using incontinence products, and maintaining good hygiene can help manage this part of care.

Assistance with Daily Living: As the person becomes increasingly dependent, caregivers must provide support with all aspects of daily life, including dressing, bathing, and grooming. Maintaining a sense of routine and letting the person participate in these activities to the best of their abilities can help preserve their dignity and sense of self.

Providing Comfort and Care:

Nonverbal Connection: When words fail, other forms of communication become important. Gentle touch, soothing music, or simply being present can convey love, comfort, and reassurance. These moments of connection, however brief, can have a profound impact on the person's well-being.

Creating a Safe and Comforting Environment: Modifying the living space to ensure safety and comfort is essential. This may involve removing tripping hazards, installing handrails, and creating a calming atmosphere with soft lighting and familiar objects. A secure and nurturing environment can help reduce agitation and promote a sense of peace.

Nutritional Support: Ensuring adequate nutrition and hydration is important in late-stage dementia. Offering small, frequent meals, using adaptive utensils, and assisting with eating can help maintain the person's health and comfort. Consulting with healthcare professionals can provide guidance on specific nutritional needs.

Preserving Dignity: Maintaining the person's dignity should lead all caregiving efforts. This includes respecting their privacy during personal care routines, involving them in decision-making to the extent possible, and treating them with the same love and respect they have always deserved.

Chapter Summary:

Late-stage dementia is a profound and challenging journey that requires immense compassion, patience, and resilience from care-givers. It is a time to focus on providing comfort, preserving dignity, and finding moments of connection and joy amidst the difficulties.

Remember, you are not alone in this journey. Seek support from health-care professionals, dementia support organizations, and caregiver communities. They can provide valuable guidance, resources, and emotional support to help you navigate this stage with love and grace.

Ultimately, late-stage dementia teaches us the power of presence, the importance of compassion, and the enduring nature of love. By embracing these qualities and finding strength in the moments of connection, we can provide the best care for our loved ones and find peace in the journey.

FREQUENTLY ASKED QUESTIONS:

1. How can I tell if someone is in the early stages of dementia, and what should I do about it? Early signs of dementia can be subtle, like forgetting recent conversations, trouble finding the right words, or changes in mood. If you notice these signs, it's important to see a healthcare professional. Early detection can make a big difference in managing the condition, planning, and accessing support. Encourage a healthy lifestyle and engaging activities to help slow progression.

2. The person I'm caring for is becoming more confused and forgetful. Are we moving into a different stage of dementia? It sounds like you might be transitioning into the middle stages of dementia. This phase can see an increase in memory loss, confusion, and difficulty with daily tasks. It's a challenging time, but adjusting your approach to care can help. Keep communication simple, maintain a routine, and ensure a safe environment. Remember, your patience and support are more important than ever.

3. I've heard the late stages of dementia can be tough. How can I prepare, and what should I expect? In the late stages, the person will probably need constant care. They may struggle with communication, mobility, and even recognizing loved ones. Focus on comfort, safety, and preserving dignity. This might involve adapting the home, considering soft foods, and finding nonverbal ways to connect. It's also a time to ensure you have support for yourself, as caregiving can be emotionally and physically taxing.

4. As a caregiver, I feel overwhelmed at times. What can I do to cope? Feeling overwhelmed is understandable. Caregiving is a demanding role, but remember, taking care of yourself is not optional—it's essential. Find time for activities you enjoy, connect with friends or support groups, and don't hesitate to seek respite care when needed. Practicing mindfulness and setting realistic goals can also help manage stress. Remember, it's okay to ask for help.

5. What can I do to support the person I'm caring for as their dementia progresses? Supporting someone with dementia means adapting to their changing needs. Engage them in activities that match their abilities, offer reassurance in moments of confusion, and maintain a calm, structured environment. Use gentle reminders and cues to help with memory, and always approach them with patience and empathy. Celebrate the good moments together and focus on what they can still do and enjoy.

Being a caregiver for someone with dementia is a journey of love, patience, and resilience. Remember, you're not alone. There are resources, communities, and professionals ready to support you every step of the way. Keep asking questions, seeking support, and taking care of yourself and the person you're caring for.

～

CASE STUDY: NAVIGATING THE JOURNEY WITH MR. JOHNSON
INTRODUCTION TO DEMENTIA: THE ESSENTIALS

MEET MR. JOHNSON, an 82-year-old widower living in a small town. A retired high school principal, Mr. Johnson was always known for his sharp wit and love for literature. However, his family began noticing changes about two years ago. His journey illustrates the essence of understanding dementia's progression and the critical role caregivers play.

Early Stage: The Subtle Onset

Mr. Johnson's first signs were subtle. He started forgetting names of former students he used to recall with pride. His daughter, Linda, first brushed it off as normal aging. However, when Mr. Johnson, a lifelong book lover, struggled to remember the plots of his favorite novels, Linda sensed something more serious.

Middle Stage: Navigating the Bumps

As the months passed, Mr. Johnson's forgetfulness evolved into significant confusion. Routine tasks like paying bills became daunting. Linda noticed her father's frustration grow as he could no longer manage his daily activities independently. It was during a family gathering that

Mr. Johnson did not recognize his cousin, leading the family to seek medical advice.

Diagnosed with Alzheimer's, the family rallied to support Mr. Johnson, with Linda taking the lead as his primary caregiver. This stage was marked by a mix of good days and challenging ones. Linda learned to celebrate the moments of clarity and navigate the confusion and agitation with patience.

Late Stage: The Need for Full Support

In the late stage, Mr. Johnson required full-time care. Verbal communication became rare, and physical abilities declined. Linda, with support from home health aides, ensured her father's comfort. She found ways to connect without words, using music from his youth to spark moments of recognition and joy.

Lessons Learned from Linda, the Caregiver:

1. **Early Detection is important:** Linda wished they had sought medical advice earlier. Recognizing the early signs of dementia can lead to better management and planning.
2. **Education and Support are Key:** Learning about dementia helped Linda understand her father's condition and what to expect. Support groups gave her coping strategies and a sense of community.
3. **Patience and Flexibility:** Linda learned that patience and flexibility were her best tools. Adapting to her father's changing needs and finding new ways to communicate and connect became part of their daily life.
4. **Importance of Self-Care:** Linda realized the importance of taking care of herself. Joining a caregiver support group and scheduling regular breaks helped her maintain her well-being.
5. **Cherishing Moments:** Despite the challenges, Linda found joy in the journey. Celebrating small victories and cherishing peaceful moments became valuable parts of her days.

Chapter Summary:

Mr. Johnson's story is a poignant reminder of the journey many families navigate with dementia. It underscores the importance of understanding the disease's progression, recognizing early signs, and the invaluable role caregivers play. Linda's experience highlights the challenges but also the profound moments of connection and love that can emerge in the face of dementia.

∾

PART TWO WRAP-UP:
ACTION ITEMS FOR THE CAREGIVER:

BASED ON LINDA'S journey with her father, Mr. Johnson, here's a tailored list of action items for caregivers navigating the progression of a loved one's dementia:

Seek a Professional Diagnosis Early: If you notice signs of cognitive decline, don't delay in consulting a healthcare professional. An early diagnosis can open up more options for management and care planning.

Educate Yourself on Dementia: Understand the types of dementia, their progression, and how they affect behavior and cognition. Knowledge empowers you to provide better care and manage expectations.

Create a Supportive Environment: Adapt your home to meet the evolving needs of your loved one, focusing on safety, comfort, and ease of navigation to reduce confusion and risks.

Establish a Routine: Consistency can help reduce confusion and anxiety for someone with dementia. Try to keep daily activities, meals, and bedtime at regular times.

Develop Communication Strategies: As dementia progresses, effective communication becomes challenging. Use simple, clear sentences, maintain eye contact, and be patient. Nonverbal cues like touch and smiles can also be comforting.

Engage in Meaningful Activities: Find activities that match their abilities and interests, such as listening to music, simple gardening, or looking through photo albums, to stimulate their mind and provide joy.

Monitor Health and Medication: Stay vigilant about their overall health, manage medications carefully, and keep regular appointments with healthcare providers.

Plan for the Future: Discuss and organize legal, financial, and long-term care planning early in the diagnosis. This preparation can alleviate future uncertainties.

Join a Support Group: Caregiving can be isolating. Support groups connect you with others in similar situations, providing a space to share experiences and advice.

Focus on Your Well-being: Caregiver burnout is real. Ensure you're taking time for self-care, whether it's exercise, hobbies, or spending time with friends. Consider respite care services to give yourself a break.

Use Community Resources: Explore local services and resources for dementia care, such as home health aides, adult day care centers, and meal delivery services.

Adapt to Changing Needs: Be ready to adjust your approach as the disease progresses. Flexibility and patience are important as their abilities and needs change.

Celebrate Small Moments: Focus on what your loved one can still enjoy and appreciate the moments of connection, however brief they may be.

Communicate with Family and Friends: Keep family and close friends informed about your loved one's condition and how they can help. It's important for everyone to be on the same page.

Seek Professional Counseling: If you or your family members struggle to cope with the emotional challenges of dementia care, consider seeking help from a therapist or counselor experienced in dementia care issues.

By following these action items, caregivers can navigate the complexities of dementia care with a balanced approach that supports both the individual with dementia and their own well-being.

∼

IN OUR NEXT PART...

In our next Part, we dig into the pivotal role of early detection and personalized care in the journey of dementia. Understanding the early signs and acting can significantly change the course of care, offering a beacon of hope for those navigating these turbulent waters. We'll explore the transformative impact of identifying dementia in its nascent stages, highlighting how early intervention can slow disease progression and enhance the quality of life for individuals and their families. This isn't just about medical treatment; it's about empowering families with the knowledge and resources to create a supportive environment that honors the individuality of their loved one's experience with dementia.

We'll focus on the importance of personalized care. Recognizing that dementia manifests differently in each individual, we emphasize the need for care plans that are as unique as the people they support. From adapting daily routines to incorporating preferred activities, we'll guide you through tailoring care strategies that respect and respond to the changing needs of your loved one. Alongside, we'll address the emotional journey for caregivers, offering strategies for self-care and maintaining emotional well-being amidst the challenges. Join us as we navigate these parts with compassion and professionalism, aiming to equip you with the tools and confidence to provide the best care for your loved one while also taking care of yourself.

∾

PART THREE
EARLY DETECTION AND PERSONALIZED CARE: NAVIGATING THE JOURNEY OF DEMENTIA

THE IMPORTANCE OF EARLY RECOGNITION IN DEMENTIA CARE

DEMENTIA IS a progressive condition that affects cognitive functions, leading to changes in memory, thinking, behavior, and the ability to perform everyday activities. Recognizing the early signs and symptoms of dementia is important for ensuring timely intervention, appropriate care, and support for individuals affected by the condition. This chapter explores the significance of early recognition in dementia care and highlights the key symptoms to look out for.

The Benefits of Early Recognition:

Early Intervention: Identifying dementia in its early stages allows for prompt interventions that may slow the progression of the disease. These interventions can include medications, lifestyle changes, and cognitive stimulation exercises aimed at maintaining cognitive function for as long as possible. Early intervention can also help manage symptoms and improve the overall quality of life for the individual.

Quality of Life: Early diagnosis enables the implementation of support systems and care plans that help individuals maintain their independence and engagement with life. By addressing the specific needs and challenges associated with dementia, caregivers can create an environment that promotes the person's well-being and preserves their dignity.

Future Planning: Recognizing dementia early provides individuals and their families with the opportunity to discuss and decide on care preferences, legal matters, and financial arrangements. This proactive planning helps reduce stress and uncertainty, making sure the person's wishes are respected and their needs are met as the condition progresses.

Safety Measures: As dementia advances, safety concerns such as wandering, driving, and managing household tasks become increasingly important. Early recognition allows for the implementation of safety measures to protect the individual's well-being and prevent accidents or injuries.

Emotional and Social Support: An early diagnosis enables individuals and their families to seek emotional support, connect with support groups, and access resources that can help them navigate the challenges associated with dementia. This support network can provide valuable information, guidance, and a sense of community during a difficult time.

Recognizing the Symptoms:

Memory Loss: One of the most common early signs of dementia is memory loss, particularly forgetting recently learned information, important dates, or events. The person may ask for the same information repeatedly or rely heavily on memory aids.

Confusion: Individuals with dementia may lose track of dates, seasons, and the passage of time. They may become confused about their location or how they arrived there.

Difficulty with Familiar Tasks: Dementia can cause challenges in planning, problem-solving, and completing familiar tasks at home or work. The person may struggle to follow recipes, manage finances, or understand visual images and spatial relationships.

Changes in Personality or Behavior: Dementia can lead to mood swings, withdrawal from social activities, and changes in personality. The person may become unusually suspicious, fearful, or anxious.

Communication Struggles: Individuals with dementia may have trouble following or joining a conversation, struggle to find the right words, or repeat themselves often.

Understanding Variability in Presentation:

The presentation of dementia symptoms can vary significantly depending on the type of dementia and the individual's unique circumstances. For example, Alzheimer's disease, vascular dementia, and frontotemporal dementia may manifest differently in terms of the specific cognitive functions affected and the rate of progression.

This variability highlights the need for personalized care and approaches tailored to the individual's specific symptoms and needs. A flexible, patient-centered approach is essential in managing dementia, focusing on enhancing the person's quality of life and supporting their independence for as long as possible.

Chapter Summary:

Early recognition of dementia is a critical step in providing effective care and support for individuals affected by the condition. By identifying the signs and symptoms early, interventions can be implemented to slow the progression of the disease, improve quality of life, and ensure planning and safety measures are in place.

Understanding the variability in the presentation of dementia symptoms is crucial for providing personalized care that addresses the unique needs of each individual. By seeking timely intervention and support, individuals and their families can navigate the challenges of dementia with greater confidence and resilience.

If you or a loved one are experiencing symptoms that may show dementia, it is important to consult with a healthcare professional for a proper evaluation and diagnosis. Early recognition and intervention can make a significant difference in the management of dementia and the quality of life for those affected by the condition.

∾

UNDERSTANDING THE COMMON SYMPTOMS OF DEMENTIA

DEMENTIA IS an umbrella term for a group of conditions characterized by the impairment of at least two brain functions, such as memory loss and judgment. While the symptoms of dementia can vary widely among individuals, there are several common signs and symptoms that may indicate the presence of the condition. Recognizing these symptoms early is important for timely diagnosis, effective management, and maintaining the best quality of life for those affected.

Key Symptoms of Dementia:

Memory Loss: One of the most common and noticeable symptoms of dementia is memory loss. Individuals may have difficulty remembering recent events, names, or faces. They may also struggle with retaining new information or rely heavily on memory aids, such as notes or reminders.

Communication and Language Difficulties: Dementia can affect a person's ability to communicate effectively. They may have trouble finding the right words, struggle to follow or join conversations, or experience a decline in their vocabulary. These challenges can lead to frustration and social withdrawal.

Impaired Focus and Attention: Individuals with dementia may find it challenging to concentrate on tasks or follow complex instructions. They may be easily distracted or have difficulty completing projects they once enjoyed.

Difficulty with Problem-Solving and Judgment: Dementia can affect a person's ability to solve problems, make decisions, or exercise good judgment. They may struggle with managing finances, making appropriate choices, or understanding the consequences of their actions.

Changes in Visual Perception: Some forms of dementia can affect visual perception, leading to difficulties with depth perception, spatial awareness, or recognizing familiar objects or faces. This can cause challenges with reading, driving, or navigating familiar environments.

Behavioral and Personality Changes: Dementia can cause changes in mood, behavior, and personality. Individuals may experience anxiety, depression, irritability, or apathy. They may also exhibit uncharacteristic behaviors, such as suspiciousness, agitation, or inappropriate social conduct.

Disorientation and Confusion: People with dementia may become disoriented, even in familiar surroundings. They may lose track of time, dates, or seasons and have difficulty understanding where they are or how they got there.

Decline in Motor Skills: As dementia progresses, individuals may experience a decline in motor skills and coordination. This can manifest as difficulty with balance, walking, or performing fine motor tasks like buttoning a shirt or writing.

Variability in Presentation:

Not everyone with dementia will experience all of these symptoms, and the severity and progression of the condition can vary significantly from person to person. The type of dementia, such as Alzheimer's disease, vascular dementia, or Lewy body dementia, can also influence the specific symptoms experienced.

If you or a loved one are experiencing several of these symptoms, it is essential to consult with a healthcare professional for a thorough evaluation. Early diagnosis allows for better management of the condition, access to appropriate treatments and support services, and the opportunity to plan for future care needs.

In addition to medical support, individuals with dementia and their caregivers can benefit from connecting with local resources, such as support groups, educational programs, and respite care services. These resources can provide valuable information, emotional support, and practical assistance in navigating the challenges of dementia.

Chapter Summary:

Recognizing the common symptoms of dementia is an important first step in seeking timely diagnosis and support. While the symptoms can vary among individuals, being aware of changes in memory, communication, problem-solving, and behavior can help prompt a conversation with a healthcare professional.

Early diagnosis and intervention can make a significant difference in managing dementia, maintaining quality of life, and accessing the resources and support. By understanding the common symptoms and seeking help when needed, individuals and families affected by dementia can navigate the journey with greater knowledge, preparedness, and resilience.

~

UNDERSTANDING DEMENTIA'S MANY FACES

DEMENTIA IS a complex condition that encompasses a wide range of disorders affecting cognitive function and daily life. While Alzheimer's disease is perhaps the most well-known form of dementia, it is important to recognize that dementia can manifest in various ways depending on the underlying cause. This chapter explores the different types of dementia and how their symptoms can vary from person to person.

Types of Dementia:

Alzheimer's Disease:

Alzheimer's disease is the most common form of dementia, accounting for 60-80% of cases. It is characterized by a gradual decline in memory, confusion, and difficulty with problem-solving and language. Individuals with Alzheimer's may struggle to remember recent events, become easily disoriented, and have trouble completing familiar tasks.

Frontotemporal Dementia:

Frontotemporal dementia (FTD) primarily affects the frontal and temporal lobes of the brain, which are responsible for behavior, personality, and language. People with FTD may show significant changes in their behavior, such as acting impulsively, displaying inappropriate social conduct, or experiencing apathy. They may also have difficulty with language, including struggling to find the right words or understanding abstract concepts.

Vascular Dementia:

Vascular dementia is caused by reduced blood flow to the brain, often due to stroke or small vessel disease. This dementia can affect a person's ability to plan, organize, and make decisions. Symptoms may include confusion, disorientation, and difficulty with problem-solving. The progression of vascular dementia can occur in a stepwise way, with periods of stability followed by sudden declines.

Lewy Body Dementia:

Lewy body dementia (LBD) is characterized by abnormal protein deposits called Lewy bodies in the brain. LBD can cause a range of symptoms, including fluctuating cognitive abilities, visual hallucinations, and Parkinson's-like motor symptoms such as tremors and rigidity. Individuals with LBD may also experience sleep disturbances and changes in attention and alertness.

Mixed Dementia:

Mixed dementia refers to more than one type of dementia in an individual. For example, a person may have both Alzheimer's disease and vascular dementia. In such cases, the symptoms may be a combination of those associated with each type of dementia, making the presentation more complex and challenging to diagnose and manage.

Variability in Presentation:

The symptoms of dementia can vary significantly from person to person, even within the same type of dementia. Factors such as age, overall health, and other medical conditions can influence how dementia manifests in an individual.

Some people may experience a gradual decline in memory and cognitive function over several years, while others may have a more rapid progression. The specific cognitive abilities affected can also differ, with some individuals struggling primarily with memory, while others may have more pronounced difficulties with language, attention, or visual-spatial skills.

Additionally, the behavioral and psychological symptoms of dementia can vary widely. Some individuals may become withdrawn and apathetic, while others may show agitation, aggression, or disinhibition. These symptoms can be challenging for caregivers to navigate and require individualized approaches to care.

Importance of Personalized Care:

Given the diverse manifestations of dementia, a one-size-fits-all approach to care is not effective. Caregivers, whether family members or professionals, must tailor their support and interventions to the unique needs and experiences of each individual with dementia.

This personalized approach involves understanding the specific type of dementia, the individual's cognitive and functional abilities, and their emotional and behavioral needs. By adapting care strategies to the person's unique challenges and strengths, caregivers can promote a higher quality of life, maintain dignity, and make sure the individual's needs are met compassionately and effectively.

Chapter Summary:

Dementia is a multifaceted condition that can present differently in each individual. Recognizing the types of dementia and the potential variability in symptoms is important for providing appropriate care and support. By understanding the unique ways dementia affects a person, caregivers can tailor their approach to best meet the individual's needs and promote their well-being.

Seek a comprehensive evaluation from a healthcare professional if you or a loved one are experiencing symptoms of dementia. An accurate diagnosis is the first step in developing a personalized care plan that addresses the specific challenges and maximizes the individual's quality of life.

Dementia may present many faces, but with knowledge, compassion, and a commitment to person-centered care, we can support individuals and families navigating this complex journey.

∼

RECOGNIZING DEMENTIA: A CAREGIVER'S GUIDE TO NOTICING THE SIGNS

As a family member or caregiver of someone with dementia, you play an important role in their care and well-being. Your close relationship and regular interactions put you in a unique position to notice changes that may show the progression of the condition or the need for more support. This guide aims to help you recognize the signs and take appropriate action to ensure the best care for your loved one.

The Importance of Regular Communication:

Maintaining open and regular communication with your loved one is important in identifying changes in their condition. Engage in conversations about their daily experiences, feelings, and any health concerns. These discussions can provide valuable insights into subtle changes that might otherwise go unnoticed.

Ask open-ended questions that encourage them to share their thoughts and feelings.

Listen actively and pay attention to any concerns or challenges they express.

Create a safe and supportive environment where they feel comfortable discussing their experiences.

Observing Changes in Daily Routines and Behaviors:

As a caregiver, you are probably familiar with your loved one's normal routines and behaviors. Pay close attention to any deviations from their usual patterns, as these changes can indicate underlying issues.

Monitor their eating habits, noting any loss of appetite or skipped meals.

Observe their engagement in favorite activities or hobbies, and notice if they lose interest or struggle to participate.

Watch for changes in sleep patterns, such as difficulty falling asleep or staying asleep, or sleeping more than usual.

Identifying Physical Changes:

Physical changes can be important indicators of your loved one's overall health and well-being. Keep an eye out for any visible signs of decline or discomfort.

Notice any changes in weight, whether it's unintended weight loss or gain.

Observe their mobility, paying attention to changes in gait, balance, or increased difficulty with movement.

Look for signs of pain or discomfort, such as wincing, grimacing, or favoring certain body parts.

Monitoring Mental Health and Cognitive Function:

Dementia can have a significant impact on mental health and cognitive function. Be attentive to changes in mood, memory, and social engagement.

Watch for signs of depression, anxiety, or apathy, such as persistent sadness, withdrawal from social interactions, or loss of interest in previously enjoyed activities.

Notice any increased forgetfulness, confusion, or difficulty with decision-making.

Pay attention to changes in communication, such as struggling to find the right words or understanding others.

Consulting with Healthcare Professionals:

If you notice any concerning changes in your loved one's physical, mental, or cognitive health, it's essential to consult with their healthcare providers promptly. Your observations and insights can provide valuable information to help in assessing their condition and adjusting their care plan.

Keep a record of the changes you've noticed, including dates and specific examples.

Share your concerns with their primary care doctor, neurologist, or other relevant healthcare professionals.

Collaborate with the healthcare team to develop strategies to address any identified issues and support your loved one's well-being.

Providing Empathy and Support:

Recognizing and addressing changes in your loved one's condition can be emotionally challenging for both you and them. Approach these situations with empathy, patience, and understanding.

Offer reassurance and support, letting them know that you are there to help them through any difficulties.

Encourage open communication and validate their feelings and concerns.

Engage in activities and conversations that promote their sense of self and maintain your emotional connection.

Chapter Summary:

As a caregiver, you have the opportunity to make a significant difference in the life of someone with dementia. By staying vigilant, observant, and proactive, you can identify changes early and make sure your loved one receives the care and support they need.

Remember, you are not alone in this journey. Contact healthcare professionals, support groups, and other resources for guidance and assistance when needed. Your dedication and compassion as a caregiver are invaluable in providing the best quality of life for your loved one.

~

THE IMPORTANCE OF
PROFESSIONAL CHECK-UPS
FOR YOUR LOVED ONE

As a caregiver for someone with dementia, you play an important role in tracking their health and well-being. Your close relationship and daily interactions let you notice changes or concerns that may require attention. When you observe something that doesn't seem right, the first and most important step is to arrange for a professional medical check-up. This chapter explores the significance of seeking a healthcare professional's evaluation and how it contributes to the best care for your loved one.

The Benefits of a Comprehensive Medical Evaluation:

Accurate Diagnosis:

A professional medical check-up assesses your loved one's specific symptoms, medical history, and other relevant factors. This detailed evaluation is essential for accurately diagnosing any new or worsening conditions. By identifying the root cause of the changes you've noticed, healthcare professionals can develop an appropriate treatment plan.

Personalized Care Planning:

Once a thorough medical evaluation is completed, the healthcare team can create a personalized care plan tailored to your loved one's specific needs. This may include a combination of medication, therapy, lifestyle changes, and other interventions to effectively manage their condition. A customized approach makes sure your loved one receives the most appropriate and targeted care.

Early Detection and Intervention:

Regular professional check-ups can help detect potential health issues early, before they become more serious or challenging to manage. Early detection is often associated with better outcomes, as it allows for prompt intervention and treatment. By catching problems early, you can help your loved one maintain their quality of life and prevent complications down the road.

Safety and Risk Reduction:

Some changes in your loved one's health may require immediate attention to ensure their safety and well-being. A professional evaluation can identify potential risks and guide you in taking necessary precautions. For example, if your loved one is experiencing increased falls or mobility issues, a healthcare provider can recommend safety measures and assistive devices to prevent accidents and injuries.

Access to Specialist Care:

Depending on your loved one's symptoms or condition, a primary care doctor may refer them to specialists for further evaluation or treatment. This may include neurologists, geriatric psychiatrists, or other experts in dementia care. Access to specialist care makes sure your loved one receives the most advanced and targeted interventions available.

The Risks of Self-Diagnosis:

While it may be tempting to try to diagnose and manage your loved one's health concerns on your own, this can be risky and potentially harmful. Without professional expertise, it's easy to misinterpret symptoms or overlook critical signs that a trained healthcare provider would recognize. Self-diagnosis and self-treatment can lead to delayed or inappropriate care, which may worsen your loved one's condition or cause more complications.

Your Role as a Caregiver:

As a caregiver, you play an important role in starting the process of seeking professional medical evaluation for your loved one. When you notice changes or concerns, it's essential to act and schedule an appointment with their healthcare provider. Be ready to share your observations, including specific examples and the duration of the changes you've noticed. Your insights and perspective are valuable in helping the healthcare team assess your loved one's condition accurately.

Chapter Summary:

Arranging a professional medical check-up for your loved one with dementia is an important step in ensuring they receive the best care. A comprehensive evaluation allows for accurate diagnosis, personalized treatment planning, early intervention, and access to specialist care when needed. By prioritizing regular check-ups and seeking professional guidance, you can significantly contribute to your loved one's health, safety, and overall quality of life.

Remember, as a caregiver, you are not alone in this journey. Collaborate closely with healthcare professionals, and please reach out for support and guidance when needed. Your dedication and proactive approach to your loved one's care can make all the difference in their well-being and comfort throughout their dementia journey.

～

AN OPEN LETTER TO FRIENDS AND FAMILY: NAVIGATING THE EMOTIONAL JOURNEY OF DEMENTIA TOGETHER

Dear Friends and Family,

As we come to terms with the early signs of dementia in our loved one, we embark on an emotional journey filled with complex and often overwhelming feelings. Witnessing changes in their memory, behavior, and overall functioning can evoke a deep sense of sadness, confusion, and even grief for the person we once knew.

It's important to acknowledge that the spectrum of emotions we experience is natural and valid. We may grapple with frustration, fear, and a profound sense of loss as we adjust to the new reality of our loved one's condition. These feelings are a testament to the deep love and connection we share with them.

In navigating this challenging path, we are not alone. Seeking the support and understanding of friends, family, and medical professionals can give us an important lifeline of strength and guidance. Sharing our experiences, concerns, and emotions with those who can empathize and offer comfort can help alleviate the sense of isolation and provide a much-needed outlet for our feelings.

As we focus on caring for our loved one, it's equally important to focus on our own well-being. Engaging in self-care practices, such as maintaining a balanced diet, getting enough rest, and finding moments of joy and relaxation, is essential for managing stress and promoting emotional resilience. Whether through meditation, physical exercise, or pursuing hobbies bring us peace, taking care of ourselves is a vital part of being present and supportive for our loved one.

Open and honest communication plays a significant role in navigating the emotional landscape of dementia. Engaging in meaningful conversations with our loved one about their condition, their wishes for the future, and their day-to-day needs can foster a deeper connection and understanding. It also provides an opportunity to express our love, offer reassurance, and plan for the road ahead together.

If the emotional burden becomes too heavy to bear alone, please seek professional support. Therapists, counselors, and support groups specializing in dementia care can offer valuable guidance, coping strategies, and a safe space to process our emotions. Reaching out for help is a sign of strength and a proactive step in caring for ourselves and our loved one.

Throughout this journey, let us strive to approach each day with patience, compassion, and understanding—both for ourselves and for our loved one. Let us cherish the moments of connection, laughter, and love that still shine through, even amidst the challenges. May we find solace in the memories we hold dear and the unwavering bond that endures.

Remember, you are not alone in this emotional journey. We, as friends and family, are here to support you, listen to you, and walk alongside you every step of the way. Together, we can face the ups and downs with resilience, love, and the strength that comes from our shared commitment to our loved one's well-being.

With heartfelt support and understanding,

Rae Stonehouse

THE IMPORTANCE OF EARLY DETECTION IN DEMENTIA CARE: EMPOWERING PATIENTS AND CAREGIVERS

EARLY DETECTION PLAYS an important role in the journey of dementia care, offering many benefits for both the individual experiencing cognitive decline and their caregivers. Recognizing the signs and symptoms of dementia in its early stages opens the door to a world of support, interventions, and resources that can significantly improve the quality of life for all involved. This chapter explores the power of early detection and how it can shape the path of dementia care.

Benefits for the Individual with Dementia:

Access to Early Interventions:

Early detection allows for timely access to interventions that can slow the progression of the disease and alleviate symptoms. This may include medications that target specific parts of cognitive decline, such as memory loss or language difficulties. Additionally, engaging in brain-stimulating activities, such as puzzles, reading, or learning new skills, can help maintain cognitive function for a longer period.

Participation in Clinical Trials:

By identifying dementia early, individuals may have the opportunity to participate in clinical trials and research studies aimed at developing new treatments or even finding a cure. This not only gives them with access to cutting-edge interventions but also contributes to the advancement of dementia research, potentially benefiting countless others.

Autonomy in Decision-Making:

Early detection empowers individuals to make important decisions about their care, finances, and legal matters while they still have the cognitive capacity to do so. This includes expressing their preferences for future care arrangements, designating a power of attorney, and ensuring their wishes are respected as the disease progresses. By being proactive, they can maintain a sense of control and dignity throughout their journey.

Benefits for Caregivers:

Access to Information and Resources:

Caregivers of individuals with dementia often face many challenges and uncertainties. Early detection provides them with access to a wealth of information and resources to better understand the condition and learn effective caregiving strategies. This may include educational materials, support groups, and training programs that offer practical advice and emotional support.

Improved Communication and Understanding:

Early detection lets caregivers develop a deeper understanding of the changes their loved one is experiencing. This knowledge can help with better communication, patience, and empathy in their interactions. By recognizing the underlying causes of certain behaviors or challenges, caregivers can respond more effectively and provide the proper level of support.

Building a Support Network:

Caring for someone with dementia can be emotionally and physically demanding. Early detection enables caregivers to connect with others going through similar experiences, forming a support network that can provide encouragement, advice, and respite when needed. This sense of community can help alleviate feelings of isolation and burnout, making sure caregivers can maintain their own well-being while providing the best care.

Promoting Early Intervention:

To maximize the benefits of early detection, it is essential to promote awareness and encourage individuals and families to seek help if they notice signs of cognitive decline. This can be achieved through public education campaigns, community outreach programs, and collaboration among healthcare professionals, social services, and local organizations.

Primary care doctors play an important role in identifying early signs of dementia during routine check-ups and referring individuals for further evaluation when necessary. Encouraging open conversations about memory concerns and cognitive changes can help reduce the stigma surrounding dementia and empower individuals to seek support sooner.

Chapter Summary:

Early detection is a powerful tool in the journey of dementia care, offering many benefits for both the individual with dementia and their caregivers. By recognizing the signs and symptoms early, individuals can access interventions, participate in decision-making, and maintain a sense of control over their lives. Caregivers, in turn, can gain valuable knowledge, support, and resources to navigate the challenges of dementia care with greater confidence and resilience.

Early intervention requires a collective effort from healthcare professionals, community organizations, and society. By raising awareness, reducing stigma, and encouraging open conversations about cognitive health, we can make sure individuals and families affected by dementia receive the support they need to live with dignity, understanding, and hope.

~

FREQUENTLY ASKED QUESTIONS:

1. How important is it to catch dementia early, and what can we do if we suspect it? Catching dementia early is important. It opens the door to interventions that can slow down its progression and significantly improves the quality of life for your loved one. If you suspect dementia, observe their behavior for consistent patterns of symptoms and consult with a healthcare professional for an assessment. Early detection enables better planning for care and support, ensuring safety, and allows for meaningful conversations about future wishes.

2. What are the signs we should watch for that might show the start of dementia? Look out for signs like noticeable memory loss, especially of recent events or conversations, confusion about times or places, difficulty completing familiar tasks, changes in mood or behavior, and struggles with communication, such as finding the right words. These symptoms can vary greatly, so note any significant changes in their usual behavior or abilities.

3. Dementia seems to affect everyone differently. How can we tailor care to meet individual needs? Dementia impacts each person uniquely, influenced by the type of dementia, their personality, and overall health. Tailor care by being attentive to their specific needs, preferences, and abilities. Engage in activities they enjoy and can participate in, adapt communication strategies, and create a safe, supportive environment. Consult with healthcare providers to develop a personalized care plan that addresses their unique challenges and promotes their independence.

4. What can we do to support our loved one in maintaining their independence and quality of life? Promote their independence by encouraging them to engage in daily tasks and activities they enjoy, with adaptations as needed. Maintain a routine to provide a sense of stability. Introduce cognitive exercises, physical activities, and social interactions suitable for their level of ability. Always focus on what they can do rather than what they cannot, and provide choices to give them a sense of control.

5. How can we, as caregivers, prepare ourselves emotionally and practically for the journey ahead with our loved one with dementia? Caring for someone with dementia is emotionally demanding. Prepare by educating yourself about the condition, joining support groups, and seeking professional advice. Practically, organize legal and financial affairs early, establish a care network, and explore local resources and services. Emotionally, allow yourself to grieve, seek emotional support, and remember to care for your own well-being. Recognizing your limits and when to seek help is a strength, not a weakness.

Remember, while the journey with dementia can be challenging, your love, patience, and support make a profound difference in your loved one's life. Keep learning, stay flexible, and lean on the community around you for support.

~

CASE STUDY: THE JOURNEY OF CAROL AND HER MOTHER, SUSAN

CAROL, a high school teacher in her early forties, began to notice subtle changes in her mother, Susan's behavior and memory. Susan, a 68-year-old retired librarian with a zest for life and a love for gardening, started forgetting names and appointments, which was out of character for her. At first, Carol attributed these lapses to the normal aging process. However, when Susan forgot her way home from the local supermarket, a route she had navigated for over 30 years, Carol realized it was time to seek help.

Early Detection: The First Step After noticing these changes, Carol encouraged her mother to see a doctor. The diagnosis was early-stage Alzheimer's disease. This early detection was important. It let them access support and start treatment that aimed to slow the progression of the disease. Carol learned the importance of early recognition and intervention, which opened doors to resources she hadn't known were available, such as support groups and access to clinical trials focusing on Alzheimer's.

Personalized Care: Tailoring Susan's Support Understanding that dementia affects everyone differently, Carol worked closely with healthcare professionals to develop a care plan tailored to Susan's needs and preferences. They incorporated cognitive exercises into Susan's daily routine, adjusted her diet, and introduced regular physical activity, which Susan enjoyed in her gardening. Carol also changed their home to make it safer and more navigable for Susan, addressing potential safety concerns proactively.

Navigating Emotional Challenges One of the most significant lessons Carol learned was the importance of caring for herself. The emotional toll of watching her mother's gradual decline was more challenging than she had expected. Carol found solace in a support group for caregivers of individuals with dementia. This group became an important outlet for her to share her experiences, learn from others, and realize she wasn't alone in her journey.

Adapting to Changes As Susan's condition evolved, so did their approach to care. Carol learned to be flexible and adapt to her mother's changing needs. Communication techniques that once worked no longer sufficed, so Carol educated herself on alternative methods to connect and engage with her mother. She also learned the value of cherishing the good days and not dwelling on the difficult ones.

Lessons Learned by Carol

- **Early detection is key**: It provides access to treatments and support systems that can improve quality of life.
- **Personalized care is essential**: Dementia manifests differently in everyone, requiring a tailored approach to care.
- **Self-care for caregivers is important**: Joining a support group and recognizing her own needs helped Carol navigate the caregiving journey.
- **Flexibility and patience**: Carol learned to adapt to her mother's evolving needs, finding new ways to communicate and connect.
- **Cherishing moments**: Embracing the good days and finding joy in small victories became a source of strength for both Carol and Susan.

Carol's journey with her mother underscores the importance of early detection, personalized care, and the need for caregiver support. By sharing their story, Carol hopes to illuminate the path for others navigating similar challenges, emphasizing that while the journey may be difficult, there is support, love, and moments of joy to be found along the way.

～

PART THREE WRAP-UP:
ACTION ITEMS FOR THE CAREGIVER:

BASED ON CAROL's journey with her mother, Susan, here's a list of action items for caregivers managing a loved one's dementia:

1. **Seek Early Diagnosis**: If you notice changes in memory, behavior, or cognitive abilities in your loved one, encourage them to see a healthcare provider for an assessment.
2. **Educate Yourself**: Learn as much as you can about dementia, including its progression, treatments, and caregiving strategies. Knowledge is power when providing the best care.
3. **Develop a Personalized Care Plan**: Work with healthcare professionals to create a care plan tailored to your loved one's specific needs, preferences, and stage of dementia.
4. **Implement Safety Measures at Home**: Evaluate your home environment and make necessary changes to ensure safety and comfort for your loved one, such as removing trip hazards and installing grab bars in the bathroom.
5. **Incorporate Cognitive and Physical Activities**: Engage your loved one in activities that promote cognitive health and physical well-being, tailored to their interests and abilities.

6. **Join a Support Group**: Connect with a support group for caregivers of individuals with dementia. Sharing experiences and receiving support can help manage the emotional toll of caregiving.

7. **Practice Self-Care**: Recognize the importance of your own health and well-being. Make time for activities that rejuvenate you, and seek respite care when needed to take breaks.

8. **Be Flexible and Patient**: Understand that dementia is a progressive condition, and your loved one's needs will change. Stay adaptable and patient as you navigate these changes together.

9. **Learn Communication Techniques**: As dementia progresses, traditional forms of communication may become less effective. Educate yourself on alternative ways to connect and communicate with your loved one.

10. **Document Care and Observations**: Keep a detailed record of your loved one's condition, care plan, and any changes you observe. This information can be valuable for healthcare providers and other family members.

11. **Legal and Financial Planning**: Discuss and arrange for the management of legal and financial matters early in the diagnosis. Planning ahead can alleviate future stresses and uncertainties.

12. **Cherish the Good Moments**: Focus on the positive aspects of caregiving and the joy that comes with spending quality time with your loved one. Celebrate small victories and meaningful moments.

13. **Seek Professional Advice**: Don't hesitate to consult with healthcare professionals, legal advisors, or dementia care specialists for guidance on care decisions and planning.

14. **Advocate for Your Loved One**: Be a strong advocate for your loved one's needs and rights, whether in healthcare settings or in the community.

By following these action items, caregivers can provide compassionate, effective care for their loved ones with dementia while also taking care of themselves.

~

IN OUR NEXT PART...

IN OUR NEXT PART, we'll guide you through the critical steps of navigating the diagnosis process for your loved one, shining a light on a path that can often feel overshadowed by uncertainty. Recognizing the signs of dementia is the beginning. From there, it's about taking actionable steps toward confirming a diagnosis, understanding what it means, and planning for the care that follows. We'll dig into the importance of professional evaluations, the many diagnostic tools available, and how to interpret and use the information they provide. This journey is about equipping yourself with knowledge and resources, ensuring you're prepared to support your loved one with compassion, understanding, and effective strategies that cater to their individual needs.

We understand the emotional weight that comes with a dementia diagnosis, not just for the individual but for their entire circle of care. So, we'll also explore the emotional parts of this journey, offering advice on how to approach conversations about dementia with sensitivity and support. We'll emphasize the strength found in numbers—how family members and caregivers can collaborate to form a strong support network, ensuring no one walks this path alone.

By fostering an environment of open communication, shared decision-making, and mutual support, you can navigate the challenges of dementia with resilience and hope, creating a care plan that respects your loved one's dignity and enhances their quality of life. Join us as we start this important Part, designed to guide, inform, and empower you through the complexities of dementia care.

~

PART FOUR

NAVIGATING THE DIAGNOSIS PROCESS FOR YOUR LOVED ONE ONCE YOU SUSPECT DEMENTIA, WHAT'S NEXT?

NAVIGATING THE PATH TO A DEMENTIA DIAGNOSIS: UNDERSTANDING THE SIGNS AND SYMPTOMS

SUSPECTING that a loved one may be showing signs of dementia can be an emotionally challenging and overwhelming experience. It marks the beginning of a journey filled with uncertainty, concern, and a search for answers. The important first step in this process is obtaining a clear and accurate diagnosis. This chapter aims to guide you through the early stages of recognizing potential dementia symptoms and the steps involved in seeking a professional evaluation.

Recognizing the Signs and Symptoms of Dementia:

Dementia is not a single specific disease but rather an umbrella term encompassing a range of symptoms that affect cognitive function, memory, and social abilities. Some common signs that may indicate dementia include:

Memory Loss:

- Forgetting recently learned information or important events
- Repeatedly asking the same questions
- Relying heavily on memory aids or family members for things they used to handle independently

Difficulty with Problem-Solving and Planning:

- Struggling to develop and follow a plan or work with numbers
- Trouble following a familiar recipe or keeping track of monthly bills
- Difficulty concentrating and taking much longer to complete tasks than before

Confusion with Time or Place:

Losing track of dates, seasons, and the passage of time

Forgetting where they are or how they got there

Having trouble understanding something if it's not happening immediately

Language and Communication Challenges:

Difficulty finding the right words or following conversations

Struggling to vocabulary or having trouble naming familiar objects

Repeating themselves or losing their train of thought mid-conversation

Changes in Mood and Personality:

- Experiencing rapid mood swings or changes in disposition
- Becoming suspicious, fearful, anxious, or easily upset
- Withdrawing from social activities or showing a lack of interest in hobbies they once enjoyed

Difficulty with Familiar Tasks:

- Struggling to complete daily tasks, such as dressing appropriately or managing personal hygiene
- Forgetting the rules or having trouble with decision-making in favorite hobbies or games
- Having trouble driving to a familiar location or remembering how to perform a routine task at work

If you notice a combination of these signs in your loved one, it's essential to seek a professional evaluation to determine the underlying cause and receive an accurate diagnosis.

Navigating the Diagnostic Process:

When you suspect that your loved one may have dementia, acting is important. Here are the steps involved in seeking a diagnosis:

Schedule a Comprehensive Medical Evaluation:

Make an appointment with a primary care doctor or a specialist, such as a neurologist or geriatrician, who has experience in assessing cognitive health.

Prepare for the appointment by noting specific examples of concerning symptoms and any changes in your loved one's behavior or abilities.

Involve Family Members and Caregivers:

Encourage family members or other caregivers to share their observations and experiences with the healthcare team.

Multiple perspectives can provide a more comprehensive picture of your loved one's condition and help identify patterns or changes that may not be apparent in a single visit.

Undergo Diagnostic Tests and Assessments:

The healthcare provider may recommend various tests, such as cognitive assessments, brain imaging scans (e.g., CT or MRI), or laboratory tests to rule out other potential causes of cognitive decline.

These tests can provide valuable information about brain structure, function, and any underlying medical conditions that may be contributing to the symptoms.

Consider Seeking a Second Opinion:

If you have concerns about the initial diagnosis or the proposed treatment plan, don't hesitate to seek a second opinion from another qualified healthcare professional.

A fresh perspective can provide more insights and help you feel more confident in the diagnosis and next steps.

Develop a Comprehensive Care Plan:

Once a diagnosis is confirmed, work closely with the healthcare team to develop a personalized care plan that addresses your loved one's specific needs and goals.

This may include medications to manage symptoms, lifestyle changes to promote brain health, and accessing support services and resources for both the person with dementia and their caregivers.

Chapter Summary:

Suspecting that a loved one may have dementia can be a daunting and emotional experience, but it's important to remember that you are not alone. By understanding the signs and symptoms to watch for and taking proactive steps to seek a professional evaluation, you can make sure your loved one receives a correct diagnosis and the proper care and support.

Throughout the diagnostic process, it's essential to involve healthcare professionals, family members, and caregivers to gather a comprehensive understanding of your loved one's condition. By working together and approaching the journey with knowledge, compassion, and a commitment to providing the best care, you can navigate the path ahead with greater confidence and hope.

Remember, an early diagnosis can open doors to interventions, support, and resources that can greatly enhance your loved one's quality of life and empower you as a caregiver. Please reach out for help and guidance every step of the way.

SUPPORTING YOUR LOVED ONE WITH DEMENTIA IN SEEKING PROFESSIONAL HELP: NAVIGATING HEALTH CONCERNS RELATED TO THE BRAIN AND NERVOUS SYSTEM

As a caregiver, one of the most important ways you can support your loved one with dementia is by encouraging them to seek professional help when navigating health concerns related to the brain and nervous system. Healthcare professionals, including doctors, neurologists, and neuropsychologists, play a crucial role in identifying the underlying causes of symptoms, providing accurate diagnoses, and developing effective treatment plans. In this chapter, we'll explore how you can assist your loved one in benefiting from the expertise of these specialists.

Recognizing the Need for Specialized Knowledge:

When your loved one with dementia experiences symptoms or changes in their cognitive functioning, it's essential to recognize the importance of seeking specialized knowledge. Healthcare professionals who specialize in brain health and neurological disorders have an in-depth understanding of the complexities of the brain and nervous system. Encourage your loved one to trust in the expertise of these professionals, who can provide accurate assessments and insights into the potential causes of their health concerns.

Facilitating Comprehensive Evaluations:

As a caregiver, you can play a vital role in facilitating comprehensive evaluations for your loved one with dementia. This may involve scheduling appointments with healthcare professionals, providing relevant medical history and information, and ensuring that your loved one attends these evaluations. During the assessment process, healthcare professionals may conduct physical examinations, neurological assessments, and specialized diagnostic tests. By supporting your loved one through this process, you enable them to receive a thorough evaluation that can lead to accurate diagnoses and targeted treatment plans.

Assisting with Differential Diagnosis:

Differential diagnosis is a critical step in identifying the true underlying cause of your loved one's health concerns. Healthcare professionals are trained to systematically consider and rule out various possibilities to arrive at the most accurate diagnosis. As a caregiver, you can assist in this process by providing detailed information about your loved one's symptoms, medical history, and any observed changes in their behavior or cognitive functioning. Your insights and observations can be valuable in helping healthcare professionals distinguish between conditions that may present similar symptoms.

Collaborating on Personalized Treatment Plans:

Once a diagnosis is established, healthcare professionals will work collaboratively with you and your loved one to develop a personalized treatment plan. This may involve medication management, therapy, lifestyle modifications, or other interventions aimed at alleviating symptoms and improving overall functioning. As a caregiver, you play a crucial role in implementing and monitoring these treatment plans. Collaborate closely with healthcare professionals, asking questions, providing feedback, and expressing any concerns you may have. Your active involvement ensures that your loved one receives the most appropriate and effective care tailored to their unique needs.

Supporting Ongoing Monitoring and Adjustments:

Navigating health concerns related to dementia is an ongoing process that requires regular follow-up and monitoring. As a caregiver, you can support your loved one by ensuring they attend regular check-ins with healthcare professionals. These appointments allow for the early detection of any new or worsening symptoms and enable prompt adjustments to the treatment plan if necessary. By staying proactive and engaged in your loved one's care, you can help prevent potential complications and optimize their well-being.

Accessing Support and Resources:

Healthcare professionals serve as valuable sources of information, support, and guidance for both you and your loved one with dementia. They can give you educational resources to better understand the condition, connect you with relevant support groups or community resources, and offer strategies for coping with the challenges of caregiving. Encourage your loved one to actively participate in these resources and support networks, as they can provide a sense of empowerment and improve overall quality of life.

Chapter Summary:

Supporting your loved one with dementia in seeking professional help is a vital aspect of their care journey. By recognizing the importance of specialized knowledge, facilitating comprehensive evaluations, assisting with differential diagnosis, collaborating on personalized treatment plans, supporting ongoing monitoring, and accessing valuable resources, you enable your loved one to receive the highest quality of care.

Remember, you are not alone on this journey. Healthcare professionals are there to support both you and your loved one every step of the way. By working together as a team, you can navigate the complexities of dementia with greater confidence, knowing that you have access to the expertise and guidance necessary to promote your loved one's well-being and quality of life.

DECODING DEMENTIA: A COMPREHENSIVE GUIDE TO DIAGNOSTIC TOOLS AND ASSESSMENTS

WHEN FACED with concerns about dementia, navigating the diagnostic process can be overwhelming and confusing. However, understanding the various tests and assessments available can provide clarity and empower individuals and their loved ones to make informed decisions about care and support. This chapter aims to shed light on the diverse tools used by healthcare professionals to diagnose and assess dementia, helping to demystify the process and pave the way for effective intervention.

Cognitive Assessments:

Cognitive assessments serve as a foundational tool in evaluating an individual's mental functions, including memory, attention, language abilities, and problem-solving skills. Commonly used tests include the Mini-Mental State Examination (MMSE) and the Montreal Cognitive Assessment (MoCA). These assessments provide healthcare professionals with a snapshot of a person's cognitive abilities, helping to identify areas of concern and establish a baseline for tracking changes.

Brain Imaging Techniques:

Advanced imaging techniques, such as Magnetic Resonance Imaging (MRI) and Computed Tomography (CT) scans, let doctors visualize the structure of the brain and detect signs of dementia-related changes. These scans can reveal brain shrinkage, the presence of abnormal proteins, or other indicators that may suggest specific types of dementia, such as Alzheimer's disease or vascular dementia. By providing a detailed view of the brain's anatomy, imaging techniques contribute to a more accurate diagnosis.

Laboratory Tests:

Blood tests play an important role in ruling out other potential causes of cognitive symptoms that may mimic dementia. These tests can identify vitamin deficiencies, thyroid disorders, infections, or other medical conditions that can affect cognitive function. By eliminating these alternative explanations, healthcare professionals can narrow down the diagnostic possibilities and focus on dementia-specific assessments.

Neuropsychological Testing:

Neuropsychological testing offers a more in-depth evaluation of an individual's cognitive abilities, providing a detailed map of strengths and weaknesses across various domains. Conducted by specialized professionals, such as neuropsychologists, these tests assess memory, language, attention, executive functioning, and other cognitive skills. The results of neuropsychological testing can help pinpoint the specific areas of the brain affected by dementia and guide personalized treatment approaches.

Genetic Testing:

In some cases, dementia may have a genetic component, particularly in early-onset forms of Alzheimer's disease or other inherited dementias. Genetic testing involves analyzing an individual's DNA to identify specific mutations or risk factors associated with these conditions. While not routinely performed for all individuals with dementia concerns, genetic testing can provide valuable information for families with a history of early-onset dementia and guide discussions about preventive measures and future care planning.

Cerebrospinal Fluid Analysis:

Analyzing cerebrospinal fluid (CSF) obtained through a lumbar puncture can provide insights into the biological markers of dementia. By measuring levels of specific proteins, such as amyloid-beta and tau, healthcare professionals can identify patterns associated with different types of dementia. CSF analysis can be useful in differentiating between Alzheimer's disease and other forms of dementia, guiding targeted treatment strategies.

Functional Assessments:

Evaluating an individual's ability to perform everyday tasks and activities of daily living (ADLs) is an important part of dementia assessment. Functional assessments may include observations of tasks such as cooking, dressing, managing medications, or handling finances. These assessments provide valuable information about the practical impact of dementia on a person's daily life and help determine the level of support and care required.

Positron Emission Tomography (PET) Scans:

PET scans are specialized imaging techniques that measure the brain's metabolic activity, including glucose and oxygen consumption. By detecting areas of reduced activity or abnormal patterns, PET scans can provide evidence of Alzheimer's disease or other dementias. Additionally, newer PET techniques using specific tracers can visualize the accumulation of abnormal proteins, such as amyloid or tau, further refining the diagnostic process.

Electroencephalography (EEG):

An EEG is a non-invasive test that measures the electrical activity of the brain using electrodes placed on the scalp. EEG can be useful in diagnosing certain types of dementia, such as Lewy body dementia or Creutzfeldt-Jakob disease, which show characteristic patterns of brain wave abnormalities. By detecting these electrical changes, EEG can contribute to a more precise diagnosis and guide treatment approaches.

Psychiatric Evaluation:

Dementia often coexists with psychiatric conditions, such as depression, anxiety, or behavioral changes. A comprehensive psychiatric evaluation is an essential part of the diagnostic process, helping to identify and address these comorbid mental health issues. By assessing mood, behavior, and overall psychological well-being, healthcare professionals can develop a holistic treatment plan that addresses both the cognitive and emotional parts of dementia.

Chapter Summary:

Decoding the complexities of dementia requires a multifaceted approach, using a range of diagnostic tools and assessments. By combining cognitive tests, brain imaging techniques, laboratory investigations, and functional evaluations, healthcare professionals can paint a comprehensive picture of an individual's cognitive health and identify the specific type and severity of dementia.

Understanding these diagnostic tools empowers individuals and their loved ones to actively participate, ask informed questions, and decide on care and support that align with their values and goals. While receiving a dementia diagnosis can be challenging, the knowledge gained through these assessments can provide a roadmap for effective interventions, personalized care planning, and access to important resources and support services.

As research continues to advance our understanding of dementia, diagnostic tools and assessments will continue to evolve, offering even greater precision and insights into this complex condition. By staying informed and partnering with healthcare professionals, individuals and families can navigate the diagnostic journey with greater confidence, ensuring the best outcomes for those affected by dementia.

～

OPENING THE CONVERSATION: TALKING ABOUT DEMENTIA WITH CARE AND COMPASSION

Discussing the possibility of dementia with a loved one can be an emotionally challenging and sensitive topic. It requires a delicate balance of compassion, understanding, and support to navigate this complex conversation effectively. While it may feel like treading on uncertain ground, having an open and honest dialogue is an important step in facing the challenges of dementia together.

This chapter provides guidance on how to approach this conversation with the care and sensitivity it deserves.

Choosing the Right Time and Place:

When starting a conversation about dementia concerns, it's essential to select a proper time and setting. Choose a moment when both you and your loved one are calm, relaxed, and free from distractions.

Choose a private and comfortable location where you can have an uninterrupted discussion. Make sure your loved one is in a receptive frame of mind and not already feeling overwhelmed or stressed by other matters.

Starting the Conversation Gently:

Begin the conversation by expressing your love, concern, and support for your loved one. Share the specific changes or behaviors you've observed that have led to your worries about their cognitive health. Use "I" statements to convey your perspective without sounding accusatory or judgmental. For example, "I've noticed that you've been having trouble remembering appointments lately, and I'm concerned about how you're doing."

Practicing Active Listening:

As your loved one responds to your concerns, focus on active listening. Give them the space to express their thoughts, feelings, and fears without interruption. Confirm their emotions and show empathy by acknowledging the challenges they may be facing. Use nonverbal cues, such as maintaining eye contact and nodding, to show your attentiveness and understanding.

Providing Information with Sensitivity:

Come prepared with accurate information about dementia, but share it in a way that is easily understandable and not overwhelming. Focus on the potential benefits of early diagnosis, such as access to appropriate medical care, support services, and the opportunity to plan. Avoid bombarding them with too many details at once, and be open to answering their questions or providing more resources as needed.

Emphasizing Your Unwavering Support:

Reassure your loved one you will be there for them throughout this journey, no matter what challenges may arise. Offer your help in attending medical appointments, gathering information, and making sense of the available options. Let them know that they are not alone and that you will support them in any way possible.

Respecting Their Autonomy:

While it's natural to have concerns and opinions about your loved one's health, it's important to respect their right to make their own choices. Avoid pressuring them into taking specific actions or making decisions they are not comfortable with. Instead, emphasize that you respect their autonomy and are there to support them in making informed decisions that align with their values and wishes.

Showing Patience and Empathy:

Recognize that processing the possibility of dementia can be emotionally overwhelming for both you and your loved one. Be prepared for a range of reactions, including denial, anger, fear, or resistance. Respond with patience, understanding, and empathy, even if the conversation becomes difficult. Remember this is a process, and it may take multiple discussions to reach a point of acceptance and readiness to act.

Chapter Summary:

Initiating a conversation about dementia with a loved one requires a thoughtful and compassionate approach. By choosing the right time and place, expressing your concerns with sensitivity, actively listening, providing gentle guidance, and emphasizing your unwavering support, you can create a safe and supportive environment for this important discussion.

Remember that the goal is not to force a specific outcome but to open the lines of communication, foster understanding, and pave the way for shared decision-making that respects your loved one's autonomy and dignity.

With patience, empathy, and a commitment to walking this path together, you can navigate the challenges of dementia as a united front, making sure your loved one receives the care, support, and understanding they need every step of the way.

$\sim$

THE STRENGTH IN NUMBERS: THE VITAL ROLE OF FAMILY AND CAREGIVERS IN THE DEMENTIA DIAGNOSIS JOURNEY

WHEN A LOVED ONE is facing the possibility of a dementia diagnosis, it can be a daunting and emotionally challenging journey. However, this should not be walked alone. Involving family members and caregivers from the beginning can provide invaluable support, insights, and advocacy throughout the diagnostic process. This chapter explores the important role that family and caregivers play and why their involvement is essential for ensuring the best outcomes for the individual affected by dementia.

Creating a Circle of Emotional Support:

Receiving a dementia diagnosis can be an emotionally overwhelming experience for both the individual and their loved ones. By involving family members and caregivers from the start, a strong circle of emotional support is established. This support network can provide comfort, understanding, and a sense of solidarity, reminding the person with dementia they are not alone in this journey. It also lets family members and caregivers lean on each other for mutual support and encouragement during challenging times.

Providing Valuable Insights and Observations:

Family members and caregivers often have unique perspectives and observations that can contribute significantly to the diagnostic process. They may notice subtle changes in behavior, memory, or daily functioning that the individual themselves may not be aware of or may not mention to healthcare professionals. By sharing these insights, family and caregivers can provide a more comprehensive picture of the person's cognitive health, aiding in accurate diagnosis and personalized care planning.

Helping with Comprehensive Care and Support:

Dementia care extends beyond medical treatment and requires a holistic approach that addresses the individual's physical, emotional, and social needs. Family members and caregivers play an important role in implementing and coordinating this comprehensive care. They can help with medication management, go to medical appointments, ensure a safe and supportive home environment, and provide practical assistance with daily activities. By being actively involved, family and caregivers can help translate the care plan into action, promoting the best quality of life for the person with dementia.

Enabling Informed Decision-Making:

Navigating the complexities of dementia diagnosis and treatment options can be overwhelming. Family members and caregivers well-informed about the condition, its progression, and resources can help make informed decisions on behalf of their loved one. They can advocate for the individual's best interests, make sure their wishes and preferences are respected, and make choices that align with their values and goals. By being knowledgeable and involved, family and caregivers can empower the person with dementia to have a voice in their own care.

Building a Supportive Community:

Dementia can be an isolating experience, but involving family and caregivers helps create a strong and supportive community around the individual. This network of care can provide various forms of help, from practical help with errands and household tasks to emotional support and companionship. By sharing the responsibilities and challenges of caregiving, family members and caregivers can prevent burnout and maintain their own well-being, making sure they can continue to provide the best care for their loved one.

Chapter Summary:

The journey of dementia diagnosis is not one that should be undertaken alone. Involving family members and caregivers from the beginning is essential for providing comprehensive support, valuable insights, and informed decision-making. By creating a circle of emotional support, helping with holistic care, and building a strong community, family and caregivers play an important role in ensuring the best outcomes for the person with dementia.

Recognizing the strength in numbers, healthcare professionals should actively encourage and help with the involvement of family and caregivers throughout the diagnostic process and beyond. By working together as a united front, the individual with dementia can receive the love, support, and advocacy they need to navigate this challenging journey with dignity and grace.

Ultimately, the involvement of family and caregivers is a powerful testament to the transformative power of love, compassion, and solidarity in the face of dementia. By walking this path together, hand in hand, we can make sure no one faces the challenges of dementia alone and that every individual receives the care and support they deserve.

$\sim$

GUIDING YOUR LOVED ONE THROUGH DEMENTIA: A CAREGIVER'S COMPASS

WHEN A LOVED ONE is diagnosed with dementia, it can feel like stepping into uncharted territory. The emotional impact of the diagnosis, combined with the practical realities of caregiving, can be overwhelming for both the person with dementia and their caregiver. As a caregiver, you may grapple with a range of emotions, from sadness and worry to a sense of responsibility and uncertainty about the future. However, with the right support, knowledge, and approach, you can navigate this journey with love, resilience, and grace, making sure your loved one receives the best care and maintains their dignity and quality of life.

Navigating the Emotional Terrain:

Witnessing the impact of dementia on someone you love can be emotionally challenging. You may experience feelings of loss, grief, and anxiety about the future. It's important to acknowledge and confirm these emotions, both for yourself and your loved one. Providing emotional support, reassurance, and a listening ear can help your loved one cope with the changes they are experiencing. At the same time, it's important to attend to your own emotional well-being by seeking support from family, friends, or support groups.

Sharing your experiences and feelings with others who understand can provide a sense of connection and help lighten the emotional burden.

Navigating the Practical Pathways:

Dementia requires significant changes in daily life, care routines, and long-term planning. As a caregiver, you may need to adapt the living environment to ensure safety and accessibility, manage medications and medical appointments, and help with daily activities such as bathing, dressing, and meal preparation. It's essential to educate yourself about dementia, its progression, and the available resources and support services in your community. Building a team of healthcare professionals, including doctors, nurses, and therapists, can provide valuable guidance and support throughout the caregiving journey.

Strategies for Navigating the Journey Together:

Lean on Others:

Recognize you need not shoulder the caregiving responsibilities alone. Contact family members, friends, and support groups for emotional and practical assistance. Delegating tasks and accepting help can prevent caregiver burnout and make sure you have the energy and resources to provide the best care for your loved one.

Educate Yourself:

Equip yourself with knowledge about dementia, its stages, and the challenges that may arise. Go to educational workshops, read books and chapters, and consult with healthcare professionals to gain a better understanding of what to expect. This knowledge can help you expect and prepare for future challenges, making the caregiving journey more manageable.

Establish a Daily Routine:

Creating a structured daily routine can provide a sense of stability and comfort for your loved one. Consistency in activities, mealtimes, and sleep schedules can reduce confusion and agitation, making caregiving tasks smoother for both of you. Incorporate activities that your loved one enjoys and that promote social engagement, cognitive stimulation, and physical activity.

Plan for the Future:

While it may be difficult to think about the future, early planning can alleviate future stresses and make sure your loved one's wishes are honored. Discuss legal and financial matters, such as power of attorney, healthcare directives, and long-term care options. Having these conversations and making necessary arrangements can provide peace of mind and let you focus on providing the best care in the present.

Prioritize Self-Care:

Caring for yourself is not a luxury, but a necessity. Engage in activities that bring you joy, help you relax, and promote your physical and mental well-being. Set aside time for hobbies, exercise, and social connections. Seeking respite care or joining a caregiver support group can provide much-needed breaks and emotional support.

Cherish the Present Moments:

Amidst the challenges of caregiving, it's important to find joy and meaning in the present moments. Engage in activities that your loved one enjoys, reminisce about happy memories, and create new ones together. Celebrate small victories and cherish the moments of connection and laughter. These positive experiences can bring a sense of purpose and strengthen your bond.

Foster Social Connections:

Encourage your loved one to maintain social connections and engage in activities that promote a sense of belonging. Participating in support groups, engaging in hobbies, or volunteering can help combat feelings of isolation and provide a sense of purpose. As a caregiver, it's also important to maintain your own social connections and seek support from others who understand your experiences.

Cultivate a Hopeful Outlook:

While the journey of dementia can be challenging, focusing on what you can control and finding strength in adaptability can help you maintain a positive perspective. Celebrate the small victories, find moments of joy and laughter, and remember that your love and dedication make a profound difference in your loved one's life. A hopeful outlook can provide the resilience needed to navigate even the toughest days.

Chapter Summary:

Guiding your loved one through the journey of dementia is a demanding yet rewarding role. As a caregiver, you will face emotional and practical challenges, but with the right support, knowledge, and approach, you can navigate this path with love, patience, and resilience. Remember that you are not alone, and there are resources and support systems available to help you along the way.

By leaning on others, educating yourself, establishing routines, planning for the future, prioritizing self-care, cherishing the present moments, fostering social connections, and cultivating a hopeful outlook, you can provide the best care for your loved one while also taking care of yourself. Your love, dedication, and compassion will make a profound difference in your loved one's life, making sure they feel respected, valued, and cared for every step of the way.

$\sim$

FORWARD THINKING: A GUIDE TO PLANNING AFTER A DEMENTIA DIAGNOSIS

RECEIVING a dementia diagnosis can be overwhelming, not only emotionally but also in terms of the practical considerations that come with planning. While it may be difficult to think about the road ahead, proactive planning is essential to make sure the individual's wishes are respected and that they receive the proper care as their condition progresses. This guide provides a roadmap to help navigate the planning process, covering legal preparations, care options, financial strategies, and the importance of building a strong support network.

Legal Preparations:

Power of Attorney:

Designating a trusted individual as your power of attorney is an important step in making sure your healthcare and financial decisions are made in accordance with your wishes, even if you become unable to make them yourself. This legal document grants the chosen person the authority to act on your behalf, making decisions that align with your values and preferences. Have open and honest conversations with your designated power of attorney to ensure they understand your desires and are ready to advocate for you when needed.

Living Will/Advance Directive:

A living will, also known as an advance directive, is a document that clearly outlines your preferences for medical care and end-of-life decisions. It serves to communicate your wishes when you may no longer be able to express them directly. This document can cover topics such as the use of life-sustaining treatments, pain management, and comfort care. By having a well-defined living will, you can make sure your healthcare team and loved ones are guided by your choices, even in difficult circumstances.

Exploring Care Options:

Researching Support Services:

As dementia progresses, the level of care required may change. Familiarize yourself with the types of support available, ranging from in-home care services to specialized dementia care facilities. In-home care can include help with daily activities, medication management, and companionship, letting the individual remain in the comfort of their own home for as long as possible. When more comprehensive care is needed, exploring options such as memory care units or skilled nursing facilities can make sure the individual receives the specialized attention and support they require.

Seeking Professional Guidance:

Navigating the complex landscape of dementia care options can be challenging. Enlisting the help of professionals, such as geriatric care managers or social workers, can provide valuable guidance and support. These experts have in-depth knowledge of local resources, can assess individual needs, and can help develop personalized care plans. They can also help with coordinating services, helping with communication between healthcare providers, and advocating for the individual's best interests.

Financial Strategies:

Financial Planning:

The costs associated with dementia care can be significant, making financial planning a critical part of the overall strategy. It's advisable to consult with a financial advisor who specializes in elder care planning to review your current financial situation and develop a comprehensive plan. This may involve analyzing income sources, evaluating assets, and exploring options such as long-term care insurance or reverse mortgages. By proactively addressing financial matters, you can help make sure the resources are available to cover care expenses and maintain the individual's quality of life.

Government Assistance Programs:

Investigating government assistance programs can provide additional financial support and access to essential services. Programs such as Medicaid, which is a joint federal and state program, can help cover the costs of long-term care for individuals with limited income and resources. Social Security Disability Insurance (SSDI) may also be available for individuals who have worked and paid into the Social Security system. Understanding the eligibility criteria and application processes for these programs can help alleviate some of the financial burden associated with dementia care.

Creating a Support Network:

Building a Team:

Surrounding yourself with a strong support network is important when navigating the journey of dementia. This network may include family members, friends, healthcare professionals, and support groups. Having a team of people to lean on can provide emotional support, practical assistance, and a sense of shared responsibility. Have open and honest conversations with your support network, expressing your needs and delegating tasks when necessary. Remember that you need not face this challenge alone, and accepting help from others can prevent caregiver burnout and make sure everyone involved receives the support they need.

Seeking Emotional Support:

Caring for someone with dementia can be emotionally taxing, and it's essential to focus on your own well-being. Joining support groups, either in-person or online, can provide a safe space to connect with others going through similar experiences. These groups offer an opportunity to share your struggles, learn from others' coping strategies, and find comfort in knowing you are not alone. Additionally, seeking individual counseling or therapy can help you process your emotions, develop coping mechanisms, and maintain your mental health throughout the caregiving journey.

Chapter Summary:

Planning after a dementia diagnosis is an act of love and empowerment. By taking proactive steps to address legal matters, explore care options, develop financial strategies, and build a strong support network, you can make sure the individual's wishes are respected and that they receive the care they need as their condition progresses. While the journey ahead may be challenging, having a well-defined plan in place can bring a sense of peace and reassurance to everyone involved.

Remember that planning is an ongoing process, and it's okay to revisit and adjust your plans as circumstances change. The most important thing is to approach the process with compassion, open communication, and a focus on the individual's well-being and dignity. By doing so, you can create a roadmap that not only addresses practical matters but also honors the unique needs and desires of the person living with dementia.

Ultimately, forward thinking and careful planning after a dementia diagnosis is a powerful way to advocate for your loved one, ensure their quality of life, and find comfort in knowing that their wishes will be carried out with love and respect.

~

FREQUENTLY ASKED QUESTIONS:

1. What's the first step if I suspect my loved one has dementia? The first step is scheduling an appointment with a healthcare professional, ideally one who specializes in cognitive disorders, such as a neurologist or geriatrician. Share your observations about your loved one's symptoms, no matter how small they seem. This information is valuable for doctors to understand the complete picture and decide on the necessary assessments or tests.

2. What kinds of tests can we expect during the diagnosis process? You can expect a combination of cognitive tests, such as the Mini-Mental State Examination (MMSE) or the Montreal Cognitive Assessment (MoCA), which assess memory, problem-solving skills, attention, language, and other mental functions. Brain imaging tests, like MRI or CT scans, may be used to look for brain changes related to dementia. Blood tests can help rule out other causes of cognitive impairment. Depending on the situation, more specialized tests like genetic testing or spinal fluid analysis might be recommended.

3. How can we prepare for our visit to the doctor? Gather information. This includes a detailed history of symptoms, any changes in behavior or personality, and how these changes impact daily life. Also, compile a list of all medications, both prescription and over-the-counter, as some substances can affect cognitive function. Bringing a family member or close friend to the appointment can help in remembering all the details and for emotional support.

4. What should we do after receiving a diagnosis of dementia? After a diagnosis, it's important to begin planning. This includes discussing care preferences, legal and financial planning, and exploring support options, such as local dementia support groups or respite care services. Educate yourself and your family about the dementia diagnosed, as this can help set realistic expectations and prepare for how the disease may progress.

5. How do we deal with the emotional impact of a dementia diagnosis? Receiving a diagnosis of dementia is challenging for both the individual and their loved ones. Allow yourself time to process the emotions. Seeking support from counseling or support groups can be beneficial. Remember, it's okay to feel a range of emotions, and seeking support is a sign of strength. Maintaining open and honest communication within the family and with healthcare providers can help navigate the emotional journey ahead.

Facing a dementia diagnosis is undoubtedly challenging, but understanding the process and knowing what steps to take can empower you to provide compassionate and effective support for your loved one. Remember, you're not alone; there are resources and communities ready to help guide you through this journey.

~

CASE STUDY: NAVIGATING THE DIAGNOSIS JOURNEY WITH MARIA AND HER FATHER, GEORGE

MARIA, a 45-year-old project manager, started noticing subtle changes in her father, George, a 72-year-old retired teacher. George, known for his sharp wit and love for literature, began forgetting names of long-time friends and misplacing his belongings more often than usual. At first, Maria chalked it up to normal aging. However, when George forgot his way back from their local park, a place he visited daily, Maria realized these were not just senior moments.

Early Signs and Seeking Diagnosis: The first step for Maria was acknowledging the potential signs of dementia in George. She remembered reading about the importance of early detection and its impact on care and management. This knowledge prompted her to schedule an appointment with a neurologist who specialized in cognitive disorders.

The Diagnostic Process: The neurologist conducted a comprehensive evaluation, including cognitive tests like the MMSE (Mini-Mental State Examination) and brain imaging studies such as MRI scans. The diagnosis confirmed early-stage Alzheimer's disease. Maria learned that early diagnosis was important. It opened up options for treatment that could slow the progression and made planning for George's care more manageable.

Creating a Support Network: One of the first lessons Maria learned was the importance of building a support network. She contacted family members, joined online support groups, and connected with local Alzheimer's associations. This network became an invaluable resource for emotional support and practical advice on navigating the care journey.

The Role of Professional Guidance: Maria quickly realized the value of turning to professionals for guidance. The neurologist helped her understand the specific aspects of George's condition and what to expect. A geriatric care manager advised on home safety changes and daily care strategies. Regular check-ups allowed for changes in George's care plan as his needs evolved.

Embracing Emotional Challenges: Navigating the emotional landscape was perhaps the most challenging part for Maria. She experienced a range of emotions, from denial and frustration to sadness. Learning to accept her feelings and discussing them in support groups helped Maria cope. She discovered that acknowledging her emotional journey was as important as managing the practical parts of George's care.

Lessons Learned by Maria:

- **Acknowledging the Signs**: Recognizing and acting on the early signs of dementia can significantly affect the care journey.
- **The Value of Early Diagnosis**: Early detection helped with access to treatments and support systems, making a difference in George's quality of life.
- **Building a Support Network**: Creating a circle of support with family, friends, and professionals gave Maria the emotional and practical support needed to navigate the challenges.
- **Turning to Professionals**: Leveraging the knowledge of healthcare professionals helped Maria understand George's condition and craft a tailored care plan.

- **Navigating Emotions**: Acknowledging and expressing her emotions was important for Maria's well-being, enabling her to be a more effective caregiver.
- **Planning for the Future**: Early planning for legal, financial, and long-term care needs helped reduce future stresses and uncertainties.

Maria's journey with her father illustrates the complexities of navigating a dementia diagnosis but also highlights the power of knowledge, support, and compassion. By taking proactive steps and leveraging available resources, Maria provided thoughtful care for George while also taking care of herself.

∾

PART FOUR WRAP-UP:

Based on Maria's journey with her father, George, here are actionable steps for caregivers navigating the dementia diagnosis process:

1. **Acknowledge Early Signs**: If you notice changes in memory, behavior, or cognitive abilities, don't dismiss them. Recognizing these signs early can lead to a more effective management plan.
2. **Schedule a Professional Evaluation**: Make an appointment with a healthcare provider specializing in cognitive disorders, such as a neurologist, to assess your loved one's condition.
3. **Educate Yourself on Dementia**: Learn about dementia, including its types, symptoms, progression, and management strategies. Knowledge is important for understanding and advocating for your loved one's needs.
4. **Build a Support Network**: Connect with family, friends, and caregiver support groups, both in-person and online. Sharing experiences and receiving support is important for navigating the caregiving journey.

onsult Multiple Professionals: Consider seeking opinions and guidance from various healthcare professionals, including geriatric care managers, for a comprehensive understanding of your loved one's condition and care needs.

6. **Participate in the Diagnostic Process**: Accompany your loved one to appointments and share observations with the healthcare team. Your insights are valuable for a complete assessment.

7. **Implement Recommended Interventions**: Follow through with recommended treatments, therapies, and lifestyle changes that can help manage symptoms and improve quality of life.

8. **Plan for Future Care Needs**: Discuss and document care preferences, legal, and financial matters early on. This proactive planning can alleviate future uncertainties.

9. **Focus on Emotional Well-being**: Recognize and address your own emotional responses to your loved one's diagnosis. Seeking support from counseling or support groups can be beneficial.

10. **Adapt to Changing Needs**: Be prepared for your loved one's needs to evolve as the disease progresses. Stay flexible and adjust care plans.

11. **Focus on Safety**: Evaluate and change the home environment to ensure safety and comfort. Consider measures to address wandering, falls, and daily living challenges.

12. **Maintain Regular Check-ups**: Keep up with regular medical appointments to track your loved one's health status and adjust care strategies as needed.

13. **Encourage Social Engagement**: Support your loved one in maintaining social connections and engaging in activities they enjoy, tailored to their abilities.

14. **Practice Self-Care**: Take care of your own health and well-being. Regular breaks, hobbies, and self-care practices are essential to sustain your ability to provide care.

15. **Celebrate the Present**: Cherish and make the most of the good days. Finding joy in small moments can provide strength and resilience for both you and your loved one.

Following these action items can help caregivers navigate the dementia diagnosis process ensuring both the caregiver and their loved one are supported throughout the journey.

∼

IN OUR NEXT PART...

IN OUR NEXT PART, we will dig into the profound emotional impact that dementia has on families. This journey, often marked by a mix of confusion, grief, and unexpected joy, reshapes the fabric of family dynamics in significant ways. We'll explore the initial shock that comes with the diagnosis, the common path of denial that many families tread, and the complex wave of emotions that follow. From the deep sadness of seeing a loved one's decline to the frustration and guilt that caregiving can stir, we aim to provide a compassionate overview of what families go through. This isn't just about understanding the emotional landscape; it's about finding ways to navigate it together, offering strategies to cope with the changes and challenges dementia brings into the lives of everyone it touches.

We'll look at how families adjust to new roles and responsibilities, a shift that can test the bonds of even the strongest family units. The transition from being a partner, child, or sibling to becoming a primary caregiver can bring about a profound change in family dynamics, often requiring a reevaluation of personal and collective strengths and limitations.

We'll offer insights into how families can maintain a sense of unity and support for one another emphasizing the importance of open communication, shared decision-making, and the need for external support. Through this exploration, our goal is to empower families to face the challenges of dementia with resilience and hope, ensuring that amidst the trials, the moments of connection and love continue to shine through, reminding us the strength found in togetherness.

∽

PART FIVE
THE EMOTIONAL IMPACT OF DEMENTIA ON FAMILIES

FEELING THE WAVES: THE EMOTIONAL JOURNEY OF DEMENTIA IN FAMILIES

A DEMENTIA DIAGNOSIS not only impacts the individual but also sends shockwaves through the entire family. As loved ones grapple with the reality of the situation, they embark on an emotional rollercoaster filled with a wide range of feelings, from shock and denial to sadness, frustration, and moments of unexpected joy. This chapter explores the complex emotional landscape that families navigate together as they support their loved one with dementia.

The Initial Shock:

Learning that a family member has dementia can be a devastating blow. It marks the beginning of a journey into uncharted territory, filled with uncertainty and a profound sense of loss. The news can leave family members reeling, struggling to come to terms with the reality of the situation. This moment forever changes the family dynamic, forcing everyone to confront the challenges that lie ahead.

Denial: A Natural Defense Mechanism:

Faced with this overwhelming news, denial often serves as a protective shield, letting family members temporarily push away the painful truth. It's a natural coping mechanism that helps individuals gradually process the amount of situation. Denial can manifest in various ways, such as downplaying the severity of the symptoms or convincing oneself that the diagnosis is a mistake. While denial can provide temporary relief, it's essential to eventually acknowledge the reality of the situation to effectively support the loved one with dementia.

Riding the Emotional Waves:

As the reality of the diagnosis sinks in, family members may ride a tumultuous wave of emotions. Sadness and grief are common companions on this journey, as loved ones mourn the gradual loss of the person they once knew. Watching someone you care about struggle with memory loss, confusion, and declining abilities can be heartbreaking. Frustration is another frequent visitor, as family members navigate the challenges of caregiving and the unpredictable nature of dementia.

The Hidden Struggles of Anger and Resentment:

Amidst the sadness and frustration, anger and resentment can also simmer beneath the surface. Caregiving can be an all-consuming task, demanding significant time, energy, and emotional resources. Family members may feel angry at the situation, resenting the changes it has brought to their lives, or even harboring frustration toward the person with dementia. These feelings are a normal part of the emotional journey, but it's important to acknowledge and address them healthily.

The Burden of Guilt:

Guilt is a heavy weight that many family members carry on their shoulders. They may feel guilty for losing patience, for needing a break from caregiving, or for not doing enough. Guilt can also arise from conflicting emotions, such as feeling relief when the person with dementia is having a good day or wishing for a respite from the constant demands of caregiving. These feelings are a testament to the love and care family members provide, but it's equally important to practice self-compassion and recognize the limits of one's own abilities.

Moments of Joy and Connection:

Despite the challenges and emotional turmoil, there are still glimmers of light along the way. Unexpected moments of clarity, laughter, and connection can bring immense joy and comfort to both the person with dementia and their family members. These precious instances serve as reminders of the enduring love and bond that exists, even amidst the trials of the disease. Cherishing these moments and finding ways to create new ones can help sustain family members through the difficult times.

Navigating the Emotional Landscape:

To effectively cope with the emotional journey of dementia, family members must prioritize their own well-being. Giving oneself permission to feel the full range of emotions, without judgment, is an important step. Seeking support from other family members, friends, or professional counselors can provide a safe space to process feelings and find solace. Joining support groups or connecting with others on a similar journey can offer a sense of community and validation.

Navigating the emotional journey of dementia as a family is undeniably challenging. From the initial shock of the diagnosis to the ongoing waves of sadness, frustration, anger, and guilt, family members are confronted with a complex tapestry of feelings. However, amidst the difficulties, there are also opportunities for growth, deepening understanding, and cherished moments of connection.

By acknowledging and confirming the wide range of emotions experienced, family members can better support one another and their loved one with dementia. Seeking support, practicing self-care, and finding healthy outlets for expressing feelings are essential parts of managing the emotional load. No one must face this journey alone, and that reaching out for help is a sign of strength, not weakness.

Ultimately, the emotional journey of dementia in families is a testament to the power of love, resilience, and the unbreakable bonds that exist within families. By navigating the waves together, family members can find solace, strength, and even unexpected moments of joy as they support their loved one through the challenges of dementia.

ADJUSTING TO NEW ROLES: THE FAMILY DYNAMICS IN DEMENTIA CARE

A DEMENTIA DIAGNOSIS not only affects the individual but also sends ripples through the entire family system. As the family navigates this uncharted territory, roles and responsibilities shift, forcing each member to find their footing in a new and unfamiliar landscape. This change period can be challenging, testing the resilience and adaptability of the family unit. This chapter explores the impact of dementia on family dynamics, the emotional toll of redefining roles, and strategies for maintaining family harmony in the face of adversity.

The Initial Shockwave:

When a family member is diagnosed with dementia, the initial reaction is often one of disbelief and denial. This natural response can temporarily cloud the family's ability to process the news and plan for the future. During this phase, tensions may arise as each family member comes to terms with the diagnosis at their own pace. Disagreements and conflicts can surface, stemming from differing perspectives on accepting the reality of the situation and determining the best course of action.

Redefining Roles and Responsibilities:

As the person with dementia's condition progresses, the need for increased care and support becomes clear. This often requires a redistribution of roles and responsibilities within the family. One family member may step into the role of the primary caregiver, while others take on tasks such as managing finances, coordinating medical appointments, or providing emotional support. This reshuffling of duties can evoke a complex mix of emotions, including resentment, guilt, and exhaustion, particularly if the caregiving burden feels disproportionately placed on certain individuals.

Navigating the Emotional Landscape:

Adjusting to these new roles and dynamics can take a significant emotional toll on family members. Feelings of guilt may arise for not doing enough or for experiencing moments of frustration and impatience. Resentment toward other family members who may not be as involved or supportive can strain relationships. The constant demands of caregiving can lead to physical and emotional exhaustion, further compounding the stress and strain on the family unit.

Navigating family dynamics in dementia care often involves managing differing opinions and approaches to caregiving. Disagreements may emerge regarding the best course of action, such as deciding on living arrangements, exploring care options, or making medical decisions on behalf of the person with dementia. These conflicts can add another layer of stress to an already challenging situation.

Strategies for Maintaining Family Harmony:

To navigate the complexities of family dynamics in dementia care, open communication, seeking external support, and focusing on self-care are essential. Here are strategies to help families find their way forward:

Foster Open Communication:

Encourage open and honest conversations among family members about the changes and challenges they are experiencing. Create a safe space for each person to express their thoughts, feelings, and concerns without judgment. Active listening and empathy can help build understanding and bridge gaps in perspectives.

Divide Responsibilities Fairly:

Work together as a family to distribute caregiving responsibilities in a way that feels equitable and manageable for everyone involved. Recognize that each family member's capacity to provide care may differ based on their individual circumstances, such as work commitments, geographical distance, or personal health. Be willing to reassess and adjust roles as needed to prevent caregiver burnout and resentment.

Seek External Support:

Please reach out for guidance and support from healthcare professionals, such as geriatric care managers, social workers, or dementia support organizations. Joining caregiver support groups can provide a platform to connect with others facing similar challenges, share experiences, and learn coping strategies. Explore respite care options to allow primary caregivers much-needed breaks and opportunities for self-care.

Prioritize Self-Care:

Encourage each family member to focus on their own physical, emotional, and mental well-being. Recognize that caregiving can be emotionally and physically draining, and emphasize the importance of setting boundaries, taking breaks, and engaging in activities that promote personal rejuvenation. Support one another in practicing self-care and seeking professional help, such as counseling or therapy, when needed.

Chapter Summary:

Adjusting to new roles and navigating family dynamics in dementia care is a challenging journey that requires patience, understanding, and resilience. The impact of a dementia diagnosis on the family unit can be profound, testing the strength of relationships and forcing a redefinition of roles and responsibilities.

While the emotional landscape can be complex, with feelings of guilt, resentment, and exhaustion intertwined, the family is not alone in this journey. By fostering open communication, dividing responsibilities fairly, seeking external support, and focusing on self-care, families can find a path forward that promotes unity, compassion, and mutual support.

Navigating the journey of dementia as a family presents an opportunity for growth, deepening connections, and discovering inner strength in the face of adversity. By working together, sharing the load, and caring for one another's well-being, families can weather the challenges and find a new sense of balance and resilience in their transformed reality.

$\backsim$

THE HEARTACHE OF
WATCHING A LOVED ONE
FADE AWAY

SEEING A LOVED one gradually lose their grip on reality due to dementia is a painful and emotionally taxing experience for families. The journey is marked by small losses that collect over time, chipping away at the person you once knew. This chapter digs into the profound heartache and complex emotions that families face as they watch their loved one slowly fade away.

The Subtle Signs:

The descent into dementia often begins with subtle changes that are easily dismissed as normal signs of aging. Misplaced keys, forgotten names, or missed appointments may be first brushed off as minor lapses in memory. However, as these incidents become more frequent and severe, the realization that something is wrong takes hold. This gradual awakening to the reality of the situation can be a deeply unsettling and emotional process for family members.

The Loss of Independence:

One of the most heartbreaking aspects of dementia is seeing the gradual loss of a loved one's autonomy and independence. The person who once thrived on self-sufficiency may now struggle with basic tasks such as dressing, bathing, or preparing meals. This shift in roles, from being the caregiver to the one needing care, can be profoundly disheartening for both the individual with dementia and their family members. It is a fundamental change in the family dynamic and can evoke feelings of sadness, helplessness, and grief.

A Whirlwind of Emotions:

As families navigate the journey of dementia, they are confronted with a complex tapestry of emotions. The constant sorrow of losing the essence of their loved one piece by piece is a heavy burden to bear. This ongoing process of mourning comes with a sense of helplessness in the face of the disease's relentless progression. The knowledge that there is no cure or way to halt the decline can be frustrating and disheartening.

The changing family roles and responsibilities add another layer of emotional complexity. Family members may find themselves thrust into unfamiliar caregiving roles, leading to a profound shift in the family dynamic. This can be challenging for adult children who care for their parents, a reversal of the nurturing roles they have always known.

The Uncertainty of the Future:

Living with the uncertainty of what lies ahead can be a source of deep anxiety and fear for families affected by dementia. Questions about the pace of decline, the level of care that will be required, and how the family will cope with the challenges to come can weigh heavily on everyone's minds. The inability to predict or control the trajectory of the disease can leave families feeling powerless and overwhelmed.

This ongoing cycle of mourning, hoping, and adapting to new realities is emotionally and mentally exhausting. Family members may find themselves in a constant state of anticipatory grief, bracing themselves for the next loss or change in their loved one's condition. The cumulative impact of this emotional roller coaster can take a significant toll on the well-being of everyone involved.

The Burden of Guilt and Resentment:

Amidst the heartache of watching a loved one fade away, guilt and resentment can also surface. Family members may experience guilt for feeling burdened by the responsibilities of caregiving or for believing they are not doing enough to support their loved one. They may also harbor feelings of resentment toward the disease itself and the drastic changes it has imposed on their lives.

These emotions can be difficult to grapple with and can strain even the strongest of family bonds. These feelings are a natural part of the grieving process and that it is essential to find healthy outlets for expressing and processing them.

Seeking Solace and Support:

Navigating the heartache of watching a loved one fade away due to dementia is a deeply personal and emotional journey. Families must lean on each other for support and to seek external resources to help them cope with the challenges they face. Finding solace in shared experiences, whether through family discussions, support groups, or professional counseling, can provide a sense of validation and understanding.

Connecting with others on a similar journey can offer comfort, practical advice, and a reminder no one must face this heartache alone. Professional guidance from healthcare providers, social workers, or counselors specializing in dementia care can also be invaluable in managing the complex emotions and practical parts of caregiving.

Chapter Summary:

The experience of watching a loved one slowly slip away due to dementia is a profound and life-altering journey for families. It is marked by small losses that gradually erode the essence of the person they once knew. The heartache of this process is compounded by the complex emotions that arise, including sorrow, helplessness, guilt, and resentment.

As families navigate this difficult path, it is essential to focus on open communication, mutual support, and self-care. Recognizing that the emotions experienced are a natural part of the grieving process and finding healthy outlets for expressing them can help prevent the strain on family relationships.

Seeking solace in shared experiences, whether through family discussions, support groups, or professional guidance, can provide a lifeline during this challenging time. It is a reminder no one must bear the weight of this heartache alone.

Ultimately, the journey of watching a loved one fade away due to dementia is a testament to the depth of love and the resilience of the human spirit. It is a journey of loss, but also one of cherishing the moments of connection and finding strength in the face of adversity. By leaning on each other and embracing the support available, families can navigate this heartache with grace, compassion, and the knowledge that they are not alone.

～

NAVIGATING THE EMOTIONAL LANDSCAPE OF DEMENTIA CARE

STEPPING into the role of a caregiver for a loved one with dementia is a journey that is as emotionally complex as it is challenging. The path is lined with many feelings, ranging from the heaviness of guilt and the grip of frustration to the profound depths of sadness. These emotions are a natural response to the immense responsibilities and the ever-changing nature of dementia care. This chapter explores the emotional landscape that caregivers must navigate, the impact on family dynamics, and the importance of seeking support to build resilience.

The Burden of Guilt:

Guilt is a persistent companion for many caregivers, casting a shadow over their efforts and magnifying every perceived shortcoming. Despite pouring their heart and soul into providing the best care, caregivers often feel like they are not doing enough. This guilt can stem from moments of frustration or exhaustion, when the weight of caregiving feels overwhelming. These feelings reflect the deep love and commitment caregivers have for their loved ones, not a measure of their adequacy or success.

The Grip of Frustration:

As dementia progresses, communication becomes increasingly challenging, and behaviors can become unpredictable. Caregivers may grapple with frustration as they try to decipher their loved one's needs and navigate the daily obstacles that arise. The feeling of running in place, striving to meet the ever-shifting demands of caregiving while also managing personal responsibilities, can be disheartening and emotionally draining. It is important to acknowledge that frustration is a natural response to the complexities of dementia care and not a sign of failure or lack of compassion.

The Depths of Sadness:

Watching a loved one gradually fade away, losing the essence of who they once were, is a profound source of sadness for caregivers. This grief is experienced in real-time, as cherished memories, shared experiences, and the ability to connect in familiar ways slowly slip away. This sorrow is compounded by the daily reminders of the relentless progression of dementia, creating a continuous cycle of mourning. Caregivers must navigate this emotional landscape while also providing practical and emotional support to their loved ones.

Shifting Family Dynamics:

Dementia has a significant impact on family dynamics, changing communication patterns, decision-making processes, and the roles and responsibilities of each family member. Caregivers may find themselves in the position of becoming the primary decision-maker, navigating not only medical and care decisions but also striving to preserve the dignity and autonomy of their loved one. This shift in dynamics can be challenging, as it requires a delicate balance of respecting the wishes of the person with dementia while ensuring their safety and well-being.

Seeking Balance:

Amidst the demands of caregiving, finding balance is important for the well-being of both the caregiver and the entire family. Caregivers must navigate the delicate dance of meeting the needs of their loved one while also attending to their own physical, emotional, and mental health. Maintaining a sense of normalcy, to whatever degree possible, becomes an important part of caregiving. This may involve finding moments of respite, engaging in self-care activities, and accepting help from others when offered. Recognizing that seeking balance is not a sign of weakness but rather an essential part of sustainable and effective caregiving is key.

The Power of Support:

Navigating the emotional landscape of dementia care can be overwhelming, but caregivers need not face these challenges alone. Seeking emotional support and guidance from others who understand the complexities of caregiving can be a lifeline. Connecting with support groups, whether online or in-person, provides a space to share experiences, learn coping strategies, and find validation for the range of emotions that come with caregiving. Professional counseling can also be invaluable in processing the grief, guilt, and stress that often go along with this journey. Building a support network is an important step in fostering resilience and finding the strength to continue providing loving care.

Chapter Summary:

Caring for a loved one with dementia is undeniably one of life's most challenging and emotionally taxing roles. The journey is marked by a complex tapestry of emotions, from the weight of guilt and the grip of frustration to the profound depths of sadness. These feelings are a natural response to the immense responsibilities and the ever-changing nature of dementia care.

As caregivers navigate this emotional landscape, seeking support and embracing the full spectrum of emotions is a sign of strength, not weakness. It is a testament to the deep love and commitment they have for their loved ones, even in the face of unimaginable challenges.

By acknowledging the impact of dementia on family dynamics, striving for balance, and leaning on the power of support, caregivers can build the resilience needed to continue this journey with grace and compassion. Amidst the trials and tribulations, there are still moments of love, connection, and profound human experience to be cherished.

Ultimately, navigating the emotional landscape of dementia care is a journey that requires patience, understanding, and an open heart. It is a path no one must walk alone. By embracing the support of others and honoring the full range of emotions that arise, caregivers can find the strength to provide the best care for their loved ones while also tending to their own well-being. In doing so, they illuminate a beacon of hope and love in the face of the challenges posed by dementia.

～

FREQUENTLY ASKED QUESTIONS:

1. How do we deal with the initial shock of a dementia diagnosis in the family? The shock of a dementia diagnosis can feel overwhelming. It's normal to experience a range of emotions, from disbelief to sadness. Give yourself and your family time to process these feelings. Open communication is key—talk about what you're going through and listen to each other's experiences and emotions. Remember, it's okay to seek support from professionals or support groups who can provide guidance and understanding during this challenging time.

2. How can we handle feelings of denial when a loved one is diagnosed with dementia? Denial is a common initial response to a difficult diagnosis like dementia. It serves as a protective mechanism to buffer the immediate shock. To move beyond denial, education is important. Learning about dementia together as a family can help you understand what to expect and how to support your loved one. Encourage each other to express feelings and concerns and consider seeking guidance from healthcare professionals or counselors who can help navigate these emotions.

3. What can we do to manage the frustration and sadness that comes with caring for a loved one with dementia? Frustration and sadness are natural responses to the challenges of caring for someone with dementia. To manage these emotions, establish a support network that includes friends, family, and caregivers who understand what you're going through. Take breaks when you need them, and don't be afraid to ask for help. Engaging in activities that bring joy and relaxation can also provide a necessary respite from caregiving duties. Lastly, focusing on the positive moments and maintaining a sense of humor can help alleviate some of the emotional burden.

4. How do we deal with guilt and resentment that may arise during the caregiving process? Guilt and resentment are common but often unspoken emotions among caregivers. Recognize these feelings are normal and don't make you a bad caregiver or family member. To combat guilt, remind yourself of the care and love you're providing, even when it's challenging. Sharing responsibilities among family members can help alleviate resentment and prevent caregiver burnout. Regularly communicating your needs and seeking external support can also maintain family harmony and ensure everyone's well-being is being considered.

5. How can we find moments of joy and connection with our loved one despite the progression of dementia? Finding joy and connection involves focusing on what your loved one can still enjoy and participate in. This might include listening to their favorite music, looking through photo albums together, or enjoying simple outdoor activities. Pay attention to the good days and cherish the moments of clarity and recognition. Adapt communication strategies to maintain a connection, using nonverbal cues and embracing the power of touch and presence. Remember, the emotional bond you share can continue to be a source of comfort and happiness for both of you.

Navigating the emotional impact of dementia on families requires patience, understanding, and compassion. This journey involves supporting each other as much as supporting the loved one affected by the disease. Remember, it's okay to seek help and take time for self-care to navigate this challenging path together.

~

CASE STUDY: THE THOMPSON FAMILY JOURNEY THROUGH DEMENTIA

Meet the Thompsons: a close-knit family grappling with their patriarch, Jack's, recent diagnosis of Alzheimer's disease. Jack, a retired school principal, has always been the cornerstone of strength and wisdom for his family. His wife, Ellen, two adult children, Sarah and Michael, and their families have started a journey none were prepared for, but together, they are learning to navigate the turbulent waters of dementia care.

The Shock and Denial: When Jack began forgetting names and missing appointments, the family joked about "senior moments." However, when he got lost driving home from his favorite golf course, reality hit hard. The diagnosis of Alzheimer's was a shock that sent waves of denial through the family. Ellen couldn't accept that the man she shared five decades with was slipping away. Sarah and Michael struggled with their invincible father becoming dependent.

Navigating the Emotional Landscape: The Thompsons experienced a rollercoaster of emotions. Ellen felt overwhelmed by sadness and guilt, questioning every impatient moment she had with Jack. Sarah grappled with frustration as her father's caregiver, feeling like she was losing parts of her own life to dementia. Michael, living in another state, wrestled with guilt for not helping more, and resentment toward his sister for what he perceived as control over their father's care.

Adjusting Roles and Responsibilities: As Jack's condition progressed, the family dynamics shifted significantly. Ellen, once the nurturer, found herself in the unfamiliar role of being cared for. Sarah took on the primary caregiver role, balancing her career and family life with her new responsibilities. Michael, feeling sidelined, struggled to find his place in the caregiving team.

Lessons Learned:

- **Open Communication is Key:** The Thompsons learned that keeping the lines of communication open was important. Family meetings became a regular part of their routine, letting everyone express their feelings, frustrations, and concerns.
- **Seeking External Support:** Ellen and Sarah joined a local support group for families dealing with dementia. The shared experiences and advice were invaluable, providing both practical tips and emotional solace.
- **Sharing the Caregiving Load:** The family realized that caregiving needed to be a shared responsibility. They enlisted the help of home health aides and explored respite care options, allowing Sarah some much-needed breaks and giving Michael specific tasks to manage from afar, like handling Jack's medical appointments and financial planning.
- **Cherishing Moments of Connection:** Amidst the challenges, the Thompsons found joy in moments of clarity and connection with Jack. They learned to live in the present, celebrating small victories and treasuring the lucid moments when Jack's humor and personality shone through.
- **Self-Care is Crucial:** Ellen and Sarah recognized the importance of taking care of themselves. Whether it was a walk in the park, a coffee with friends, or simply taking time to read a book, finding moments for themselves helped them recharge and continue to give Jack the love and care he needed.

Chapter Summary: The Thompson family's journey through dementia is a testament to the power of love, resilience, and shared commitment. By facing the emotional challenges together, adjusting to new roles with grace, and seeking support, they've navigated Jack's dementia with dignity and strength. Their story underscores the importance of community, the value of each moment, and the enduring strength of family bonds in the face of adversity.

$\sim$

PART FIVE WRAP-UP:
ACTION ITEMS FOR THE CAREGIVER:

BASED on the Thompson family's journey through dementia care, here are action items for caregivers:

1. **Help with Open Communication**: Establish regular family meetings to discuss care plans, emotional challenges, and responsibilities. Ensure everyone involved has a chance to voice their feelings and concerns.
2. **Join Support Groups**: Seek local or online support groups for families and caregivers dealing with dementia. Sharing experiences and advice with others in similar situations can provide invaluable support and practical tips.
3. **Divide Caregiving Responsibilities**: Distribute caregiving tasks among family members according to their abilities and availability. Consider creating a schedule that outlines who does what and when to avoid misunderstandings and burnout.
4. **Use Professional Care Services**: Research and engage home health aides or respite care services to provide professional care for your loved one and relief for the primary caregiver.
5. **Focus on the Present**: Cherish moments of clarity and

connection with your loved one. Celebrate the small victories and enjoy the time spent together, despite the challenges.

6. **Focus on Self-Care**: Recognize the importance of self-care for caregivers. Engage in activities that rejuvenate your spirit, such as exercise, hobbies, or spending time with friends.

7. **Educate Yourself and Your Family**: Learn as much as you can about dementia, including its progression, management strategies, and how to communicate effectively with someone with dementia.

8. **Plan for the Future**: Discuss and document legal, financial, and long-term care preferences early in the diagnosis. Consult with professionals as needed to ensure all affairs are in order.

9. **Seek External Resources**: Explore resources offered by local health services, Alzheimer's associations, and community organizations for more support and information.

10. **Implement Home Safety Measures**: Evaluate and change the home environment to ensure safety and accessibility for your loved one. Consider installing grab bars, removing tripping hazards, and putting security measures into practice for wandering.

11. **Monitor Health Regularly**: Keep up with regular medical appointments for your loved one to track their health status and adjust care plans as needed.

12. **Encourage Involvement in Activities**: Support your loved one in engaging in activities they enjoy and can manage, such as listening to music, simple gardening, or looking through photo albums, to stimulate their mind and maintain a sense of normalcy.

13. **Maintain Emotional Health**: Acknowledge and address the emotional toll dementia care can take on caregivers. Consider seeking counseling or therapy to help manage stress, guilt, and other complex emotions.

14. **Adapt to Changing Needs**: Be ready to adjust caregiving approaches as your loved one's condition evolves. Stay flexible and open to changing care strategies to meet their evolving needs.

By following these action items, caregivers can navigate the complexities of dementia care with greater confidence, compassion, and resilience, ensuring the best quality of life for their loved one and themselves.

~

IN OUR NEXT PART...

IN OUR NEXT PART, we will explore the art and heart of communicating effectively with someone with dementia. It's about more than just exchanging words; it's about building bridges to their world, ensuring they feel understood, respected, and loved. We'll dig into practical tips and strategies that can help you connect more deeply with your loved one, even as they face the challenges that come with cognitive decline. From the importance of clear, simple language to the power of nonverbal cues like eye contact and touch, we'll cover the do's and don'ts that can make every interaction more meaningful. This is about enhancing your communication skills to strengthen your bond, making each moment count.

We recognize this journey can be as challenging as it is rewarding. Thus, we'll also focus on the emotional part of caregiving, offering insights on how to navigate your own feelings as well as those of your loved one. Patience, empathy, and understanding are key, and we'll provide guidance on how to maintain your emotional well-being while being an effective caregiver. By embracing these principles, you can create a nurturing environment for your loved one, where they feel safe, valued, and connected. Join us as we explore these important parts of dementia care, empowering you to be the best caregiver you can be, filled with hope, strength, and compassion.

∾

PART SIX
COMMUNICATING EFFECTIVELY WITH SOMEONE WITH DEMENTIA

BUILDING BRIDGES: EFFECTIVE COMMUNICATION WITH LOVED ONES LIVING WITH DEMENTIA

Communicating with a loved one with dementia can be a challenging and ever-changing landscape. It is not just about the words we use but also about the way we connect and maintain that important link to their world. Effective communication is the bridge that lets us enter their reality, making sure they feel heard, understood, and valued. This chapter explores essential strategies and guidelines for enhancing communication and strengthening the bond with loved ones living with dementia.

The DOs:

Speak Clearly and Calmly:

When communicating with someone with dementia, it is important to use a calm and soothing tone of voice. The way we deliver our message is as important as the words we choose. Speaking clearly and at a measured pace helps to make sure our loved one can process and understand what we are saying. By maintaining a gentle and reassuring tone, we create a safe and comfortable environment for communication.

Keep It Simple and Straightforward:

Simplicity is key when engaging in conversations with individuals with dementia. Using straightforward sentences and avoiding complex language helps to make the exchange more accessible and less overwhelming. By breaking down information into manageable chunks and focusing on one topic at a time, we can help with better understanding and reduce the likelihood of confusion or frustration.

Maintain Eye Contact and Open Body Language:

Nonverbal communication plays a significant role in creating a positive and engaging interaction. Making eye contact and maintaining an open and relaxed body language shows our presence and attentiveness. It conveys that we are fully engaged in the conversation and value the thoughts and feelings of our loved one. This level of connection and validation is essential for fostering a sense of trust and comfort.

Use Visual Aids:

Sometimes, words alone may not convey a message or idea. Incorporating visual aids, such as pictures, objects, or gestures, can help to clarify and reinforce our points. These tangible representations can serve as anchors for memory and understanding, making it easier for our loved one to grasp and retain the information being shared.

Exercise Patience and Allow Time:

Patience is a fundamental virtue when communicating with someone with dementia. Give them ample time to process what has been said and to formulate their own thoughts and responses. Rushing or interrupting can lead to frustration and disengagement. By allowing for pauses and moments of silence, we create a space for our loved one to express themselves at their own pace, fostering a sense of respect and understanding.

Use Familiar and Respectful Language:

Familiarity and respect are essential parts of effective communication. Using terms, names, and references that our loved one recognizes helps to create a sense of comfort and connection. Address them by their preferred name and to use language that honors their dignity and life experiences. By speaking with respect and avoiding patronizing or infantilizing language, we affirm their worth and maintain their sense of self.

Encourage and Listen to Their Voice:

Meaningful conversations involve not only speaking but also actively listening. Encouraging our loved one to share their thoughts, feelings, and memories is a powerful way to confirm their experiences and maintain their sense of identity. By asking open-ended questions, showing genuine interest, and practicing active listening, we create opportunities for them to express themselves and feel heard.

The DON'Ts:

Avoid Talking Down or Using Patronizing Language:

Individuals with dementia are adults with a lifetime of experience and deserving of dignity and respect. Avoiding patronizing language or a condescending tone is essential for maintaining their sense of self-worth. Instead, we should communicate with them as we would with any other adult, using a respectful and age-appropriate manner.

Don't Rush or Interrupt:

Patience is paramount when communicating with someone with dementia. Rushing or interrupting them can lead to frustration, confusion, and withdrawal. Allow them the time and space to process their thoughts and express themselves at their own pace. By resisting the urge to fill silences or complete their sentences, we show our respect for their autonomy and ability to communicate.

Simplify, Don't Complicate:

While it is important to engage in meaningful conversations, it is equally important to avoid using jargon, abstract ideas, or complex ideas that may confuse or overwhelm our loved one. Simplifying our language and breaking down information into manageable pieces helps to ensure better understanding and retention. By focusing on concrete, tangible topics and using clear, concise language, we can help with more effective communication.

Avoid Arguments and Confrontations:

When a loved one with dementia expresses a belief or memory that is not grounded in reality, it is tempting to correct them or challenge their perception. However, arguing or confronting them about their understanding of reality can cause distress, agitation, and a breakdown in communication. Instead, it is often more compassionate and productive to meet them where they are, validate their emotions, and gently redirect the conversation if necessary.

Minimize Distractions:

A calm and quiet environment can greatly enhance communication with someone with dementia. Distractions, such as background noise, multiple conversations, or visual clutter, can make it difficult for them to focus and engage in the interaction. By finding a peaceful setting and reducing potential disruptions, we can create a more conducive atmosphere for meaningful dialogue.

Avoid Information Overload:

Providing too much information at once can be overwhelming and counterproductive when communicating with a loved one with dementia. Break down complex topics into smaller, more manageable pieces and to focus on one idea at a time. By presenting information gradually and allowing for processing time, we can help our loved one better understand and keep the key points of the conversation.

Limit Multiple Questions:

Asking multiple questions in rapid succession can be confusing and overwhelming for someone with dementia. It is more effective to ask one question at a time and to allow for a response before moving on to the next topic. By keeping our inquiries simple, direct, and focused, we can help with clearer communication and reduce the likelihood of confusion or frustration.

Chapter Summary:

Building bridges of effective communication with loved ones living with dementia requires patience, understanding, and a willingness to adapt our approach. By embracing the dos and don'ts outlined in this chapter, we can enhance the quality of our interactions and strengthen the emotional connection we share.

The key to successful communication lies in creating a supportive and respectful environment where our loved one feels seen, heard, and valued. By speaking clearly, using simple language, maintaining eye contact, and allowing ample time for processing and response, we can foster a sense of trust and understanding.

It is equally important to avoid communication pitfalls, such as patronizing language, rushing, complicating information, arguing, and overwhelming our loved one with too much stimuli or questions. By meeting them where they are, validating their emotions, and gently guiding the conversation, we can navigate the challenges of dementia-related communication with compassion and grace.

Ultimately, effective communication is about maintaining that important bridge to our loved one's world, making sure they feel connected, supported, and loved. By approaching each interaction with patience, respect, and an open heart, we can create moments of meaningful connection that transcend the boundaries of dementia and affirm the enduring power of love and human connection.

$\sim$

SIMPLE STEPS FOR TALKING TO SOMEONE WITH DEMENTIA

ENGAGING in conversation with someone living with dementia may seem challenging at first, but by following a few simple guidelines, you can create meaningful and positive interactions. The key is to approach communication with compassion, patience, and a focus on clarity and simplicity. This chapter outlines practical strategies for effective communication and highlights the importance of maintaining a respectful and supportive environment.

What to Do:

Keep it Simple and Clear:

When communicating with someone with dementia, it is essential to use simple language and short, straightforward sentences. Avoid complex vocabulary or abstract concepts that may cause confusion. By expressing your thoughts and ideas clearly, you help with better understanding and reduce the likelihood of misinterpretation or frustration.

Maintain Eye Contact and Use a Kind Tone:

Nonverbal communication plays a significant role in creating a positive and supportive atmosphere. Making eye contact and using a warm, friendly tone of voice conveys your attentiveness and care. It helps to establish a sense of connection and reassurance, making your loved one feel safe and valued. Remember that the way you deliver your message is as important as the words you choose.

Exercise Patience and Allow Time for Response:

Patience is a fundamental part of effective communication with someone with dementia. It is important to give them ample time to process what you have said and to formulate their own thoughts and responses. Avoid rushing or interrupting, as this can lead to frustration and disengagement. By allowing for pauses and moments of silence, you show your respect for their pace and ability to express themselves.

Use Visual Aids and Gestures:

Sometimes, words alone may not convey a message or idea. Incorporating visual aids, such as pictures, objects, or simple hand gestures, can help to clarify and reinforce your points. These real representations can serve as anchors for understanding and memory, making it easier for your loved one to grasp and retain the information being shared.

Encourage Participation and Inclusion:

Engaging your loved one in conversations and activities is a powerful way to promote a sense of belonging and purpose. Invite them to join in discussions, ask for their opinions, and involve them in decision-making processes. By seeking their participation, you affirm their value and help maintain their sense of identity and self-worth.

What to Avoid:

Refrain from Arguing or Correcting:

If your loved one with dementia expresses a belief or memory that is inaccurate, it is important to avoid arguing or correcting them. Challenging their perception of reality can lead to distress, agitation, and a breakdown in communication. Instead, focus on confirming their emotions and gently redirecting the conversation if necessary. Remember that their subjective experience is their reality, and it is more important to focus on their emotional well-being than to insist on factual accuracy.

Avoid Information Overload:

When communicating with someone with dementia, it is important to avoid overwhelming them with too much information at once. Stick to one idea or topic at a time and break down complex ideas into smaller, more manageable pieces. By presenting information gradually and allowing for processing time, you can help your loved one better understand and keep the key points of the conversation.

Minimize Background Noise and Distractions:

A calm and quiet environment can greatly enhance communication with someone with dementia. Background noise, such as television, radio, or multiple conversations, can make it difficult for them to focus and engage in the interaction. Try to find a peaceful setting where distractions are reduced, allowing your loved one to concentrate on the conversation at hand.

Don't Rush or Pressure:

Rushing or pressuring someone with dementia to communicate or respond quickly can be counterproductive and stressful. It is essential to allow them the time and space to process their thoughts and express themselves at their own pace. By adopting a patient and unhurried approach, you create a supportive environment that encourages open and comfortable communication.

Avoid Criticism and Negative Language:

When communicating with someone with dementia, it is important to use positive and encouraging language. Avoid criticism, sarcasm, or negative comments that can make them feel sad, frustrated, or devalued. Instead, focus on offering praise, validation, and reassurance. By maintaining a positive and supportive tone, you foster a sense of trust and emotional safety.

Chapter Summary:

Communicating with someone with dementia requires a thoughtful and compassionate approach. By following these simple steps, you can create meaningful and positive interactions that reinforce your bond and ensure your loved one feels understood and respected.

The key is to keep things simple, clear, and kind. Use easy words, short sentences, and visual aids to clarify your points and avoid confusion. Maintain eye contact, use a friendly tone, and allow ample time for processing and response. Encourage participation and inclusion, and avoid arguing, overwhelming them with information, or rushing the conversation.

Remember, the goal is to maintain a strong connection and to focus on your loved one's emotional well-being. By approaching each interaction with patience, respect, and a focus on simplicity, you can navigate the challenges of dementia-related communication with grace and understanding.

Ultimately, effective communication is about creating a supportive and loving environment where your loved one feels valued, heard, and understood. With a little patience and these simple strategies, you can have meaningful conversations that affirm the enduring power of human connection and the importance of compassion in the face of dementia.

~

HOW TO CONNECT THROUGH CONVERSATION WITH SOMEONE WITH DEMENTIA

ENGAGING in conversation with a loved one living with dementia requires a gentle, patient, and thoughtful approach. By employing a few simple strategies, you can create a more supportive and meaningful communication experience, making sure your loved one feels heard, valued, and connected.

This chapter explores practical tips for effective communication and highlights the importance of maintaining a respectful and compassionate environment.

Do This:

Keep it Simple and Clear:

When communicating with someone with dementia, it is essential to use simple language and short, easy to understand sentences. Avoid complex vocabulary or abstract ideas that may cause confusion or frustration. By expressing your thoughts and ideas clearly, you help with better understanding and reduce the likelihood of misunderstandings.

Maintain a Calm and Supportive Tone:

The way you deliver your message is as important as the words you choose. Use a gentle, reassuring tone that conveys your support and understanding. Speaking calmly and patiently helps to create a safe and comforting environment, encouraging your loved one to feel more at ease and open to communication.

Exercise Patience and Allow Ample Response Time:

Patience is a fundamental part of effective communication with someone with dementia. It is important to give them plenty of time to process what you have said and to formulate their own thoughts and responses. Avoid rushing or pressuring them, as this can lead to anxiety and disengagement. By allowing for pauses and moments of silence, you show your respect for their pace and ability to express themselves.

Maintain Eye Contact and Use Nonverbal Cues:

Eye contact is a powerful way to show your attentiveness and interest in the conversation. It helps to establish a sense of connection and engagement, making your loved one feel valued and heard. Additionally, using nonverbal cues such as smiles, nods, and gentle gestures can reinforce your message and provide reassurance and comfort.

Incorporate Visual Aids and Tactile Cues:

Sometimes, words alone may not convey a message or idea. Incorporating visual aids, such as pictures, objects, or simple hand gestures, can help to clarify and reinforce your points. Similarly, a gentle touch on the hand or arm can provide comfort and a sense of connection, enhancing the overall communication experience.

Encourage Sharing of Memories and Stories:

Engaging your loved one in conversations about their experiences, cherished memories, or favorite stories can be a wonderful way to connect and provide comfort. Reminiscing about positive moments can evoke feelings of joy and familiarity, strengthening your bond and creating a sense of shared history and understanding.

Avoid Doing This:

Refrain from Using Complex Language:

When communicating with someone with dementia, it is important to avoid using difficult vocabulary, professional jargon, or complex sentence structures. Stick to simple, everyday language easy to understand and process. Using complicated words or ideas can lead to confusion, frustration, and disengagement.

Don't Rush or Interrupt:

Rushing or interrupting your loved one while they are speaking can make them feel anxious, undervalued, and unheard. It is essential to allow them the time and space to express themselves at their own pace, even if there are pauses or moments of silence. By showing patience and active listening, you create a supportive environment that encourages open and comfortable communication.

Maintain Composure and Avoid Showing Frustration:

If your loved one struggles to communicate or expresses thoughts that are confusing or inaccurate, it is important to maintain your composure and avoid showing irritation or frustration. Raising your voice or displaying impatience can heighten their anxiety and shut down communication. Instead, remain calm, supportive, and understanding, acknowledging that they are doing their best to express themselves.

Avoid Information Overload:

When communicating with someone with dementia, it is important to avoid overwhelming them with too much information at once. Stick to one idea or topic at a time, and break down complex ideas into smaller, more manageable pieces. By presenting information gradually and allowing for processing time, you can help your loved one better understand and engage in the conversation.

Treat Them with Respect and Dignity:

Always communicate with your loved one in a way that preserves their dignity and respects their ability to understand and contribute to the conversation. Avoid talking about them as if they are not present or cannot comprehend what is being said. Instead, talk to them directly, value their input, and maintain a respectful and inclusive tone throughout your interactions.

Prioritize Connection Over Correction:

If your loved one with dementia expresses a belief or memory that is inaccurate, it is important to avoid arguing or correcting them. Challenging their perception of reality can lead to distress, agitation, and a breakdown in communication. Instead, focus on confirming their emotions and maintaining the connection you share. Remember that the goal is to foster a positive and supportive relationship, rather than insisting on factual accuracy.

Chapter Summary:

Connecting through conversation with a loved one living with dementia requires a thoughtful, patient, and compassionate approach. By using simple strategies such as using clear language, maintaining a calm tone, exercising patience, and incorporating nonverbal cues, you can create a more supportive and meaningful communication experience.

It is equally important to avoid communication pitfalls such as using complex language, rushing or interrupting, showing frustration, overwhelming them with information, or disregarding their dignity and ability to understand. By focusing on connection over correction and focusing on creating a respectful and inclusive environment, you foster a stronger bond and ensure your loved one feels supported and valued.

Remember, the goal is to maintain that precious connection and to provide comfort and reassurance through every interaction. By keeping these tips in mind and approaching each conversation with patience, kindness, and understanding, you can navigate the challenges of dementia-related communication with grace and compassion.

Ultimately, effective communication is about creating moments of shared understanding, love, and connection. By using these strategies and maintaining a respectful and supportive approach, you can make sure your loved one feels heard, valued, and cherished, reinforcing the enduring power of human connection in the face of dementia.

∽

ENHANCING CONNECTION: THE ROLE OF NONVERBAL COMMUNICATION IN DEMENTIA CARE

IN DEMENTIA CARE, effective communication goes beyond the spoken word. Nonverbal cues, such as gestures, facial expressions, and touch, play an important role in fostering understanding, connection, and emotional well-being. When words may fail or become confusing, these alternative forms of communication can bridge gaps and create a more supportive and meaningful interaction. This chapter explores the importance of nonverbal communication in dementia care and provides practical strategies for enhancing connection through these powerful tools.

Do's:

Keep Language Simple and Clear:

When communicating with someone living with dementia, it is essential to use simple, straightforward language. Short sentences and clear, concise words help to clarify your point and reduce the likelihood of confusion or misunderstanding. By expressing your thoughts and ideas in a direct and uncomplicated manner, you help with better understanding and create a more accessible communication environment.

Exercise Patience and Allow Ample Response Time:

Patience is a fundamental part of effective communication in dementia care. It is important to give your loved one ample time to process what you have said and to formulate their own thoughts and responses. Rushing or pressuring them can lead to increased stress and anxiety, hindering the communication process. By allowing for pauses, moments of silence, and a relaxed pace, you create a supportive atmosphere that encourages open and comfortable interaction.

Maintain Eye Contact and a Calm Demeanor:

Eye contact is a powerful way to establish a sense of connection and attentiveness. It conveys your genuine interest and engagement in the conversation, helping your loved one feel seen and heard. Pairing eye contact with a soothing voice tone and a calm demeanor can create a reassuring and comforting atmosphere. By projecting a sense of tranquility and understanding, you foster a more positive and supportive communication experience.

Leverage Nonverbal Cues:

Nonverbal cues, such as gestures, smiles, and gentle touch, can often convey meaning and emotion more effectively than words alone. These cues can help bridge gaps in understanding and provide more context and support. Using hand gestures to illustrate a point, offering a warm smile to convey affection, or providing a gentle touch on the hand or arm can communicate compassion, reassurance, and connection. By incorporating nonverbal cues into your interactions, you enhance the overall communication experience and create a more meaningful bond.

Approach with Empathy and Respect:

Every interaction with someone living with dementia should be approached with kindness, empathy, and a genuine attempt to understand their perspective. It is essential to confirm their feelings and experiences, even if their perception of reality may differ from your own. By showing respect for their thoughts and emotions, you create a safe and supportive environment that encourages open communication and fosters a deep sense of connection.

Don'ts:

Avoid Arguments and Corrections:

When communicating with someone living with dementia, it is important to avoid arguing or correcting them, even if their statements or beliefs may not align with reality. Challenging their perception or engaging in debates can lead to confusion, agitation, and a breakdown in communication. Instead, focus on confirming their emotions and maintaining a supportive and understanding approach. Remember, the goal is to focus on their emotional well-being and the connection you share, rather than insisting on factual accuracy.

Refrain from Loud or Patronizing Talk:

Always communicate with your loved one in a way that preserves their dignity and respects their ability to understand and engage in the conversation. Avoid speaking in a loud or patronizing tone, as this can be perceived as disrespectful or condescending. Instead, use a calm, clear, and age-appropriate voice that conveys respect and understanding. By treating them as an equal partner in the conversation, you foster a sense of self-worth and maintain a positive communication dynamic.

Simplify Information and Avoid Overload:

When communicating with someone living with dementia, it is important to avoid overwhelming them with too much information at once. Stick to one idea or topic at a time, and break down complex ideas into smaller, more manageable pieces. By presenting information gradually and allowing for processing time, you can help your loved one better understand and engage in the conversation. Simplifying your messages and avoiding information overload creates a more accessible and less stressful communication environment.

Allow Them to Express Themselves:

It is essential to give your loved one the space and time to express themselves, even if it takes longer than usual or if their words may not always make perfect sense. Interrupting or finishing their sentences can make them feel unheard or dismissed. Instead, practice active listening and show genuine interest in their thoughts and feelings. By letting them communicate at their own pace and in their own way, you show respect for their autonomy and create a more inclusive and supportive conversation.

Be Attuned to Nonverbal Signals:

Pay close attention to your loved one's body language and facial expressions, as these nonverbal signals can provide valuable insights into their emotional state and unspoken needs. Changes in posture, eye contact, or facial expressions can show discomfort, confusion, or a desire to communicate something that words may not convey. By being attuned to these nonverbal cues, you can respond with empathy, adjust your approach, and provide the necessary support and understanding.

Chapter Summary:

Nonverbal communication plays an important role in enhancing connection and understanding when caring for someone living with dementia. By embracing the do's and don'ts outlined in this chapter, you can create a caring and supportive environment that fosters meaningful interactions and deepens your bond.

The key is to approach communication with patience, respect, and a focus on simplicity and clarity. Use short sentences, maintain eye contact, and leverage nonverbal cues to convey meaning and emotion. Exercise patience, allow ample response time, and avoid arguments or corrections. Simplify information, avoid overload, and allow your loved one the space to express themselves at their own pace.

Remember, the goal is not just to communicate but to connect on a profound level. By being attuned to nonverbal signals and responding with empathy and understanding, you can navigate the challenges of dementia-related communication with grace and compassion.

Ultimately, effective communication in dementia care is about creating moments of shared understanding, love, and connection. By embracing the power of nonverbal communication and approaching each interaction with kindness and respect, you can make sure your loved one feels supported, valued, and deeply connected, even when words may fail. Through these meaningful connections, you can provide comfort, reassurance, and a sense of belonging, reinforcing the enduring power of human connection in the face of dementia.

❧

FOSTERING MEANINGFUL CONVERSATIONS WITH DEMENTIA PATIENTS

ENGAGING in meaningful conversations with individuals living with dementia requires a compassionate, patient, and thoughtful approach. By adopting specific communication strategies and creating a supportive environment, you can enhance the quality of your interactions and foster a deeper connection with your loved one. This chapter explores practical techniques for navigating conversations, promoting understanding, and focusing on emotional well-being in dementia care.

Steer Clear of Corrections:

When communicating with someone living with dementia, it is essential to avoid correcting or arguing with them, even if their perception of reality differs from your own. Challenging their beliefs or memories can lead to confusion, agitation, and a breakdown in communication. Instead, focus on meeting them where they are, validating their emotions, and maintaining a supportive and understanding approach. By prioritizing their emotional well-being over factual accuracy, you create a safe and nurturing environment that encourages open and comfortable dialogue.

Cultivate a Peaceful Setting:

Creating a calm and peaceful environment is important for fostering meaningful conversations with individuals living with dementia. By reducing distractions, such as background noise or visual clutter, you help them focus and feel more at ease during the interaction. A serene setting promotes relaxation, reduces stress, and enhances their ability to engage in the conversation. Consider finding a quiet, comfortable space where you can sit together and communicate without interruptions or overwhelming stimuli.

Simplify Your Language:

When communicating with someone living with dementia, it is important to use straightforward, uncomplicated language to ensure your message is easily understood. Avoid using complex vocabulary, idioms, or abstract ideas that may cause confusion or frustration. Instead, choose clear, concise sentences that convey your thoughts and ideas directly and accessibly. By simplifying your language, you help with better understanding and reduce the likelihood of misunderstandings or communication breakdowns.

Maintain Eye Contact and Speak Clearly:

Eye contact is a powerful way to show your attentiveness and engagement in the conversation. It helps establish a sense of connection and reassures your loved one you are present and interested in what they have to say. Additionally, speaking slowly and enunciating clearly can greatly aid their understanding. By taking the time to articulate your words deliberately and distinctly, you allow them to process the information more effectively, reducing the risk of confusion or misinterpretation.

Practice Active Listening:

Active listening is a fundamental part of fostering meaningful conversations with individuals living with dementia. Give them your undivided attention and allow them the time and space to express themselves at their own pace. Avoid interrupting or rushing them, even if there are pauses or moments of silence. By showing patience and genuine interest in their thoughts and feelings, you confirm their experiences and show that their contributions are valued and respected.

Empathize and Be Patient:

Empathy and patience are essential qualities when communicating with someone living with dementia. Show compassion for their struggles and acknowledge the challenges they may be facing. By maintaining a patient and understanding demeanor, you create a safe and supportive environment that encourages them to open up and share their thoughts and emotions. Remember that their communication abilities may vary from day-to-day, and it is important to adapt your approach, accordingly, always focusing on their comfort and well-being.

Incorporate Visuals and Gestures:

Nonverbal communication, such as visuals and gestures, can be effective in enhancing understanding and reinforcing your messages. When words alone may not be enough, consider using pictures, objects, or simple hand gestures to clarify your points and provide more context. These visual cues can serve as anchors for understanding and memory, making it easier for your loved one to grasp and retain the information being shared.

Choose Positive Phrasing:

The way you frame your words can have a significant impact on the tone and atmosphere of the conversation. When communicating with someone living with dementia, it is important to use positive, encouraging language that promotes a sense of comfort and reassurance. Avoid using negative phrases or commands that could be perceived as harsh or confrontational. Instead, choose supportive and affirming statements that convey warmth, understanding, and respect.

Respect and Validate Emotions:

Acknowledging and confirming the feelings and experiences of individuals living with dementia is important for fostering meaningful connections. Show respect for their emotions, even if they may not align with your own perspective or the objective reality. By recognizing and affirming their emotional state, you build trust, promote comfort, and create a safe space for them to express themselves freely. Remember that their subjective experience is their reality, and it is important to honor and support their emotional journey.

Keep Questions and Information Simple:

When engaging in conversations with someone living with dementia, it is essential to avoid overwhelming them with too many questions or complex information. Stick to simple, open-ended questions or statements that let them respond at their own pace and in their own way. Bombarding them with rapid-fire inquiries or presenting an overload of details can lead to confusion, anxiety, and disengagement. By keeping your interactions focused and manageable, you create a more comfortable and accessible communication environment.

Follow Their Lead:

Allow your loved one to take the lead in conversations. By following their cues and interests, you create opportunities for them to discuss topics that are meaningful and important to them. This approach not only fosters a sense of autonomy and self-expression but also provides valuable insights into their thoughts, feelings, and unique perspectives. By being attentive to their lead and adapting your communication accordingly, you show respect for their individuality and create a more personalized and engaging interaction.

Chapter Summary:

Fostering meaningful conversations with individuals living with dementia requires a compassionate, patient, and adaptable approach. By steering clear of corrections, cultivating a peaceful setting, simplifying language, maintaining eye contact, practicing active listening, and incorporating visuals and gestures, you create a supportive communication environment that focuses on their emotional well-being and promotes understanding.

Additionally, choosing positive phrasing, respecting and confirming emotions, keeping questions and information simple, and following their lead further enhances the quality of your interactions and strengthens the bond you share.

Remember, the goal is to create moments of connection, comfort, and shared understanding. By adopting these guidelines and approaching each conversation with empathy, patience, and respect, you can navigate the challenges of dementia-related communication with grace and compassion.

Ultimately, fostering meaningful conversations with your loved one living with dementia is about focusing on their needs, honoring their experiences, and nurturing the profound connection you share. By creating a supportive and inclusive communication environment, you make sure they feel heard, valued, and deeply cared for, reinforcing the enduring power of human connection in the face of dementia.

∽

COMMUNICATION ESSENTIALS: CONNECTING WITH LOVED ONES WITH DEMENTIA

ENGAGING in effective communication with a loved one living with dementia is a crucial part of providing compassionate care and maintaining a strong, supportive relationship. By using strategies that focus on clarity, empathy, and respect, you can foster meaningful interactions that ensure your loved one feels heard, valued, and understood. This chapter explores essential guidelines for enhancing communication and navigating the unique challenges that dementia may present.

Do's for Effective Communication:

Speak Clearly and Simply:

When communicating with a loved one with dementia, it is important to use simple words and sentences to help with understanding. Speak slowly and clearly, allowing them ample time to process the information. Avoid complex vocabulary or convoluted explanations that may cause confusion or frustration. By expressing yourself clearly, you create a more accessible and comfortable communication environment.

Maintain Eye Contact and Friendly Nonverbal Cues:

Eye contact is a powerful way to establish a personal connection and convey your attentiveness. It shows you are fully present and engaged in the conversation, helping your loved one feel seen and heard. Combine eye contact with friendly nonverbal cues, such as smiles, nods, and gentle gestures, to communicate warmth, reassurance, and support. These nonverbal signals can enhance the overall quality of your interaction and foster a sense of comfort and connection.

Practice Active Listening:

Active listening is a fundamental part of effective communication, particularly when interacting with a loved one with dementia. Give them your undivided attention and listen to what they are saying. Allow them the time and space to express themselves at their own pace, without rushing or interrupting. By showing genuine interest and patience, you confirm their thoughts and feelings, showing that their input is valued and respected.

Empathize and Validate Their Experiences:

Empathy and validation are essential when communicating with a loved one with dementia. Acknowledge their feelings and experiences, even if their perception of reality may differ from your own. Show compassion for their struggles and affirm their emotions, letting them know that they are heard and understood. By creating a supportive and non-judgmental environment, you foster a sense of safety and encourage open and honest communication.

Encourage Reminiscing and Positive Conversations:

Conversations about the past can be a meaningful and enjoyable experience for individuals with dementia. Reminiscing about cherished memories, significant life events, or beloved hobbies can stimulate memory and bring joy to your interactions. Encourage your loved one to share their stories and experiences, actively listening and showing interest in their recollections. These positive conversations can provide comfort, boost self-esteem, and strengthen your emotional bond.

Don'ts to Remember:

Avoid Complex Language and Professional Jargon:

When communicating with a loved one with dementia, it is important to steer clear of complicated words, technical terms, or professional jargon. These complex expressions can be confusing and overwhelming, leading to frustration or disengagement. Instead, choose simple, everyday language that is easily understood and relatable. By using familiar words and ideas, you create a more accessible and inclusive communication environment.

Refrain from Correcting or Arguing:

If your loved one with dementia remembers something incorrectly or expresses a belief that does not align with reality, it is generally best to avoid correcting or arguing with them. Challenging their perception or engaging in debates can cause unnecessary stress, agitation, and a breakdown in communication. Instead, focus on confirming their emotions and maintaining a supportive and understanding approach. Focus on their emotional well-being over factual accuracy, recognizing that their subjective experience is their reality.

Allow Conversations to Flow at Their Pace:

When communicating with a loved one with dementia, it is important to let conversations unfold at a pace that is comfortable for them. Avoid rushing or pressuring them to remember specific details or respond quickly. Rushing can cause undue stress and hinder effective communication. Instead, provide them with ample time to process information, formulate their thoughts, and express themselves in their own way. By respecting their pace, you create a more relaxed and supportive environment that encourages open and meaningful dialogue.

Reduce Distractions and Create a Calm Environment:

To enhance communication with a loved one with dementia, it is essential to reduce distractions and create a calm, peaceful setting for conversations. Choose a quiet space with minimal background noise or visual clutter, as these distractions can interfere with their ability to focus and comprehend. A serene environment promotes relaxation, reduces stress, and enables them to engage more fully in the interaction. By reducing distractions, you create a conducive atmosphere for effective communication and connection.

Always Treat Them with Respect and Dignity:

Despite the stage of dementia or the challenges in communication, it is important to always treat your loved one with the utmost respect and dignity. Never patronize or speak to them in a condescending way, as this can be hurtful and damaging to their self-esteem. Instead, approach each interaction with compassion, patience, and a genuine desire to understand their perspective. By honoring their inherent worth and respecting their autonomy, you foster a relationship built on trust, love, and mutual appreciation.

Chapter Summary:

Effective communication is a cornerstone of providing compassionate care and maintaining a strong, supportive relationship with a loved one living with dementia. By implementing the essential do's and don'ts outlined in this chapter, you can enhance your interactions, making sure your loved one feels heard, valued, and understood.

Remember to speak clearly and simply, maintain eye contact, practice active listening, empathize and confirm their experiences, and encourage positive reminiscing. Simultaneously, avoid complex language, refrain from correcting or arguing, let conversations flow at their pace, reduce distractions, and always treat them with the respect and dignity they deserve.

Every person with dementia is unique, and what works for one may not work for another. The key is to approach each interaction with love, patience, and a willingness to adapt to their individual needs and communication styles. By remaining flexible, compassionate, and attuned to their emotional well-being, you can foster meaningful connections that enhance their quality of life and strengthen your bond.

Ultimately, effective communication with a loved one with dementia is an ongoing journey that requires dedication, understanding, and a commitment to focusing on their dignity and well-being. By using these essential strategies and approaching each interaction with an open heart and a compassionate spirit, you can navigate the challenges of dementia-related communication with grace, making sure your loved one feels cherished, supported, and deeply connected throughout their journey.

~

STRENGTHENING BONDS: COMMUNICATION GUIDE FOR DEMENTIA CARE

DEMENTIA CARE EXTENDS beyond addressing physical needs; it encompasses the important task of maintaining a heartfelt connection through thoughtful, empathetic communication. By adopting effective communication strategies, you can foster meaningful interactions with your loved one living with dementia, making sure they feel seen, heard, and valued. This chapter provides a comprehensive guide to nurturing these precious bonds, focusing on the do's and don'ts of communication in dementia care.

Do's for Nurturing Connection:

Speak Clearly and Calmly:

When communicating with your loved one living with dementia, it is essential to use straightforward language and maintain a gentle, soothing tone. Choose simple sentences and avoid complex vocabulary or abstract ideas that may cause confusion or frustration. By speaking clearly and calmly, you create a more accessible and comfortable communication environment, helping with understanding and fostering a sense of security and trust.

Use Eye Contact and Gestures:

Nonverbal cues play an important role in reinforcing your words and conveying care and affection. Maintain warm eye contact to establish a personal connection and show your attentiveness. Combine this with gentle gestures, such as a reassuring smile, a soft touch on the hand, or a comforting embrace. These nonverbal signals speak volumes, communicating your love, support, and presence in a way that transcends the limitations of language.

Practice Patience in Listening:

Active listening is a fundamental part of nurturing meaningful connections with your loved one living with dementia. Allow ample time for them to process your words and formulate their responses, resisting the urge to rush or interrupt. Give them your undivided attention, showing genuine interest in their thoughts and feelings. By practicing patience and providing a supportive, non-judgmental space for communication, you confirm their experiences and reinforce the importance of their voice.

Focus on the Positive:

When engaging in conversations with your loved one, make a conscious effort to highlight their abilities, achievements, and the positive aspects of their life. Steer the dialogue toward what they can do rather than dwelling on limitations or challenges. Celebrate their successes, no matter how small, and express appreciation for their unique qualities and contributions. By focusing on the positive, you boost their self-esteem, foster a sense of purpose, and create a more uplifting and affirming communication environment.

Encourage Reminiscing and Shared Memories:

Sharing stories and memories from the past can be a powerful tool for sparking joy, connection, and engagement in conversations with your loved one living with dementia. Encourage them to reminisce about cherished moments, significant life events, or beloved hobbies. Actively listen to their recollections, showing genuine interest and enthusiasm. By digging into shared memories, you create opportunities for bonding, emotional resonance, and a sense of continuity in your relationship.

Don'ts to Keep in Mind:

Avoid Talking Down or Patronizing:

Always communicate with your loved one as the adult they are, treating them with the respect and dignity that every individual deserves. Refrain from using a condescending tone or infantilizing language, as this can be hurtful and damaging to their self-esteem. Instead, approach each interaction with patience, empathy, and a genuine desire to understand their perspective. By honoring their inherent worth and respecting their autonomy, you foster a relationship built on trust, love, and mutual appreciation.

Simplify Questions and Offer Choices:

When communicating with your loved one living with dementia, it is important to avoid overwhelming them with open-ended questions or complex decision-making. Instead, simplify your inquiries and offer clear choices or prompts to guide the conversation gently. For example, instead of asking, "What would you like to wear today?" you could present two options: "Would you prefer the blue shirt or the green one?" By providing manageable choices, you reduce confusion and empower them to express their preferences more easily.

Steer Clear of Arguments and Corrections:

If your loved one makes statements or recalls events that are inaccurate or inconsistent with reality, it is often more beneficial to agree or gently redirect the conversation rather than engaging in arguments or corrections. Challenging their perception or insisting on factual accuracy can lead to frustration, agitation, and a breakdown in communication. Instead, focus on their emotional well-being and focus on maintaining a supportive, understanding atmosphere. Remember, the goal is to foster connection and comfort, not to prove a point.

Keep Language Uncomplicated and Clear:

When communicating with your loved one living with dementia, it is important to use language that is easily understood and relatable. Avoid complex terms, professional jargon, or slang that might confuse or alienate them. Aim for clarity and simplicity in your dialogue, using familiar words and ideas that resonate with their experiences. By keeping your language uncomplicated, you create a more accessible and inclusive communication environment that promotes understanding and engagement.

Practice Patience and Remain Calm:

Communicating with a loved one living with dementia can sometimes be challenging, requiring a lot of patience and understanding. If interactions become difficult or frustrating, take a moment to breathe deeply and center yourself. Remember that your loved one is not intentionally trying to be difficult; they are navigating the complexities of dementia. By remaining calm and patient, you provide a stable, supportive presence that offers comfort and reassurance beyond words.

Chapter Summary:

Strengthening the bonds with your loved one living with dementia through effective communication is a vital part of providing compassionate care and maintaining a meaningful connection. By consistently practicing the do's and don'ts outlined in this guide, you can significantly enhance the quality of your interactions and make sure your loved one feels seen, heard, and valued.

Remember to speak clearly and calmly, use eye contact and gestures, practice patience in listening, focus on the positive, and encourage reminiscing and shared memories. Simultaneously, avoid talking down or patronizing, simplify questions and offer choices, steer clear of arguments and corrections, keep language uncomplicated, and practice patience and remain calm in challenging moments.

Communication in dementia care is an ongoing journey that requires flexibility, empathy, and a willingness to adapt to your loved one's evolving needs. By consistently approaching interactions with compassion, understanding, and a commitment to nurturing connection, you can navigate the challenges of dementia-related communication with grace and love.

Ultimately, the power of your presence, the warmth of your touch, and the sincerity of your words have the capacity to create a comforting and loving world for your loved one, even amidst the difficulties of dementia. By focusing on thoughtful, empathetic communication, you reinforce the unbreakable bond you share and make sure your loved one feels cherished, supported, and deeply connected throughout their journey.

~

FREQUENTLY ASKED QUESTIONS:

1. How do I start a conversation with my loved one with dementia without confusing or upsetting them? Start by choosing a quiet, comfortable place to reduce distractions. Use their name to get their attention and establish eye contact. Speak calmly, using simple, straightforward sentences and familiar words. Introduce one topic at a time and allow them plenty of time to process the information and respond. It's also helpful to approach conversations with a positive attitude and patience, focusing on the connection rather than the content of the conversation.

2. My loved one often repeats the same stories or questions. How should I handle this? Repetition is common in individuals with dementia, often stemming from a need for reassurance or memory challenges. When they repeat stories or questions, respond with patience and understanding each time. Avoid showing irritation or pointing out the repetition. Instead, listen and engage as if hearing it for the first time, or gently guide the conversation in a new direction if needed. This approach confirms their feelings and maintains a positive interaction.

3. What should I do when my loved one becomes upset or agitated during a conversation? When agitation occurs, remain calm and speak in a soothing tone. Try not to take their upset personally, as it's a symptom of the disease, not a reflection of their feelings toward you. Acknowledge their emotions and offer reassurance. If specific topics consistently trigger agitation, it might be best to avoid them. Sometimes, a change in activity or environment can help soothe them. Remember, your presence and reassurance can be comforting.

4. How can I effectively communicate with my loved one who's in the later stages of dementia and has trouble understanding or speaking? In the later stages, focus more on nonverbal communication. Maintain eye contact, smile, and use gentle touches to convey your presence and care. Use simple, clear words for necessary communication, accompanied by visual cues or gestures. Playing their favorite music, reading aloud, or sharing photo albums can also be effective ways to connect and communicate without relying only on speech.

5. What strategies can I use to improve communication and make my loved one feel more understood and respected? To improve communication, always approach your loved one with empathy, patience, and respect. Use their name, involve them in conversations even if their responses are limited, and listen actively, showing you value their input. Encourage them to express themselves, whether through words, gestures, or expressions, and confirm their feelings. Focusing on their abilities, rather than limitations, and maintaining a positive, supportive tone can significantly enhance your connection.

Communicating with a loved one with dementia can be challenging, but it's also an opportunity to strengthen your bond through patience, understanding, and creative strategies. Each interaction is a chance to show love and support, making a positive difference in their quality of life.

～

CASE STUDY: EMMA AND HER MOTHER, JUNE

EMMA, a 38-year-old graphic designer, found herself in the role of primary caregiver for her mother, June, who was diagnosed with early-stage Alzheimer's disease at the age of 72. Navigating this new reality, Emma faced challenges she never expected, especially when communicating effectively with her mother. Through trial and error, empathy, and patience, Emma learned valuable lessons on connecting with June, enhancing both their lives amidst the journey with dementia.

Early Challenges in Communication: Initially, Emma found conversations with her mother to be increasingly fraught with confusion and frustration. June struggled to find the right words and often lost her train of thought. Emma, in her desire to help, would finish June's sentences or correct her when she misspoke, which only led to more distress and withdrawal from June.

Adopting New Strategies: Emma realized she needed a new approach after attending a workshop on dementia care communication strategies. She learned the importance of simple, clear language and the power of patience in allowing her mother time to express herself. Emma started using visual aids to help June understand complex ideas and made a conscious effort to maintain eye contact, offering physical cues of support and understanding.

The Do's and Don'ts in Practice:

- **Do Speak Clearly and Calmly:** Emma tried to use simple sentences and a soothing tone, which helped reduce June's anxiety during conversations.
- **Don't Correct or Argue:** Emma learned that correcting June's inaccuracies often led to agitation. Instead, she found it more effective to enter June's reality, affirming her feelings rather than focusing on factual accuracy.
- **Do Use Nonverbal Communication:** Nonverbal cues like smiles, nods, and gentle touches became key in Emma's communication toolkit, often conveying more than words could.
- **Don't Overwhelm with Choices:** Emma discovered that offering too many options confused June. Instead, she presented one choice at a time, making decisions easier for her mother.

Lessons Learned by Emma:

- **Patience is Invaluable:** Giving June time to respond without rushing or interrupting allowed for more meaningful exchanges and less frustration for both.
- **Listening is as Important as Speaking:** Active listening, showing genuine interest in what June had to say, reinforced her sense of self-worth and engagement.
- **Flexibility Enhances Communication:** Adapting her communication style to meet June's changing needs helped Emma maintain a strong connection with her mother.
- **Self-Care is important:** Emma recognized the importance of caring for her own emotional well-being. Joining a support group for caregivers gave her a sense of community and understanding, crucial for sustaining her capacity to care for June.

Chapter Summary: Emma's journey with her mother taught her that effective communication in dementia care is built on patience, empathy, and understanding. By focusing on connecting with June in ways that respected her mother's experience and emotions, Emma found a path through the challenges of Alzheimer's. This case study illustrates that, with the right approach, caregivers can foster meaningful interactions that honor their loved ones' dignity and strengthen their bond, even in the face of dementia.

~

PART SIX WRAP-UP:

BASED ON EMMA'S experience in caring for her mother, June, with Alzheimer's disease, here's a list of action items for caregivers to enhance communication and connection with loved ones living with dementia:

Action Items for the Caregiver:

1. **Adopt Clear and Simple Communication**: Use straightforward language and short sentences to make it easier for your loved one to understand and respond.
2. **Practice Patience in Conversations**: Allow ample time for your loved one to process information and express themselves without rushing them.
3. **Use Nonverbal Cues**: Incorporate gestures, facial expressions, and touch to convey messages and emotions when words fall short.
4. **Maintain Eye Contact**: Ensure you have your loved one's attention by maintaining eye contact, which also shows you are present and engaged.
5. **Avoid Correcting Mistakes**: Focus on the emotion behind the

communication rather than correcting inaccuracies, which can lead to frustration and distress.

6. **Reduce Environmental Distractions**: Choose a quiet and calm setting for conversations to help your loved one focus and engage more effectively.

7. **Offer Choices Simplistically**: When presenting options, keep them limited and straightforward to avoid overwhelming your loved one.

8. **Engage in Active Listening**: Show you value their thoughts and feelings by listening attentively and responding with empathy.

9. **Use Visual Aids When Necessary**: use pictures or objects to help clarify ideas and help with better understanding.

10. **Encourage Reminiscing**: Stimulate positive memories and emotions by discussing familiar topics and sharing stories from the past.

11. **Seek Support and Education**: Join caregiver support groups and participate in workshops to learn more about effective dementia care strategies.

12. **Focus on Self-Care**: Take care of your own emotional and physical well-being to maintain your ability to provide compassionate care.

13. **Create a Supportive Environment**: Adjust the living environment to be more dementia-friendly, ensuring safety and comfort for your loved one.

14. **Document Effective Strategies**: Keep a record of successful communication techniques and strategies that resonate with your loved one for future reference.

15. **Stay Flexible and Adaptable**: Be ready to adjust your communication methods as the disease progresses, remaining open to finding new ways to connect.

By following these action items, caregivers can foster a more positive and effective communication experience with their loved ones, making sure they feel heard, understood, and valued throughout their journey with dementia.

IN OUR NEXT PART...

IN OUR NEXT PART, "Creating a Safe and Supportive Environment at Home," we'll tackle how to make your living space safer for the elderly, especially those living with dementia. We will take a page out of my book, "MAKE IT SAFE! A FAMILY CAREGIVER'S HOME SAFETY ASSESSMENT GUIDE FOR SUPPORTING ELDERS@HOME," to guide you through assessing potential hazards in your home. Like child-proofing, but with a twist, we're focusing on accessibility and avoiding risks that come with lower mobility and memory issues. It's all about making sure your home isn't just a place where they live but a space where they can do so safely and with independence.

We'll dive into the 3 As of Personal Safety: Awareness, Assessment, and Action. First up, awareness – recognizing the everyday hazards that might not have been a concern before but now pose a risk to your elderly loved one. Then, we'll move on to assessment, conducting a thorough walkthrough of their living environment, much like a home inspector, to spot these hazards.

And finally, action – trying to resolve these issues, whether it's as simple as rearranging furniture or as involved as making significant home changes. Alongside practical advice, we'll explore installing safety features, improving lighting, and organizing the home to reduce risks and promote a sense of independence. By the end of this Part, you'll have a solid foundation for creating a home environment that supports your loved one's safety and well-being.

~

PART SEVEN
CREATING A SAFE AND SUPPORTIVE ENVIRONMENT AT HOME:

ASSESS POTENTIAL HAZARDS IN THE HOME AND FOCUS ON SAFETY MEASURES BASED ON THE SPECIFIC NEEDS OF YOUR LOVED ONE

THE CONTENT for this Part is excerpted from my book **MAKE IT SAFE! A FAMILY CAREGIVER'S HOME SAFETY ASSESSMENT GUIDE FOR SUPPORTING ELDERS@HOME.**

While that book is directed at caregivers supporting elders living in their home, the same principles apply to us as caregivers to those living with dementia.

HOME SAFETY OVERVIEW

IF YOU ARE A PARENT, you will probably remember what it was like to make your home safe for your children.

Many of the same principles apply when making your home safe for elders. Whereas, with children you are usually protecting them from accessing something that could be hazardous and could cause them harm, when making the home safe for elders, you will also think about accessibility, accommodating decreased mobility and memory deficits.

At the same time, you need to support the elder in maintaining their independence if you can and as long as they are able.

In this Part we look at making your home safer for an elder to live with you or making adaptations to the elder's current home, allowing them to live independently, with your support.

Throughout the book I use the terms 'elder', 'senior' and 'loved one' interchangeably. While this book is written from the perspective of helping an older person to live safely either independently or semi-independently in their own home, or yours, the same safety principles apply to caring for someone who is not elderly.

To do so, we will draw from the field of <u>personal safety</u> to organize ourselves.

~

INTRODUCING THE 3 AS OF PERSONAL SAFETY... AWARENESS, ASSESSMENT AND ACTION.

Awareness: As we go about the activities of our daily life, we likely encounter many situations or conditions that are hazardous. I hope we have learned how to avoid or prevent negative results from these hazards.

This is your awareness. You realize a particular situation could be hazardous to you, so you take avoidant or corrective actions to prevent harm or injury.

This Part on home safety will raise your awareness on how the safety needs of an elder can be greater than what we may be used to.

I would suspect upon completion of this book you will identify hazards in your home needing rectifying to help your entire family, not just an elderly person as I did when developing this program.

Assessment: At a basic level, assessment is where you will do a walk-about inspection of the elder's living environment.

Much the same as a home inspector would investigate a home you were considering purchasing... letting you know what is right or wrong with the house, you will conduct a safety inspection of the elder's home.

As we work our way through the book, we will explore a collection of safety-related questions, focusing on different areas of the home.

The chapters are organized in main areas common to most homes and suggestions are given to the questions posed.

As you work your way through the content, you will notice there are specific hazards common to many areas of the home. They will be identified in the chapter you are reading. To draw attention to their importance, some will have their own specific chapter examples: Fire Safety and Electrical Safety.

Home Safety Assessment Form: I have created a set of question sheets you can print and carry with you to complete your inspection. You can download a copy of the form at https://BookHip.com/SXGMBT

It is helpful to use a clipboard when performing your safety inspection.

Action: It helps nobody if you identify a hazard and do nothing to resolve it.

Resolving a problem may mean taking a piece of equipment such as a toaster with a faulty cord out of service, repairing a hazard or maybe undergoing a major renovation to accommodate the elder's needs.

Create a Safety Upgrade Budget.

There are several steps to creating a budget for safety upgrades.

Some fixes you may do fairly quickly. Others may take time to organize and to raise the funds to pay for the upgrades.

Once you identify a safety hazard needing improving, you need to research the options available and determine a cost.

Also, are you able to make the improvements yourself, or will you require a professional tradesperson to make the improvements? This will affect the costs involved in the home improvement.

While we complete our safety inspection, we will keep track of items that may require a budget to rectify.

Depending on where you live, there may be government or NGO (non-government organizations) funds you could access to offset the costs of home safety improvements.

Safety Assessment Question: Is the home safe for a professional caregiver to visit the home?

Here are some sample assessment questions from **MAKE IT SAFE! A FAMILY CAREGIVER'S HOME SAFETY ASSESSMENT GUIDE FOR SUPPORTING ELDERS@HOME**

Rationale: Professional caregivers are trained to consider their own health and safety first. If the home presents a potential hazard to their personal safety, they may deny service until the hazard has been rectified.

If the elder is a smoker, they may have to refrain from smoking for a specific amount of time to reduce the hazards of second-hand smoke to the caregiver.

Action Item: if the elder requires the services of a professional caregiver who provides services within the elder's home, speak to the caregiver about their requirements and/or health & safety needs.

Safety Assessment Question: Are emergency numbers posted?

Considerations: Emergency numbers include: poison control, doctors, most responsible family member, 911 for police, fire or ambulance, an involved neighbor, etc.

Action Items:

1. If an Emergency Number List hasn't been created, make one.
2. Post the list in an easily accessible location such as the refrigerator.

Safety Assessment Question: Is there a designated danger zone in the home to store hazardous chemicals or products?

Rationale: People with dementia forget the purpose of things and how to use them. They may think wiper fluid is juice or be unaware that the grill is hot.

Action Items:

1. Designate a danger zone.
2. To make the home safer, turn the garage, workroom, closet, outdoor shed, recycled TV armoire or a large cabinet into a storage place for:

- cleaning products
- bleach
- mothballs
- insecticide
- paint, turpentine, stain
- sharp knives, scissors, box cutters, blades
- alcohol
- tobacco products, including chewing tobacco
- hand and power tools

Better still, remove these products completely from the home and find alternative storage. You could then bring them with you when you visited the home if you required them.

1. Install key or combination locks on rooms and other storage places containing potentially dangerous items. In addition, use childproof doorknob covers or cabinet locks.

Safety Assessment Question: Is there good lighting in stairways & hallways?

Considerations: Make home lighting brighter but prevent glare.

Action Item: Provide good lighting where required.

Safety Assessment Question: Are bookshelves anchored to walls to prevent toppling over?

Action Item: Ensure bookshelves are anchored to walls. Heavy duty anti-tip furniture straps are readily available for purchase at your local hardware store.

Further home locations requiring assessment are included in **MAKE IT SAFE! A FAMILY CAREGIVER'S HOME SAFETY ASSESSMENT GUIDE FOR SUPPORTING ELDERS@HOME** and are:

- Indoors General
- Assessing Fall Hazards
- Hallways & Stairwells
- Kitchen
- Bathrooms
- Bedrooms
- The Great Outdoors
- Home Use Medical Devices
- Electrical Safety
- Fire Safety & Prevention

Here are more safety strategies to consider:

Install safety features such as grab bars, non-slip mats, and handrails in key areas to prevent falls and promote independence.

Creating a safe and supportive environment for your loved one at home is essential for their well-being. One of the key aspects of this is ensuring safety measures are in place to prevent accidents and promote independence. Here are tips on how to create a safe and supportive environment at home:

Install safety features: Installing grab bars in the bathroom, non-slip mats in the shower and handrails along staircases can greatly reduce the risk of falls and accidents. These simple additions can provide stability and support, especially for older adults or individuals with mobility issues.

Remove hazards: Identify and remove any potential hazards in the home, such as loose rugs, cluttered walkways, or slippery surfaces. Keeping the living space clear and free of obstacles can help prevent accidents and ensure a safe environment for your loved one.

Improve lighting: Proper lighting is important for safety at home. Make sure all areas of the house are well-lit, especially in hallways, staircases, and bathrooms. Consider installing motion-sensor lights or night lights to provide added visibility during nighttime.

Organize and label items: Keep commonly used items within easy reach and label them for easy identification. This can help your loved one navigate their living space more independently and reduce the risk of accidents or confusion.

Seek professional help: If you're unsure about how to best adapt your home for safety, consider seeking the advice of a professional, such as an occupational therapist or a home care specialist. They can provide recommendations tailored to your loved one's specific needs and help create a safe and supportive environment.

By taking these steps to create a safe and supportive environment at home, you can help protect your loved one from harm and promote their overall well-being and independence. Remember, ensuring safety first is key to providing a comfortable and secure living space for your loved one.

~

ORGANIZE FURNITURE AND BELONGINGS IN A WAY THAT IS EASY TO NAVIGATE AND REDUCES THE RISK OF ACCIDENTS OR INJURIES

HERE ARE tips for creating a safe and supportive environment at home:

Remove tripping hazards: Keep floors clear of clutter, loose rugs, and wires to reduce the risk of falls.

Install handrails: If your loved one has difficulty with balance or mobility, consider installing handrails along staircases and in bathrooms to provide more support.

Adequate lighting: Make sure that the home is well-lit to help prevent falls and improve visibility.

Secure rugs and mats: Use non-slip mats or rugs with anti-slip backings to prevent slipping accidents.

Organize belongings: Keep commonly used items within easy reach to avoid unnecessary bending or reaching.

Maintain smoke detectors and fire extinguishers: Regularly check and replace batteries in smoke detectors and keep fire extinguishers in accessible areas in case of emergencies.

Accessibility: Ensure that your home is easily accessible, with ramps or stairlifts if necessary for those with mobility issues.

Emergency numbers: Keep a list of emergency contact numbers in a visible place in case of medical emergencies.

By following these safety precautions and adjusting your home, you can create a safe and supportive environment where your loved one can feel secure and comfortable.

Create designated spaces for necessary medical equipment and supplies, ensuring easy access and efficient organization.

Additionally, promote a sense of independence and confidence by encouraging your loved one to participate in daily activities to the best of their abilities. Provide opportunities for social interaction and mental stimulation to maintain their emotional well-being.

Establish a routine that includes regular check-ins and communication to address any concerns or changes in their condition promptly. Make sure emergency contact information is easily accessible and understood by all household members.

Finally, foster a supportive and understanding atmosphere by being patient, empathetic, and responsive to your loved one's needs. Encourage open communication and active involvement in decision-making to maintain a sense of autonomy and dignity.

By creating a safe and supportive environment at home, you can help your loved one feel secure, cared for, and empowered to navigate their daily life with confidence and peace of mind.

~

FREQUENTLY ASKED QUESTIONS:

CREATING a safe and supportive environment at home for a loved one with dementia is paramount. Here are five frequently asked questions to guide you in making your home a safer place.

1. How do I begin assessing my home for potential hazards to my loved one with dementia?

Start with a thorough walk-around of your home, similar to how a home inspector would assess a property. Look for anything that could pose a risk, like loose rugs, cluttered walkways, or sharp objects. Pay particular attention to areas where your loved one spends the most time. It's about spotting anything that might cause harm and figuring out how to fix it.

2. My loved one has a tendency to wander. How can I ensure they stay safe at home?

Wandering is a common concern. Consider installing door alarms or locks that are out of their direct line of sight. GPS trackers can also be a lifesaver, literally. These devices help track their location, giving you peace of mind while respecting their autonomy.

3. What changes should I consider to prevent falls at home?

Good lighting and clear walkways are essential. Install grab bars and railings in critical areas like the bathroom and along stairs. Non-slip mats in the bathroom and kitchen can prevent slips. Also, consider furniture arrangement that allows ample space for movement without obstacles.

4. How can I make the kitchen safer for someone with dementia?

Consider safety locks for cabinets and appliances that could pose a danger. Store hazardous materials, like cleaning supplies or sharp tools, in a locked cabinet. You might also want to invest in appliances that automatically shut off after a certain period of inactivity to prevent accidents.

5. What can I do to ensure emergency numbers are easily accessible if my loved one needs help?

Create a large print list of emergency contacts, including family members, close neighbors, and local emergency services. Place it in several easily visible locations throughout the house, such as on the refrigerator or by the main phone. Consider programming these numbers into a landline or cell phone with speed dial to make it easier for them to call for help if needed.

By addressing these key areas, you can create a safer environment for your loved one with dementia. Remember, the goal is not only to protect them from harm but also to support their independence for as long as possible.

~

CASE STUDY: MAKING HOME SAFE FOR JOHN WITH DEMENTIA

JOHN, an 82-year-old widower with early-stage dementia, lived independently until his condition began to present safety concerns. His daughter, Marie, noticed during visits that John had forgotten to turn off the stove twice in one week. Concerned for his safety, Marie acted.

Awareness and Assessment: Marie started with a thorough walk-through of her father's home, noting potential hazards like loose rugs that could cause tripping, poor lighting in hallways, and the cluttered living space that made navigation difficult for John.

Action:

- **Decluttering and Rearrangement:** Marie first tackled the clutter, clearing walkways and organizing the home to make it easier for John to move around safely.
- **Safety Features:** She installed grab bars in the bathroom and handrails along the stairs. Non-slip mats were placed in the shower and beneath area rugs to prevent falls.
- **Lighting:** Additional lighting was installed in dim areas, and night lights were placed in hallways and John's bedroom to help him navigate at night.

- **Kitchen Safety:** The stove knobs were covered with safety covers, and Marie arranged for meals to be delivered, reducing John's need to cook.
- **Emergency Preparedness:** Marie posted emergency contact numbers on the refrigerator and gave John a wearable emergency button to call for help if needed.

Through these interventions, Marie created a safer living environment for John, letting him maintain his independence while ensuring his safety.

Case Study 2: Emma's Transition to Safer Living

Emma, a 76-year-old with advanced dementia, lived with her son, Alex. As her dementia progressed, Emma's mobility decreased, and she began experiencing falls. Alex realized the need for a safer home environment to support Emma's well-being.

Awareness and Assessment: Acknowledging the increased risk of falls, Alex conducted a safety inspection of their home, identifying areas like the bathroom and kitchen as high-risk zones for Emma.

Action:

- **Bathroom Safety:** Alex installed grab bars near the toilet and in the shower. A shower chair was added to let Emma bathe safely.
- **Removing Hazards:** Loose rugs were removed, and furniture was rearranged to create clear pathways for Emma to walk without obstacles.
- **Medication Safety:** All medication was moved to a locked cabinet to prevent accidental ingestion by Emma, who sometimes forgot what her medications were for.
- **Danger Zone:** Recognizing Emma's inability to recognize hazardous substances, Alex designated a locked area for cleaning supplies and sharp objects.
- **Professional Caregiver Safety:** To ensure the home was safe for professional caregivers, Alex made sure all areas Emma

and the caregivers would use were free of hazards and well-lit. He also established a smoke-free environment to accommodate the health and safety of visiting caregivers.

Through thoughtful changes and ongoing attention to safety, Alex provided a secure and supportive home environment for Emma, ensuring her comfort and reducing the risk of accidents.

~

PART SEVEN WRAP-UP:

HERE's a list of action items that can guide caregivers in creating a safer home environment for loved ones with dementia:

1. **Walkthrough Safety Check**: Take a stroll through your home with a keen eye for potential hazards. Look out for loose rugs, cluttered pathways, and anything else that might pose a risk.
2. **Secure Rugs and Mats**: Make sure all rugs and mats are securely fixed to the floor with non-slip backing to prevent slips and falls.
3. **Install Grab Bars and Handrails**: Place grab bars in the bathroom, particularly near the toilet and shower, and install handrails along staircases to provide extra support and stability.
4. **Improve Home Lighting**: Brighten up the home to ensure visibility is ideal. Add extra lighting to dark hallways, staircases, and rooms. Nightlights can be helpful in preventing nighttime falls.
5. **Organize and Label**: Keep everyday items within easy reach and clearly label them. This reduces frustration for your loved one and aids in their navigation around the house.

6. **Reduce Kitchen Risks**: Cover stove knobs or invest in an automatic shut-off device to prevent accidents. Consider meal delivery services if cooking becomes too risky.

7. **Create a Safe Zone for Hazardous Materials**: Lock away cleaning supplies, sharp objects, and any hazardous materials in a designated safe zone, out of reach of your loved one.

8. **Emergency Contacts List**: Compile a list of emergency numbers, including poison control, family doctors, and a responsible family member. Post this list prominently in the home, like on the fridge.

9. **Medication Safety**: Ensure medications are stored safely and are organized so they can be administered correctly.

10. **Assess Furniture Stability**: Make sure bookshelves and other large pieces of furniture are anchored to walls to prevent them from tipping over.

11. **Evaluate Accessibility**: Consider the need for ramps or stairlifts if your home has steps or levels to ensure your loved one can move around easily.

12. **Professional Caregiver Requirements**: If employing professional caregivers, ensure the home environment meets their safety requirements to protect both them and your loved one.

13. **Regular Check-Ins**: Establish a routine that includes regular check-ins and communication to quickly address any concerns or changes in your loved one's condition.

14. **Encourage Independence Safely**: Find ways to support your loved one's independence in safe, manageable ways, such as using assistive devices or simplifying tasks.

15. **Plan for Home Adjustments**: Set aside a budget for necessary safety upgrades. Research any available community or government assistance programs that might help cover costs.

By taking these actions, you can greatly improve the safety and comfort of your home for a loved one living with dementia, ensuring their well-being and your peace of mind.

IN OUR NEXT PART...

IN OUR NEXT PART, we'll dive into "Grace Under Pressure: Managing Tough Moments in Dementia Care," focusing on the inevitable challenges that arise when caring for a loved one with dementia. This journey is filled with moments that test our patience, understanding, and emotional resilience. We'll explore the underlying causes of challenging behaviors, such as agitation, and how they often stem from the individual's struggle to communicate their needs or discomfort. Understanding these triggers is the first step toward addressing them effectively and compassionately.

We'll provide you with practical strategies and techniques to create a calm and supportive environment, emphasizing the importance of setting clear boundaries, using effective communication, and using de-escalation techniques. This Part aims to equip you with the tools to navigate these difficult moments with grace, ensuring the well-being of both you and your loved one.

We'll discuss the significance of patience, empathy, and compassion as your best allies in this journey. Recognizing that every challenging behavior is a form of communication will change how you respond to these situations, reinforcing the bond of trust between you and your loved one. We'll also highlight the value of seeking professional insight and leaning on support networks to share experiences and find solace in the shared journeys of others. Creating safety and security for your loved one with dementia is about more than managing the moment; it's about fostering a feeling of understanding and care that transcends the challenges. Join us as we navigate these tough times together, offering insights and strategies to manage challenging behaviors with understanding, dignity, and love, making every interaction more meaningful.

~

PART EIGHT
GRACE UNDER PRESSURE: MANAGING TOUGH MOMENTS IN DEMENTIA CARE

Caring for a loved one with dementia is a journey filled with both profound love and unique challenges. As the disease progresses, it is common to encounter difficult behaviors and moments of agitation that can test even the most patient and compassionate caregivers. However, by understanding the underlying causes of these behaviors and equipping yourself with a toolkit of effective strategies, you can navigate these tough times with grace, empathy, and resilience.

This Part explores the art of managing challenging moments in dementia care, focusing on fostering a calm environment, promoting understanding, and focusing on the well-being of both your loved one and yourself.

～

DIGGING DEEPER: UNDERSTANDING THE CAUSES

To EFFECTIVELY ADDRESS challenging behaviors in dementia care, it is essential to understand the root causes behind them. Often, these behaviors are a manifestation of the person's struggle to communicate their needs, discomfort, or emotional state. Agitation, for example, could be a sign of physical discomfort, confusion, frustration, or fear. By adopting the role of a compassionate detective, you can uncover the underlying factors contributing to the behavior and tailor your response.

Consider These Potential Triggers:

Physical discomfort: Is your loved one experiencing pain, hunger, thirst, or fatigue?

Environmental factors: Is the surrounding environment overstimulating, unfamiliar, or unsettling?

Emotional distress: Is your loved one feeling anxious, afraid, or overwhelmed?

Communication difficulties: Is your loved one struggling to express their needs or understand others?

By identifying the specific trigger, you can address the root cause more effectively and provide targeted support to alleviate the distress.

Building a Calm Environment: Strategies for Caregivers

Creating a calm and supportive environment is important in managing challenging behaviors in dementia care. Here are key strategies for caregivers:

Set Clear Boundaries:

While flexibility is important, establishing consistent rules and routines helps create a sense of structure and safety for your loved one. Communicate expectations and boundaries in a gentle, respectful manner. Predictability and familiarity can reduce anxiety and the likelihood of challenging behaviors arising.

Effective Communication is Key:

The way you communicate with your loved one can significantly affect their behavior and emotional state. Use simple, reassuring language and speak in a calm, soothing tone. Avoid rushing or raising your voice, as this can escalate agitation. Keep your body language open and relaxed, maintaining eye contact and using gentle gestures to convey understanding and support. By fostering effective communication, you can prevent misunderstandings and ease tension.

De-escalation Techniques:

When moments of agitation or challenging behavior arise, having a repertoire of de-escalation techniques can be invaluable. One powerful tool is distraction. Gently redirecting your loved one's attention to a different activity, topic, or sensory experience can help diffuse stress and refocus their energy. This could involve engaging them in a favorite hobby, looking through old photographs, or listening to soothing music. The key is to find activities that resonate with your loved one and bring them a sense of comfort and joy.

Patience, Empathy, and Compassion:

Above all, approaching challenging moments with patience, empathy, and compassion is essential. Recognize that your loved one's behavior reflects their struggle and distress, not a personal attack on you. Take a deep breath, remain calm, and respond with kindness and understanding. Validate their feelings, even if you don't fully understand them, and offer reassurance you are there to support them. By leading with compassion, you can often calm fears, reduce agitation, and strengthen the bond of trust between you.

Seeking Professional Insight:

Managing challenging behaviors in dementia care can be complex and emotionally taxing. Please reach out to healthcare professionals, such as geriatric psychiatrists, neurologists, or counselors experienced in dementia care. They can offer valuable insights, specific strategies, and support tailored to your loved one's unique needs. Collaborating with a multidisciplinary team can provide a comprehensive approach to managing difficult behaviors and ensuring the best care.

Support Networks:

Caring for a loved one with dementia can be isolating and overwhelming. Remember, you are not alone in this journey. Connecting with support networks, whether in person or online, can provide a invaluable space to share experiences, exchange strategies, and find solace in the understanding of others who have walked a similar path. Support groups, caregiver forums, and local organizations dedicated to dementia care can offer a sense of community, validation, and practical guidance.

Creating Safety and Security:

At the heart of managing challenging behaviors in dementia care is the goal of fostering a deep sense of safety and security for your loved one. Recognize these behaviors are a form of communication, a signal that something is amiss in their world. By responding with understanding, patience, and care, you are not merely managing the moment—you are reinforcing the main bond of trust and love between you.

Consider these strategies to promote a sense of safety and security:

- Maintain a consistent routine and familiar environment.
- Ensure basic needs, such as comfort, nutrition, and hydration, are met.
- Provide reassurance through gentle touch, soothing words, and a calm presence.
- Adapt the environment to reduce potential triggers or hazards.
- Offer choices and opportunities for autonomy.

By creating a haven, both physically and emotionally, you lay the foundation for more positive interactions and a higher quality of life for your loved one.

Navigating the Tough Times Together:

Managing challenging behaviors and moments of agitation in dementia care requires a delicate balance of strategy, understanding, and heart. It is a journey that demands patience, resilience, and an unwavering commitment to preserving the dignity and well-being of your loved one. Remember, it is not just about getting through the tough moments; it is about doing so in a way that upholds their humanity, promotes understanding, and strengthens the bond you share.

As you navigate these challenges, be kind to yourself. Recognize that you are doing your best in a profoundly difficult situation. Seek support when needed, take moments for self-care, and celebrate the small victories along the way. By approaching each moment with grace, compassion, and a willingness to adapt, you can weather the storms and continue to provide the loving, effective care your loved one deserves.

Faced with dementia's challenges, your love, dedication, and unwavering support are the anchors that provide comfort, security, and a profound sense of connection. Trust in the strength of your bond and the power of your presence. Together, you can navigate the tough times with grace, finding moments of joy, meaning, and love amidst the struggles. Remember, your love and care make all the difference in your loved one's world.

∾

PROACTIVE CARE: STAYING AHEAD OF DIFFICULT MOMENTS IN DEMENTIA CARE

CARING for a loved one with dementia often involves navigating challenging behaviors and moments of agitation. While these situations can be stressful and emotionally taxing, adopting a proactive approach can significantly improve the management of difficult moments. By recognizing early signs, understanding triggers, and using effective strategies for calm resolution, caregivers can stay ahead of potential crises and foster a more supportive and compassionate care environment. This section explores the art of proactive care in dementia, focusing on spotting warning signs, adapting to triggers, and implementing techniques for peaceful resolution.

Spotting the Signs and Understanding Triggers:

One of the key aspects of proactive care in dementia is the ability to recognize the early warning signs of agitation or difficult behavior. By identifying these indicators, caregivers can intervene before the situation escalates, potentially preventing more severe or prolonged episodes of distress. Common signs to look out for include:

1. Restlessness or pacing
2. Increased confusion or disorientation

3. Irritability or short-tempered responses
4. Changes in sleep patterns or appetite
5. Verbal or physical aggression

In addition to recognizing these signs, it is important to understand the triggers that may contribute to challenging behaviors. Every individual with dementia is unique, and their triggers can vary. However, some common factors that may precipitate difficult moments include:

1. Loud noises or overstimulating environments
2. Crowded or unfamiliar spaces
3. Changes in routine or schedule
4. Physical discomfort or pain
5. Unmet needs, such as hunger, thirst, or toileting

By identifying and addressing these triggers proactively, caregivers can create a more conducive environment that reduces the likelihood of agitation or difficult behaviors.

Strategies for Calm Resolution:

When faced with challenging behaviors or moments of agitation, caregivers must remain calm and composed. Reactive or impulsive responses can inadvertently escalate the situation, leading to further distress for both the individual with dementia and the caregiver. Instead, using strategies for calm resolution can help de-escalate the situation and promote a more positive outcome. Consider these approaches:

Active Listening and Empathy:

Often, the key to de-escalating a difficult moment lies in showing genuine understanding and empathy. Take the time to listen attentively to your loved one, even if their communication is fragmented or confused. Confirm their feelings and show you are trying to comprehend their perspective. Respond with compassion and reassurance, letting them know that you are there to support them. By creating a safe and empathetic space, you can help alleviate their distress and foster a sense of connection.

Clear Boundaries and Communication:

Establishing and communicating clear boundaries and expectations can help create a predictable and structured environment for your loved one with dementia. Consistency and predictability can reduce confusion and frustration, as they provide a sense of security and familiarity. Be clear and concise in your communication, using simple language and avoiding complex or abstract ideas. Gently remind them of established routines, boundaries, and expectations, while remaining patient and understanding if they struggle to remember or adhere to them.

Consistent Consequences:

While it is important to approach challenging behaviors with empathy and understanding, it is equally important to maintain consistency in consequences. This does not mean punishing or reprimanding your loved one, but rather gently and firmly reinforcing established boundaries and expectations. Consistent consequences help provide a sense of structure and predictability, which can be reassuring for individuals with dementia. However, always make sure the consequences are appropriate, proportionate, and delivered with love and respect.

Empowering the Individual:

Involve your loved one with dementia in discussions and decisions about managing their challenging behaviors. Empowering them to have a voice in their care can help maintain their sense of autonomy and dignity. Ask for their input on strategies that may help them feel more calm and secure. Collaborate with them to identify potential triggers and develop coping mechanisms together. By including them, you show respect for their experiences and promote a sense of control and participation in their own care.

Seeking Professional and Community Support:

Managing challenging behaviors in dementia care can be emotionally and physically demanding. You need not face these challenges alone. Contacting mental health professionals, such as geriatric psychiatrists or counselors specializing in dementia care, can provide valuable insights, strategies, and support. They can offer personalized guidance tailored to your loved one's specific needs and help you develop a comprehensive care plan.

In addition to professional support, connecting with community resources and support groups can be immensely beneficial. Joining a dementia caregiver support group, either in person or online, lets you share experiences, learn from others who have faced similar challenges, and find solace in knowing you are not alone. These communities can offer practical advice, emotional support, and a sense of belonging during difficult times.

Chapter Summary:

Navigating challenging behaviors and moments of agitation in dementia care requires a proactive, compassionate, and resilient approach. By staying attuned to early warning signs, understanding individual triggers, and using strategies for calm resolution, caregivers can effectively manage difficult situations and promote the well-being of their loved ones.

Remember to focus on active listening and empathy, establish clear boundaries and communication, maintain consistent consequences, empower the individual, and seek professional and community support when needed.

These strategies, coupled with a calm and patient demeanor, can help mitigate the impact of challenging behaviors and foster a more supportive care environment.

Caring for a loved one with dementia is a demanding and often emotionally charged journey. It is important to focus on your own self-care and well-being alongside the needs of your loved one. Recharge, engage in activities that bring you joy, and lean on the support of family, friends, and professionals when needed. By nurturing your own resilience and emotional well-being, you can continue to provide the compassionate and effective care your loved one deserves.

Remember, proactive care is not about perfection; it is about approaching each moment with love, understanding, and a commitment to finding peaceful resolutions. Trust in the power of your connection, the strength of your compassion, and the resilience of your spirit.

Together, you can navigate the challenges of dementia care with grace, empathy, and unwavering dedication to your loved one's well-being.

∼

NAVIGATING THE STORM: CALMING STRATEGIES FOR DIFFICULT MOMENTS

CARING for a loved one with dementia is a journey filled with both tender moments and challenging storms. As the disease progresses, it is common to encounter episodes of agitation, confusion, and difficult behaviors that can test the resilience of even the most dedicated caregivers. In these moments, having a repertoire of de-escalation techniques and calming strategies can be a lifeline, helping you navigate the tempest with grace and compassion. This section explores practical approaches to diffusing tense situations, fostering a sense of calm, and focusing on the well-being of both your loved one and yourself amidst the challenges of dementia care.

Maintain Your Composure:

Faced with agitation or difficult behaviors, one of the most powerful tools at your disposal is your own composure. By remaining calm, centered, and collected, you set the tone for the interaction and create an atmosphere of peace and security. Your serene presence can be contagious, helping to soothe your loved one's anxiety and agitation. Breathe deeply, ground yourself, and approach the situation with a clear and compassionate mindset. Remember, your loved one is not acting out deliberately; their behavior reflects their struggle with the disease. By embodying calmness, you offer a sanctuary of stability and understanding amidst the chaos.

Engage in Active Listening:

When your loved one is experiencing distress or agitation, it is important to give them your full, undivided attention. Engage in active listening, focusing not only on their words but also on the emotions and needs beneath the surface. Often, simply feeling heard and understood can significantly reduce a person's distress, making them more receptive to calming down. Put aside any distractions, maintain gentle eye contact, and give them the space to express themselves. Avoid interrupting or rushing to provide solutions; instead, let them know that you are there to listen and support them. By creating a safe and confirming space for their concerns, you foster a sense of connection and trust that can help de-escalate the situation.

Validate Their Feelings:

Validation is a powerful tool in dementia care, as it acknowledges the reality and significance of your loved one's emotional experience. When they express fear, anger, or confusion, let them know that their feelings are valid and taken seriously. This doesn't mean agreeing with incorrect statements or endorsing challenging behaviors; rather, it means recognizing the underlying emotions as real and important.

Use phrases like, "I can see how upsetting this is for you," or "It's understandable to feel frustrated in this situation." By validating their feelings, you convey empathy, respect, and a willingness to understand their perspective. This validation can help diffuse the intensity of their emotions and create a bridge of connection between you.

Employ Supportive Nonverbal Communication:

In moments of agitation or distress, the way you communicate nonverbally can be as important as the words you use. Maintain gentle, consistent eye contact to convey attention and engagement. Speak in a calm, measured tone, even if your loved one's voice becomes loud or aggressive. Use open, relaxed body language, with uncrossed arms and a posture that signals openness and receptivity. Offer reassuring touches, such as holding their hand or placing a comforting hand on their shoulder, if they are receptive to physical contact. These nonverbal cues of support and safety can help regulate their emotional state and de-escalate the situation.

Extend a Helping Hand:

When your loved one is struggling with a task or experiencing frustration, offer assistance in a way that respects their autonomy and dignity. Instead of jumping in and taking over, ask if they would like help or suggest working on the task together. By extending a helping hand, you show you are there to support them while still honoring their sense of independence. Sometimes, a simple offer of help can shift the dynamic from one of conflict to cooperation, diffusing the tension and fostering a sense of teamwork.

Clearly Define Boundaries:

While it is essential to approach challenging behaviors with empathy and understanding, it is equally important to communicate the limits of acceptable conduct. Clearly define boundaries firmly but kindly, using simple, direct language. For example, you might say, "I understand that you're upset, but it's not okay to yell at me. Let's take a moment to calm down together." By setting clear boundaries, you create a sense of structure and safety for both your loved one and yourself. It helps establish a predictable environment where expectations are understood, reducing the likelihood of escalation.

Redirect Focus:

When agitation or difficult behaviors arise, gently shifting the focus to a more neutral or positive topic can be an effective de-escalation strategy. Distraction can be a powerful tool in redirecting energy away from the source of stress and toward a more calming activity or conversation.

Consider engaging your loved one in a favorite hobby, looking through old photographs, or listening to soothing music. The key is to find activities that resonate with them and bring a sense of comfort and enjoyment. By redirecting their attention, you create an opportunity for the intense emotions to subside and for a more peaceful interaction to emerge.

Propose a Pause:

In the heat of the moment, when emotions are running high, proposing a short break can be beneficial for everyone involved. Suggest taking a few minutes to breathe, collect thoughts, and regain composure. This pause can provide the necessary space for tensions to dissipate and for a fresh perspective to emerge. You might say, "Let's take a moment to step back and catch our breath. We can come back to this discussion when we both feel calmer." By offering a temporary respite, you create an opportunity for emotions to settle and for a more constructive dialogue to resume.

Chapter Summary:

Navigating the storms of dementia care requires a delicate balance of patience, empathy, and skill. Mastering the art of de-escalation is an ongoing process, as each person with dementia is unique, and what works in one situation may not be effective in another. The key is to approach each challenge with an open heart, a compassionate mind, and a willingness to adapt your strategies to meet the needs of the moment.

By maintaining your composure, engaging in active listening, validating feelings, using supportive nonverbal communication, extending a helping hand, defining clear boundaries, redirecting focus, and proposing pauses, you cultivate a toolkit of calming techniques. These strategies can help create a more peaceful environment for your loved one, reducing stress and enhancing the quality of your interactions.

Remember, caring for someone with dementia is a journey that requires immense resilience, self-compassion, and support. Focus on your own well-being alongside the needs of your loved one, seeking respite and assistance when needed. Surround yourself with a network of understanding individuals who can offer guidance, encouragement, and a listening ear.

As you navigate the storms of dementia care, hold fast to the power of love, the strength of your bond, and the unwavering commitment to your loved one's dignity and well-being. With each challenging moment, you have the opportunity to deepen your connection, to grow in empathy, and to find moments of grace amidst the tempest. Trust in your resilience, lean on the support of others, and know that your loving presence is the most precious gift you can offer your loved one on this journey.

～

CRAFTING PEACE: STRATEGIES FOR COMMUNICATING THROUGH CHALLENGING BEHAVIORS

Communicating effectively with a loved one experiencing dementia-related challenging behaviors is a delicate dance that requires patience, empathy, and a strategic approach. It goes beyond merely managing difficult moments; it's about forging a connection that honors the dignity and needs of the person in your care.

Effective communication serves as a bridge of understanding, helping to navigate the choppy waters of agitation and confusion. This section explores key strategies for developing and using communication techniques that can transform challenging situations into opportunities for connection and peace.

Stay Centered and Calm:

The foundation of managing challenging behaviors lies in your ability to maintain a calm and centered presence. Faced with agitation or confusion, it's essential to take a moment to breathe deeply and ground yourself before responding. This brief pause allows you to collect your thoughts, regulate your own emotions, and approach the situation with a clear and compassionate mindset.

Remember, your loved one is not acting out deliberately; their behavior reflects the disease's impact on their brain. By embodying calmness, you create an environment that is more conducive to positive interactions and reduces the likelihood of escalation. Your composed demeanor can have a ripple effect, influencing the emotional state of your loved one and helping to diffuse tension.

Listen With Heart and Mind:

Active and empathetic listening is a powerful tool in dementia care communication. When faced with challenging behaviors, it's important to look beyond the surface and seek to understand the feelings and needs driving the actions. Often, these behaviors are expressions of unmet needs, discomfort, or underlying emotions that your loved one may struggle to articulate. By listening with both your heart and mind, you can begin to decipher the message behind the behavior.

Give your full attention, maintain eye contact, and use nonverbal cues like nodding and gentle touches to show you are present and engaged. Avoid the temptation to interrupt or rush to provide solutions; instead, create a safe space for them to express themselves.

By genuinely listening, you can identify the root cause of the behavior and address it more effectively, demonstrating that their concerns are heard and valued.

Communicate Clearly and Simply:

When communicating with a loved one experiencing dementia, clarity and simplicity are key. As the disease progresses, it can affect language comprehension and processing, making complex instructions or questions challenging to understand. To help with effective communication, use straightforward, concise language and break down information into smaller, more manageable pieces.

Speak slowly and calmly, allowing time for your loved one to process and respond. Avoid using abstract ideas or figurative language, as these can be confusing. Instead, choose concrete, descriptive words that paint a clear picture. Use short sentences and ask one question at a time, allowing them to answer before moving on. By communicating clearly and simply, you reduce the likelihood of frustration and agitation arising from misunderstandings or confusion.

Validate Emotions:

Validating the emotions behind challenging behaviors is a powerful way to de-escalate tense situations and foster a sense of connection. When your loved one expresses anger, fear, or sadness, acknowledge and confirm their feelings, even if you don't agree with the content of their statements. This validation sends a message that their emotions are real, understood, and respected. Use phrases like, "I can see how frustrating this must be for you," or "It's understandable to feel scared in this situation."

By validating their emotions, you create a safe and supportive space where they feel heard and valued. This emotional attunement helps build trust and rapport, making future interactions more positive and cooperative. Remember, validation is not about agreeing with false beliefs or endorsing challenging behaviors; it's about recognizing and honoring the human experience beneath the surface.

Set Boundaries with Compassion:

While empathy and validation are essential in dementia care communication, it's equally important to set clear boundaries around acceptable behavior. Establishing and consistently enforcing these boundaries helps create a sense of structure and predictability, which can be comforting for someone navigating the uncertainties of dementia.

When communicating boundaries, use a firm but kind tone, explaining the limits in simple, direct language. For example, you might say, "I know you're feeling angry, but it's not okay to hit. Let's take a deep breath together and find a different way to express your frustration." By setting boundaries with compassion, you provide a framework of safety and respect for both your loved one and yourself. It's a delicate balance of understanding their challenges while also maintaining a healthy and secure environment for all involved.

Strategies in Practice:

De-escalation: When agitation or challenging behaviors start to escalate, use de-escalation techniques to prevent further intensification. Gently redirect the conversation to a more neutral or calming topic or suggest a change in activity. Distraction can be a valuable tool in diffusing tension and shifting focus away from the source of stress. Engage your loved one in a favorite hobby, reminisce about happy memories, or introduce a sensory experience like listening to soothing music or looking at beautiful pictures. The goal is to create a positive diversion that lets the intense emotions subside naturally.

Problem-Solving Together: Whenever possible, involve your loved one in finding solutions to challenges or conflicts that arise. Rather than imposing a decision or taking over completely, engage them in a collaborative problem-solving process. Ask for their input, opinions, and ideas on how to approach the situation.

This inclusive approach empowers them, reduces feelings of helplessness or frustration, and promotes a sense of control over their environment. By working together, you foster a spirit of partnership and respect, strengthening your bond and reducing the likelihood of resistance or agitation.

Seek Understanding, Not Correction: In the midst of confusion or disorientation, it's common for individuals with dementia to make inaccurate statements or hold false beliefs. While it is tempting to correct these inaccuracies, it's often more productive to focus on the emotion being expressed rather than the factual content.

Avoid arguing or insisting on correcting their perception, as this can lead to further agitation and distress. Instead, validate the underlying feeling and respond with empathy and understanding. For example, if they insist on going home when they are already home, acknowledge their desire for comfort and security, and gently redirect the conversation to a soothing topic or activity.

Routine as a Tool: Establishing and maintaining a consistent daily routine can be a powerful tool in reducing anxiety, confusion, and challenging behaviors. Predictability and structure provide a sense of comfort and security for individuals with dementia, helping them navigate the challenges of memory loss and disorientation.

Create a daily schedule that includes regular times for meals, activities, rest, and personal care. Use visual cues like written reminders or pictorial schedules to reinforce the routine. Be flexible and adaptable when necessary, but strive to maintain the overall structure.

By incorporating routines into your communication strategies, you can help prevent challenging behaviors before they arise and create a more peaceful and manageable care environment.

Professional Support: Navigating the complexities of dementia care communication can be overwhelming, and you need not do it alone. Don't hesitate to seek guidance and support from healthcare professionals experienced in dementia care, such as geriatric specialists, dementia care coaches, or social workers.

These experts can offer personalized strategies tailored to your loved one's unique needs and provide valuable insights into effective communication techniques. They can also connect you with local resources, support groups, and educational programs that can further enhance your skills and resilience as a caregiver.

Remember, seeking professional support is a sign of strength and dedication to providing the best possible care for your loved one.

Chapter Summary:

Communicating effectively through the challenges of dementia requires a heart full of compassion, a mind open to understanding, and a toolbox of strategic approaches. By staying centered and calm, listening with empathy, communicating clearly and simply, validating emotions, and setting boundaries with kindness, you can create an environment that fosters connection, respect, and peace.

Remember, each interaction is an opportunity to build trust, offer comfort, and affirm the dignity of your loved one. By using de-escalation techniques, engaging in collaborative problem-solving, focusing on understanding rather than correction, leveraging the power of routines, and seeking professional support when needed, you equip yourself with a comprehensive set of strategies to navigate even the most challenging behaviors.

As you start this journey of dementia care, hold fast to the power of patience, the strength of your love, and the resilience of your spirit. Your commitment to effective communication, even in the face of difficulty, is a testament to the depth of your devotion and the beauty of your relationship. With each day, you have the opportunity to craft moments of peace, connection, and understanding that will forever enrich both your lives.

∽

STAYING ANCHORED: MINDFULNESS AND SELF-REGULATION IN DEMENTIA CARE

CARING for a loved one with dementia is a journey that often presents moments of intense challenge and emotional turbulence. As a caregiver, you may navigate a sea of complex behaviors, agitation, and confusion, which can take a toll on your own well-being and ability to provide effective care. In these times of stress and uncertainty, mindfulness and self-regulation techniques emerge as invaluable tools, offering a lifeline of calm and clarity amidst the chaos.

By integrating these practices into your caregiving approach, you can cultivate a greater sense of presence, resilience, and compassion, both for yourself and the person in your care. This section explores the power of mindfulness and self-regulation in dementia care, providing practical strategies to help you stay anchored and centered, even in the most challenging of moments.

Embrace Mindfulness:

Mindfulness, the practice of being fully present and aware in the moment, is a transformative tool in dementia care. When faced with difficult situations or intense emotions, it's easy to become caught up in a whirlwind of reactivity and stress. However, by embracing mindfulness, you can learn to navigate these challenges with a clearer perspective and a more grounded presence.

Mindfulness teaches you to observe your thoughts and emotions without judgment, letting you respond to the situation with intention and compassion, rather than simply reacting on autopilot. Pause, tune into your breath, and notice the sensations in your body. By cultivating this state of present-moment awareness, you create a space between the trigger and your response, enabling you to choose a more thoughtful and effective course of action.

Deep Breathing:

In moments of heightened stress or agitation, our breath can serve as a powerful anchor, bringing us back to the present moment and calming both the mind and body. When we're overwhelmed, our breathing usually becomes shallow and rapid, perpetuating a state of anxiety and tension.

However, by consciously shifting to deep, mindful breathing, we can activate the body's natural relaxation response and restore a sense of equilibrium. Try taking a deep, slow inhale through your nose, letting your belly expand as you fill your lungs with air. Hold the breath briefly, and then exhale slowly through your mouth, releasing any tension or stress. Repeat this process several times, focusing your attention on the sensation of the breath moving in and out of your body. This simple yet potent practice can help you find your center of calm, even in the midst of chaos.

Recognize Triggers:

Understanding the triggers that lead to challenging behaviors in your loved one with dementia is a crucial part of effective caregiving. By becoming attuned to the specific circumstances, environments, or activities that usually precipitate agitation or confusion, you can proactively manage these situations and reduce their impact. Common triggers may include changes in routine, overstimulation, fatigue, or unmet physical needs such as hunger or discomfort.

Note patterns and observations and use this knowledge to adapt your approach and create a more supportive and predictable environment. For example, if you notice that late afternoon is usually a time of increased agitation (often called "sundowning"), you can plan soothing activities or adjust the lighting and noise levels to promote a sense of calm. By recognizing and addressing triggers preemptively, you can help prevent or mitigate challenging behaviors before they escalate.

Positive Self-Talk:

The internal dialogue we have with ourselves plays a significant role in shaping our emotional state and resilience. When caring for someone with dementia, it's common to experience feelings of self-doubt, frustration, or helplessness.

However, by consciously engaging in positive self-talk, you can reframe your perspective and maintain a more supportive and compassionate mindset. Notice the thoughts that arise in challenging moments, and practice replacing self-critical or negative statements with affirmations of your strength, dedication, and resilience.

Remind yourself that you are doing your best, that your efforts matter, and that you are making a profound difference in your loved one's life. Cultivating a narrative of self-compassion and encouragement can help you stay motivated, empowered, and emotionally balanced, even in the face of difficult circumstances.

Permission to Pause:

Caregiving is a demanding and often all-consuming role, and it's essential to recognize when you need a break to recharge and refocus. Giving yourself permission to pause and step away briefly is not a sign of weakness or selfishness, but rather a necessary act of self-care that ultimately helps both you and the person you're caring for.

When you feel overwhelmed or depleted, take a moment to assess your own needs and focus on your well-being. This may involve taking a few minutes to engage in a soothing activity, such as listening to music, practicing a relaxation technique, or simply stepping outside for some fresh air. It could also mean reaching out for support and respite, whether from family members, friends, or professional caregiving services.

Remember, taking care of yourself is not a luxury, but a critical part of sustainable and effective caregiving.

Lean on Your Support System:

Dementia care is a journey no one must navigate alone. Surrounding yourself with a strong support system is important for maintaining your own well-being and resilience. Contact family members, friends, or support groups who can offer a listening ear, practical assistance, or a shoulder to lean on.

Sharing your experiences, challenges, and emotions with others who understand can provide a profound sense of validation, connection, and relief. Consider joining a local or online caregiver support group, where you can exchange insights, strategies, and encouragement with others walking a similar path.

Additionally, please seek professional support from a counselor or therapist who specializes in caregiver well-being. They can provide personalized guidance, coping strategies, and a safe space to process your emotions and experiences.

Chapter Summary:

Mindfulness and self-regulation are essential anchors in the stormy seas of dementia care. By integrating these practices into your caregiving approach, you can navigate challenging moments with greater clarity, compassion, and resilience.

Embracing mindfulness lets you remain present and grounded, even in the face of intense emotions or difficult behaviors. Deep breathing serves as a powerful tool for calming the mind and body, while recognizing triggers enables you to proactively manage and mitigate potential sources of agitation.

Cultivating positive self-talk and self-compassion helps you maintain a supportive and empowering mindset, while giving yourself permission to pause and focus on self-care is essential for sustainable and effective caregiving. Leaning on your support system, whether through family, friends, support groups, or professional help, provides an important lifeline of connection, validation, and practical assistance.

Remember, caring for someone with dementia is a profound act of love and dedication, but it is also a journey that requires immense patience, adaptability, and self-awareness. By staying anchored in mindfulness and self-regulation, you can weather the storms with greater grace, find moments of joy and connection amidst the challenges, and provide the highest quality of care for your loved one.

As you navigate this path, hold fast to the power of your presence, the strength of your compassion, and the resilience of your spirit. Trust in your ability to find calm in the chaos, to respond with kindness and understanding, and to make a meaningful difference in your loved one's life. And always remember, you are not alone in this journey – there is support, guidance, and hope every step of the way.

~

TEAMING UP TO TACKLE
DEMENTIA CHALLENGES

NAVIGATING the complexities of dementia care, particularly when faced with challenging behaviors and agitation, can feel like an overwhelming and isolating experience. However, you are not alone in this journey.

By harnessing your own inner resilience, using clear communication strategies, and leveraging a strong network of support, you can chart a course through these turbulent waters with greater confidence and effectiveness. This section explores how to optimally use the resources at your disposal, both internal and external, to manage the challenges of dementia care with compassion, skill, and resilience.

Stay Centered:

When confronted with agitation or challenging behaviors, it's essential to maintain your own emotional equilibrium. In the heat of the moment, it is tempting to react with frustration, anger, or helplessness. However, by staying centered and grounded, you can approach the situation with the calmness and clarity it requires. Pause, close your eyes, and focus on your breath. Inhale deeply, letting the air fill your lungs and anchor you in the present moment. Exhale slowly, releasing any tension or stress you may be holding in your body.

This simple act of conscious breathing can help you regain your composure, enabling you to respond to your loved one's needs with patience, understanding, and compassion.

Clear Communication:

Effective communication is a key part of managing challenging behaviors in dementia care. When interacting with your loved one, focus on simplicity and clarity in your language. Use short, direct sentences that convey your message straightforwardly. Avoid complex or abstract language, as this can be confusing or overwhelming for someone with cognitive impairment.

Additionally, pay attention to your tone of voice and nonverbal cues. Speak in a calm, soothing, and reassuring manner, even if the content of your words is firm or directive. Your tone and demeanor can have a powerful impact on your loved one's emotional state, helping to de-escalate tension and promote a sense of safety and security.

Consistent Boundaries:

Establishing and maintaining clear boundaries is a crucial part of managing challenging behaviors in dementia care. Consistency in your approach helps create a predictable and structured environment, which can reduce the likelihood of triggers that may lead to agitation or confusion.

Clearly communicate your expectations and limits, using simple and direct language. For example, if your loved one becomes agitated when faced with too many choices, limit the options presented and guide them toward a specific decision. If certain behaviors, such as wandering or aggression, pose safety risks, calmly and firmly redirect your loved one to a safer activity or environment. By providing consistent boundaries and structure, you can help your loved one feel more secure and grounded, reducing the potential for challenging behaviors to escalate.

Understand the Triggers:

Gaining insight into the specific triggers that precipitate challenging behaviors can be a powerful tool in dementia care. Observe and document the circumstances, environments, or interactions that usually precede episodes of agitation or confusion.

Common triggers may include changes in routine, overstimulation, fatigue, pain or discomfort, or unmet needs such as hunger or thirst. By identifying these triggers, you can proactively adapt your approach to reduce their impact. For example, if you notice that your loved one becomes agitated in crowded or noisy environments, you can plan outings or activities during quieter times of the day or in more peaceful settings.

If unmet physical needs are a frequent trigger, you can establish a consistent routine for meals, hydration, and comfort measures. By understanding and addressing triggers preemptively, you can create a more supportive and conducive environment for your loved one's well-being.

Professional Allies:

When facing the challenges of dementia care, you need not navigate this path alone. Seeking the guidance and support of healthcare professionals experienced in dementia care can be an invaluable resource.

Please reach out to your loved one's primary care doctor, neurologist, or geriatric specialist for advice and assistance. These experts can provide personalized recommendations based on your loved one's specific needs, medical history, and stage of dementia. They may offer insights into medication management, behavioral interventions, or environmental changes that can help alleviate challenging behaviors. Additionally, consider enlisting the support of dementia care specialists, such as occupational therapists, speech therapists, or behavioral health professionals. These experts can assess your loved one's abilities and challenges, providing targeted strategies and techniques to enhance communication, engagement, and overall quality of life.

Lean on Your Network:

Surrounding yourself with a strong support network is important for maintaining your own well-being and resilience as a caregiver. Contact family members, friends, or neighbors who can offer practical assistance, emotional support, or simply a listening ear.

Sharing the responsibilities of caregiving, even in small ways, can help alleviate the burden and provide much-needed respite. Consider joining a caregiver support group, either in-person or online, where you can connect with others who understand the unique challenges of dementia care. These groups offer a safe space to share experiences, exchange ideas, and receive validation and encouragement from those who have walked a similar path.

Additionally, explore community resources such as adult day programs, respite care services, or in-home support, which can provide valuable breaks and assistance when needed.

Embrace Coping Mechanisms:

Developing and practicing effective coping mechanisms is essential for both you and your loved one in navigating the challenges of dementia care. Identify strategies that help promote relaxation, reduce stress, and enhance overall well-being. This may include mindfulness exercises, such as deep breathing, meditation, or yoga, which can help you stay grounded and present in the moment.

Establishing structured routines and engaging in meaningful activities, such as music therapy, art projects, or gentle exercise, can provide a sense of purpose and enjoyment for your loved one, while also helping to manage challenging behaviors. Additionally, finding healthy outlets for your own emotions, such as journaling, talking with a trusted friend or therapist, or engaging in hobbies or self-care activities, can help you maintain your resilience and emotional equilibrium.

Chapter Summary:

Tackling the challenges of dementia care, particularly when faced with agitation and difficult behaviors, requires a collaborative and multifaceted approach. By staying centered in moments of stress, using clear and compassionate communication, setting consistent boundaries, understanding triggers, seeking professional guidance, leaning on your support network, and embracing effective coping mechanisms, you can navigate this journey with greater skill, resilience, and grace.

Remember, you are not alone in this endeavor. By engaging with healthcare professionals, tapping into the strength of your personal relationships, and using the resources available within your community, you can create a powerful support system that helps you manage the day-to-day challenges of dementia care with confidence and compassion.

As you start this path, hold fast to the power of your love, the depth of your commitment, and the resilience of your spirit. Trust in your ability to adapt, to learn, and to find moments of joy and connection amidst the challenges. And always remember, by providing loving and skilled care to your loved one, you are making an immeasurable difference in their life and honoring the profound bond you share.

~

PROACTIVE PEACEKEEPING: AVERTING AGITATION IN DEMENTIA CARE

IN THE COMPLEX landscape of dementia care, proactive strategies emerge as powerful tools for reducing episodes of agitation and managing challenging behaviors. By expecting and addressing the underlying causes of these behaviors, caregivers can cultivate a more serene and supportive environment for both themselves and their loved ones. This proactive approach involves a combination of emotional attunement, clear communication, trigger identification, positive reinforcement, and strategic redirection.

By putting these strategies into practice consistently and with compassion, caregivers can navigate the complexities of dementia care while fostering a sense of calm, security, and well-being for their loved ones.

Cultivate Calmness:

As a caregiver, your emotional state can have a profound impact on the person you're caring for. Individuals with dementia are often highly attuned to the moods and energy of those around them, and they may mirror or react to the emotions they perceive.

So, it's important to approach each interaction and situation with a sense of tranquility and composure. When you feel your patience waning or your stress levels rising, take a moment to pause, regroup, and engage in deep, intentional breathing. By consciously regulating your own emotional state, you create a calming presence that can help diffuse potential agitation and promote a more peaceful environment.

Set Clear Boundaries:

Establishing and maintaining clear boundaries is an essential part of managing challenging behaviors in dementia care. Define what behaviors are acceptable and which ones are not and communicate these boundaries in a compassionate yet firm manner. Use simple, direct language and a calm tone of voice to convey your expectations and limits.

Consistency is key in reinforcing these boundaries, as it helps create a predictable and stable environment for your loved one. When challenging behaviors arise, gently remind your loved one of the established boundaries and redirect them to a more appropriate activity or response.

Detect and Deter Triggers:

Proactively identifying and addressing the triggers that precede challenging behaviors is a powerful strategy in dementia care. Keep a keen eye on the circumstances, environments, or interactions that usually precipitate episodes of agitation or distress.

Common triggers may include changes in routine, overstimulation, fatigue, pain or discomfort, or unmet needs such as hunger or thirst. By recognizing these triggers, you can try to either avoid them altogether or develop targeted coping strategies to mitigate their impact. For example, if you notice that your loved one becomes agitated in noisy or crowded settings, you can plan activities and outings during quieter times or in more peaceful environments.

Encourage Positive Actions:

Positive reinforcement is a powerful tool in shaping behavior and promoting a sense of well-being in dementia care. Make a conscious effort to notice and praise your loved one's positive actions, no matter how small they may seem.

This acknowledgment not only boosts their self-esteem but also encourages the continuation of such behaviors. When you catch your loved one engaging in a constructive activity, expressing kindness, or showing a moment of clarity, offer specific and heartfelt praise. This positive feedback helps create a nurturing and supportive environment that fosters a sense of accomplishment and purpose.

Provide Reassurance:

Individuals with dementia often experience fear, confusion, and anxiety, which can manifest as challenging behaviors. In these moments, offering reassurance and validation can be a powerful antidote to their distress. When your loved one expresses agitation or upset, respond with a comforting word, a gentle touch, or a listening ear.

Acknowledge their feelings and let them know that you understand and empathize with their experience. Use simple, calming language to convey a sense of safety and security. Reassure them you are there to support them and that everything will be okay. This emotional attunement and validation can help reduce their distress and promote a greater sense of connection and trust.

Distraction and Redirection:

When you sense that agitation or challenging behaviors are building, using techniques of distraction and redirection can be highly effective in defusing potential upsets. Gently steer your loved one's attention to a more soothing activity or topic, using their interests and preferences as a guide.

This could involve engaging them in a favorite hobby, looking through old photos, listening to calming music, or taking a short walk in nature. By skillfully redirecting their focus to a positive and engaging activity, you can help break the cycle of agitation and promote a more peaceful and enjoyable experience for both of you.

Professional Insight:

While proactive strategies can significantly reduce the frequency and intensity of challenging behaviors, sometimes, persistent or severe behaviors require expert intervention. Please reach out to healthcare professionals who specialize in dementia care, such as geriatric psychiatrists, neurologists, or dementia care consultants.

These experts can provide personalized guidance and strategies tailored to your loved one's specific needs, medical history, and stage of dementia. They may offer insights into medication management, behavioral interventions, environmental changes, or other targeted approaches to address complex behavioral challenges.

Chapter Summary:

Proactive peacekeeping is a powerful approach to averting agitation and managing challenging behaviors in dementia care. By cultivating a calm and compassionate presence, setting clear boundaries, identifying and addressing triggers, encouraging positive actions, providing reassurance, using distraction and redirection techniques, and seeking professional guidance when needed, caregivers can create a supportive and nurturing environment that promotes well-being and reduces distress.

Caring for someone with dementia requires patience, empathy, and a willingness to adapt and learn. It's a journey that demands both strength and tenderness, resilience and flexibility. By embracing proactive strategies and approaching each moment with compassion and understanding, you can navigate the complexities of dementia care while maintaining a sense of peace and connection with your loved one.

Remember, you are not alone in this journey. Reach out for support from family, friends, and professional resources when needed. Take care of yourself, both physically and emotionally, so you can bring your best self to the caregiving role. And always hold fast to the power of love, the strength of your commitment, and the knowledge that your presence and care make an immeasurable difference in your loved one's life.

~

FREQUENTLY ASKED QUESTIONS:

1. How can I calm my loved one when they become agitated or upset? First, try to identify any immediate causes of their agitation, such as physical discomfort or a change in their environment. Once any physical needs are addressed, use a calm and soothing tone, maintain eye contact, and offer reassurance. Distraction can be effective; gently redirect their focus to a favorite activity or memory. Remember, your presence and a calm demeanor can be comforting.

2. What should I do if my loved one shows challenging behaviors, like aggression? Safety is the top priority. Ensure there is no immediate physical risk to them or others. Try to identify triggers for the behavior and avoid or change these situations. Respond with patience, avoiding confrontation. Speak calmly, and give them space if needed. It's also helpful to consult with healthcare professionals for tailored strategies that can prevent or reduce these behaviors.

3. How can I effectively communicate with my loved one when they are confused or disoriented? Maintain a simple, clear way of speaking and use short, reassuring sentences. Avoid open-ended questions; instead, offer choices or use yes/no questions. Nonverbal communication, such as gentle touching (if appropriate) and maintaining eye contact, can also convey your message and support. Confirm their feelings to help them feel heard and understood, even if you need to redirect the conversation gently.

4. How do I handle my own feelings of frustration or sadness during these tough moments? Acknowledging your emotions is important. Give yourself permission to feel frustrated or sad; these are natural responses to a challenging situation. Take breaks when you need them, seek support from friends, family, or caregiver support groups, and consider professional counseling to manage these feelings. Practicing self-care and mindfulness can also help maintain your emotional balance.

5. What are some preventive strategies to avoid tough moments? A routine can provide a sense of stability and security for your loved one. Pay attention to their environment, removing stressors or sources of confusion when possible. Engage them in activities they enjoy, which can also serve as a distraction from potential triggers of challenging behaviors. Stay informed about their condition, as understanding the progression of dementia can help expect and mitigate difficult situations.

Navigating the journey of dementia care with your loved one involves understanding, patience, and a toolbox of strategies for those tough moments. Remember, it's okay to seek help, and taking care of yourself is as important as caring for your loved one.

~

CASE STUDY: THE JOURNEY OF CAROL AND HER FATHER, DAVID

CAROL, a 52-year-old high school teacher, became the primary caregiver for her father, David, an 80-year-old with advancing Alzheimer's disease. Their journey through the maze of dementia care was marked by moments of both profound challenge and unexpected grace. This case study explores how Carol navigated difficult moments with her father, using strategies that maintained his dignity and their bond.

Background: David was a retired engineer with a passion for classical music and woodworking. As his Alzheimer's progressed, he began exhibiting challenging behaviors, including agitation in the evenings and resistance to assistance with daily tasks. Carol struggled to manage these moments, feeling both frustrated and heartbroken over her father's distress.

Challenging Behaviors: One of the first significant challenges Carol faced was her father's sundowning syndrome, which led to increased confusion and agitation as the day progressed. David would become restless, pacing the house, and occasionally, became verbally aggressive. Additionally, he started resisting Carol's attempts to help him with personal care, insisting he could manage on his own, despite his declining ability to do so.

Adopting New Strategies: Carol realized she needed a new approach after a tough evening. She began researching and attending workshops on dementia care, where she learned valuable strategies for managing challenging behaviors.

Key Strategies and Lessons Learned:

- **Understanding the Causes:** Carol learned to see her father's behaviors as attempts to communicate his needs or discomfort. Recognizing that his agitation might stem from physical discomfort, confusion, or a disrupted routine helped her address the root causes rather than the symptoms.
- **Creating a Calm Environment:** Carol made changes to create a more soothing environment for David, especially in the evenings. She introduced a predictable routine, played soft classical music he loved, and ensured the house was well-lit to reduce shadows that could cause confusion.
- **Effective Communication:** Carol adopted a calm, reassuring tone when speaking to David. She learned to use simple, clear sentences and to give him time to process information and respond. Nonverbal communication, such as gentle touches and maintaining eye contact, became important in conveying her care and presence.
- **De-escalation Techniques:** Redirecting David's attention to familiar and comforting activities became Carol's go-to strategy for managing moments of agitation. She found that involving him in simple woodworking projects or looking through old photo albums together helped to calm him.
- **Patience, Empathy, and Compassion:** Carol discovered the power of patience and empathy in her role as a caregiver. Approaching each difficult moment with understanding and compassion made a significant difference in how David responded.

- **Seeking Professional Insight and Support:** Realizing she didn't have to do this alone, Carol contacted healthcare professionals for advice on managing challenging behaviors and connected with a support group of fellow caregivers, which became an invaluable source of comfort and practical tips.
- **Creating Safety and Security:** Ensuring David felt safe and secure became Carol's primary goal. She learned to communicate the limits of acceptable behavior gently but firmly, providing reassurance and reducing his anxiety.

Chapter Summary: Carol's journey with her father taught her that grace under pressure in dementia care comes from knowledge, understanding, and heart. By using strategies that addressed the causes of challenging behaviors, creating a calm environment, and communicating effectively, she managed difficult moments with dignity. The lessons Carol learned—about patience, empathy, the importance of seeking support, and the power of a calm and loving approach—transformed their caregiving journey into one of deeper connection and mutual respect.

~

PART EIGHT WRAP-UP:
ACTION ITEMS FOR THE CAREGIVER:

BASED ON CAROL'S journey with her father, David, here are actionable steps for caregivers navigating similar challenges with loved ones living with dementia:

1. **Seek to Understand the Root Causes of Challenging Behaviors**: Recognize that behaviors such as agitation or resistance may signal unmet needs or discomfort. Investigate potential physical, emotional, or environmental triggers.
2. **Establish a Predictable Routine**: Create a daily schedule that incorporates familiar and comforting activities to reduce confusion and provide a sense of security.
3. **Optimize the Environment for Calm**: Use soft lighting, reduce background noise, and play soothing music to create a peaceful setting, especially during known difficult times of the day, like evening hours.
4. **Communicate Clearly and Calmly**: Use simple, straightforward language. Speak slowly, maintain eye contact, and use gentle, reassuring tones to convey messages effectively.

5. **Employ Nonverbal Communication Techniques**: Utilize touch, gestures, and facial expressions to convey care and support, especially when verbal communication may not be effective.
6. **Master De-escalation Strategies**: Learn and apply techniques such as distraction, redirection to a favorite activity, or changing the environment to manage and soothe agitation.
7. **Practice Patience and Empathy**: Approach each situation with patience, trying to empathize with your loved one's experience, recognizing that their reality may differ from yours.
8. **Connect with Healthcare Professionals**: Don't hesitate to seek advice from doctors, nurses, or dementia care specialists for strategies tailored to your loved one's specific needs and behaviors.
9. **Join Support Groups**: Engage with caregiver support communities, both in-person and online, to share experiences, gain insights, and find emotional support.
10. **Educate Yourself on Dementia Care**: Go to workshops, read chapters, and gather information on dementia to better understand the condition and care techniques.
11. **Create a Safe and Secure Environment**: Implement safety measures at home to prevent falls, wandering, or other risks. Consider using specialized dementia care products as needed.
12. **Regularly Evaluate and Adapt Care Strategies**: As dementia progresses, needs and behaviors change. Continuously assess the effectiveness of your strategies and be willing to adjust your approach.
13. **Take Care of Your Own Well-being**: Recognize the importance of self-care. Ensure you're getting enough rest, eating well, and finding time for activities that rejuvenate you.
14. **Set Clear but Compassionate Boundaries**: Communicate the limits of acceptable behavior in a way that is firm but kind, ensuring your loved one understands expectations while feeling respected.

15. **Celebrate the Good Moments**: Focus on and cherish the positive interactions and moments of clarity, no matter how small, to foster joy and connection in your caregiving journey.

By following these action items, caregivers can navigate the complexities of dementia care with greater confidence and compassion, enhancing the quality of life for both themselves and their loved ones.

∾

IN OUR NEXT PART...

IN OUR NEXT PART, titled "Enhancing Dignity in Personal Care: A Guide for Caregivers," we'll dig into the delicate balance between providing necessary personal care and maintaining the dignity and autonomy of those in our care. This journey of caregiving is deeply personal and requires a blend of compassion, respect, and practical skill.

We'll explore strategies for establishing a comforting routine that not only addresses the physical needs of personal hygiene but also respects the emotional and psychological comfort of our loved ones. From setting a regular schedule that fosters predictability and security to engaging in open communication that involves them in their care plan, we aim to give you actionable steps to navigate these essential tasks with empathy and efficiency.

Flexibility and adaptability are key in responding to the daily needs and moods of those we care for, ensuring their comfort is always at the forefront. We'll discuss the importance of breaking down personal care activities into manageable steps, using visual supports for those with cognitive challenges, and encouraging participation in self-care to promote a sense of independence and self-worth.

Our goal is to empower you, the caregiver, with the knowledge and tools to approach personal care tasks with confidence, making sure each interaction upholds the dignity of your loved one and strengthens the bond between you. Join us as we navigate the complexities of personal care with sensitivity and a deep commitment to enhancing the well-being and dignity of those we serve.

～

PART NINE
ENHANCING DIGNITY IN PERSONAL CARE: A GUIDE FOR CAREGIVERS

Personal care and hygiene assistance are among the most intimate and sensitive parts of caregiving. These essential tasks require a delicate balance of compassion, respect, and efficiency to ensure the dignity and comfort of those receiving care.

Establishing a consistent routine, maintaining open communication, and promoting autonomy are key elements in creating a supportive and empowering care environment. This guide provides practical strategies for caregivers to navigate personal care activities with empathy, adaptability, and a focus on preserving the dignity of those they serve.

Set a Regular Schedule:

Creating a consistent and predictable routine is a cornerstone of effective personal care. By conducting hygiene and grooming activities at similar times each day, you establish a sense of familiarity and structure that can greatly help those in your care. This predictability can help ease anxiety, reduce confusion, and foster a sense of security, especially for individuals with cognitive impairments.

When developing a care schedule, consider their natural preferences and daily rhythms, such as their typical waking and sleeping times, meal schedules, and energy levels throughout the day. Consistency in routine not only promotes comfort but also helps maintain a sense of normalcy and control in their lives.

Keep Communication Open:

Open and respectful communication is essential in personal care. Involve the person you're caring for in discussions about their care plan, seeking their input and preferences. This dialogue not only respects their autonomy but also reinforces their importance in the decision-making process. Take the time to explain each task or activity, using clear and simple language, and ensure they understand what to expect. Listen actively to their concerns, questions, or hesitations, and address them with patience and empathy.

By maintaining open lines of communication, you create a collaborative and trusting care relationship that focuses on their dignity and well-being.

Embrace Flexibility:

While routines are important, it's equally important to embrace flexibility in personal care. Recognize that no two days are exactly the same, and be ready to adjust care plans in response to the individual's daily needs, moods, and preferences. Some days, they may require more support or time to complete tasks, while on other days, they may be more independent or eager to participate.

Be attuned to their verbal and nonverbal cues and adapt your approach. This flexibility shows respect for their autonomy and makes sure their comfort and well-being remain the top priority. By responding to their changing needs, you create a person-centered care environment that values their individuality and dignity.

Simplify Tasks:

Personal care activities, such as bathing, dressing, or grooming, can sometimes feel overwhelming or daunting, especially for those with physical or cognitive limitations. To promote a more manageable and less stressful experience, consider breaking down these tasks into smaller, more achievable steps. This approach can help prevent feelings of being overwhelmed and foster a sense of accomplishment and control.

For example, when helping to dress, focus on one piece of clothing at a time, providing clear and concise instructions for each step. Similarly, during bathing, guide them through the process step by step, offering assistance as needed while encouraging their participation to the extent possible. By simplifying tasks and providing gentle guidance, you create a supportive environment that promotes dignity and independence.

Visual Supports:

For individuals with cognitive challenges, such as dementia or memory loss, visual aids can be powerful tools in supporting personal care routines. Consider creating picture schedules or checklists that outline the steps involved in each task, such as the sequence of dressing or the steps in dental hygiene.

These visual supports serve as helpful reminders and cues, reducing confusion and anxiety while promoting a sense of structure and predictability. Use clear, simple images or photographs that are easily recognizable and place them in prominent locations, such as on the bathroom mirror or near the wardrobe. Visual aids not only help with memory recall but also foster a sense of independence and control, as individuals can refer to them for guidance and self-directed care.

Promote Self-Care:

Encouraging participation in personal care activities, to whatever extent possible, is a powerful way to promote dignity and autonomy. Even if an individual requires significant assistance, finding opportunities for them to engage in self-care can have a profound impact on their self-esteem and sense of purpose.

This may involve simple tasks such as choosing their own clothing, brushing their own hair, or applying lotion to their hands. By promoting self-care, you reinforce the message that their abilities and contributions are valued and respected. This empowerment can significantly boost self-worth, contribute to a positive self-image, and enhance overall well-being. Remember to provide praise and positive reinforcement for their efforts, celebrating the small victories and progress along the way.

Gentle Encouragement:

When memory issues or cognitive impairments are present, providing gentle reminders and encouragement can help maintain structure and routines without causing distress. Use a calm and reassuring tone when prompting individuals about personal care activities, offering clear and concise instructions.

Avoid rushing or pressuring them, as this can lead to anxiety or resistance. Instead, allow ample time for each task and be patient if they require multiple reminders or repetition. If they express frustration or confusion, respond with empathy and validation, acknowledging their feelings while gently redirecting them to the task at hand. By offering gentle encouragement and support, you create a nurturing care environment that focuses on their emotional well-being and dignity.

Offer Choices:

Providing choices, whenever possible, is a simple yet effective way to respect preferences and promote autonomy in personal care. This can involve offering options in clothing selection, letting them choose between two outfits or accessories. Similarly, regarding the order of tasks, allow them to decide whether they prefer to start with dental hygiene or hair brushing, for example.

By offering choices, you engage them in the care process, fostering a sense of control and self-determination. This approach also helps tailor care to their individual preferences, making sure their unique needs and desires are respected and met. Remember, even small choices can have a significant impact on their sense of dignity and overall satisfaction with their care experience.

· · ·

Chapter Summary:

Enhancing dignity in personal care requires a compassionate, respect-ful, and person-centered approach. By establishing regular schedules, maintaining open communication, embracing flexibility, simplifying tasks, using visual supports, promoting self-care, offering gentle encouragement, and providing choices, caregivers can create a care environment that focuses on the dignity and autonomy of those they serve.

Remember, personal care is not just about completing tasks; it's an opportunity to foster connection, trust, and empowerment. By approaching these intimate moments with empathy, patience, and a focus on individual needs and preferences, you can transform daily routines into opportunities for nurturing relationships and promoting overall well-being.

As caregivers, it's essential to also focus on self-care and seek support when needed. Caring for others can be emotionally and physically demanding, and it's important to maintain your own well-being to provide the best care. Contact family, friends, or professional resources for guidance, respite, and emotional support.

Ultimately, by putting these strategies into practice and leading with compassion, you can make a profound difference in the lives of those you care for, making sure their dignity is upheld and their quality of life is enhanced every step of the way.

∽

ENHANCING COMMUNICATION IN PERSONAL CARE

EFFECTIVE COMMUNICATION IS the foundation of providing compassionate, respectful, and dignified personal care and hygiene assistance. It goes beyond mere words and encompasses a holistic approach that considers the individual's unique needs, preferences, and comfort levels.

By fostering open dialogue, respecting personal boundaries, and empowering the individual's autonomy, caregivers can create a positive and supportive care environment. This guide explores key communication strategies that not only reinforce the individual's dignity but also promote their active participation and well-being throughout the personal care process.

Routine Reinforcement:

Establishing and maintaining a consistent routine is important in personal care communication. Engage the individual in planning their care schedule, considering their preferences and daily rhythms. This collaborative approach fosters a sense of involvement and control, letting them have a say in their care routine.

Consistently communicate the steps and timing of each care activity, providing gentle reminders and cues as needed. This predictability brings comfort and reduces anxiety, as the individual knows what to expect and can mentally prepare for each task. By reinforcing the routine through clear communication, you create a structured and supportive environment that enhances their overall well-being.

Empathy and Respect:

Approach every personal care activity with empathy and respect, recognizing the intimate nature of these tasks. Use a gentle, reassuring tone of voice and maintain a respectful demeanor throughout the process. Acknowledge that personal care can be uncomfortable or vulnerable for some individuals, and confirm their feelings.

Emphasize that their comfort and dignity are your top priorities, and that you are there to support them every step of the way. Respect their privacy by ensuring appropriate draping or covering during care tasks and avoiding unnecessary exposure. By communicating with empathy and respect, you build trust and create a safe space where the individual feels heard, valued, and cared for.

Understanding Nonverbal Signals:

Nonverbal communication plays a significant role in personal care. Pay close attention to the individual's body language, facial expressions, and gestures, as they can provide valuable insights into their comfort level and understanding. If you notice signs of discomfort, such as tensing up, flinching, or avoiding eye contact, pause and gently ask about their feelings.

Respect their personal boundaries and adjust your approach. For example, if they seem hesitant about a particular task, offer other options or break it down into smaller, more manageable steps. By being attuned to nonverbal cues, you can proactively address any concerns and ensure a more positive and comfortable care experience.

Empowering Choices:

Empowering the individual with choices is a powerful way to enhance their sense of autonomy and dignity in personal care. Offer options such as choosing between different toiletry products, selecting their preferred clothing, or deciding the order of care tasks. This gives them a voice in their care routine and reinforces their role as an active participant.

When presenting choices, use clear and concise language, and provide visual cues if helpful. Be patient and allow them time to process the options and decide. Respect their choices, even if they differ from your own preferences, as this confirms their autonomy and promotes a sense of control over their care.

Patience is Paramount:

Personal care tasks may take longer than expected, especially for individuals with physical limitations or cognitive impairments. Communicate your willingness to adapt to their pace and focus on their comfort throughout the process. Use a calm and unhurried tone, avoiding any signs of frustration or impatience.

If the individual becomes tired or agitated, offer breaks or suggest returning to the task later. Convey there is no rush and that you are there to support them for as long as needed. By exhibiting patience and understanding, you create a stress-free environment that lets the individual feel respected and valued.

Clarity in Communication:

When discussing personal care tasks, use clear, simple, and easy to understand language. Avoid medical jargon or complex terminology that may confuse or overwhelm the individual. Break down each task into step-by-step instructions, providing guidance and reassurance along the way.

Use visual aids, such as pictures or diagrams, to supplement verbal explanations if needed. Encourage questions and clarify any doubts or concerns. By communicating with clarity and simplicity, you make sure the individual understands the process and feels more at ease during personal care activities.

Open to Feedback:

Create an open and safe space for the individual to express their preferences, concerns, or any discomfort they may experience during personal care. Actively listen to their feedback and confirm their feelings. Ask open-ended questions to gain a deeper understanding of their needs and desires. For example, ask about their preferred water temperature during bathing or any specific products they enjoy using.

Encourage them to voice any pain, discomfort, or emotional distress they may be experiencing. By being receptive to feedback, you can tailor the care approach to their individual needs and ensure a more positive and comfortable experience.

Involving Loved Ones:

In some cases, involving family members or other trusted caregivers in personal care discussions can provide valuable insights and support. This is helpful when the individual has difficulty communicating their needs or preferences. Collaborate with loved ones to gather information about the individual's routines, habits, and any specific considerations.

Encourage open dialogue between all parties involved to ensure continuity of care and a shared understanding of the individual's needs. However, always focus on the individual's privacy and autonomy, and seek their consent before involving others in their personal care decisions.

Honoring Boundaries:

Respecting the individual's personal boundaries is essential in maintaining a dignified and comfortable care environment. Communicate openly about any discomfort or concerns they may have during personal care tasks. Ask for permission before touching or helping with intimate areas and explain each step of the process to ensure their understanding and consent.

If the individual expresses discomfort or wishes to stop a particular task, honor their request and explore alternative approaches or accommodations. By honoring their boundaries, you show respect for their autonomy and create a trusting and secure care relationship.

Positive Encouragement:

Provide positive encouragement and recognition for the individual's cooperation and efforts in participating in their personal care. Acknowledge their strengths and progress, no matter how small they may seem. Use phrases like "You're doing a great job" or "I appreciate your patience and cooperation."

This positive reinforcement can boost their self-esteem, promote a sense of accomplishment, and encourage their continued involvement in their care routine. Celebrate milestones and successes together, fostering a positive and supportive care environment.

Chapter Summary:

Enhancing communication in personal care is a multifaceted approach that focuses on the individual's dignity, comfort, and autonomy. By integrating strategies such as routine reinforcement, empathy and respect, understanding nonverbal signals, empowering choices, patience, clarity in communication, openness to feedback, involving loved ones, honoring boundaries, and providing positive encouragement, caregivers can create a supportive and respectful care environment.

Remember, effective communication goes beyond words and encompasses active listening, empathy, and a genuine desire to understand and meet the individual's unique needs. By fostering open dialogue, respecting personal boundaries, and empowering the individual's participation in their care, you not only enhance their sense of dignity but also promote their overall well-being and quality of life.

As a caregiver, it's essential to continually reflect on your communication approach and adapt it to the individual's evolving needs and preferences. Seek guidance and support from healthcare professionals, such as occupational therapists or social workers, who can provide more strategies and resources tailored to your specific care situation.

Ultimately, by focusing on effective communication in personal care, you build trust, foster a positive care relationship, and make sure the individual receives the compassionate, respectful, and dignified care they deserve.

~

UPHOLDING DIGNITY IN PERSONAL CARE: A CAREGIVER'S GUIDE

PERSONAL CARE and hygiene assistance are among the most intimate and sensitive parts of caregiving. As a caregiver, it is important to approach these tasks with the utmost respect, compassion, and sensitivity to uphold the dignity and privacy of the person in your care.

This guide provides essential strategies and principles to make sure personal care routines are conducted in a way that focuses on the individual's comfort, autonomy, and sense of self-worth. By incorporating these practices into your caregiving approach, you can create a supportive and respectful environment that enhances the overall well-being of the person you are caring for.

Transparent Communication:

Open and honest communication is the foundation of dignified personal care. Before beginning any care task, take the time to explain what you will do and why. Use clear, simple language and avoid medical jargon that may confuse or overwhelm the individual. Seek their consent and permission before moving forward, allowing them to ask questions or express any concerns.

This transparent approach respects their autonomy, helps them mentally prepare for the task, and establishes trust in the caregiving relationship. Remember to maintain an open dialogue throughout the care routine, checking in with the individual and responding to any discomfort or preferences they may express.

Ensure Privacy:

Maintaining privacy is paramount in upholding dignity during personal care tasks. Conduct care routines in a private space, such as a bathroom or bedroom, with the door closed or a privacy screen in place. This makes sure the individual's body is not exposed unnecessarily and reduces any potential embarrassment or vulnerability.

When helping to dress or undress, provide a robe or towel for coverage and only expose the necessary areas of the body for the specific task at hand. By focusing on privacy, you show respect for the individual's personal boundaries and create a comfortable and secure environment for care.

Empower with Choices:

Offering choices throughout the personal care routine is a powerful way to promote the individual's sense of control and dignity. While the overall care plan may be predetermined, there are often opportunities to provide options within each task. For example, you can ask the individual if they prefer a particular type of soap, shampoo, or lotion, or give them a choice between different clothing items.

These small decisions may seem insignificant, but they can have a profound impact on the individual's sense of independence and self-determination. By empowering them with choices, you acknowledge their preferences and involve them as active participants in their own care, enhancing their overall sense of dignity.

Be Mindful of Personal Space:

Respecting personal space is important in maintaining the individual's comfort and dignity during personal care tasks. Always be mindful of their physical boundaries and avoid any unnecessary or prolonged touch. Before making physical contact, explain what you are about to do and seek their permission. Use gentle, respectful touch and be attentive to any signs of discomfort or resistance.

If the individual expresses a preference for certain areas of their body to be avoided or handled specifically, honor their wishes. By being mindful of personal space, you show respect for their bodily autonomy and create a safe and trusting care environment.

Maintain Confidentiality:

Upholding the individual's privacy extends beyond the physical aspects of personal care. It is essential to treat any information related to their care with the utmost confidentiality. This includes details about their health status, personal preferences, and any sensitive or private matters discussed during care routines.

Only share necessary information with those directly involved in their care, such as healthcare professionals or immediate family members. Avoid discussing the individual's care in public spaces or with individuals who do not legitimately need to know. By maintaining confidentiality, you protect the individual's privacy, foster trust, and show respect for their personal information.

Adopt Respectful Language:

The language you use during personal care tasks can significantly affect the individual's sense of dignity and self-esteem. Always address the person by their preferred name or title, avoiding any diminutive or infantilizing terms. When discussing care tasks, use clear, respectful language that is free from judgment or embarrassment.

For example, instead of using childlike or demeaning terms for body parts or functions, use proper anatomical terms or neutral descriptors. Be mindful of your tone of voice, speaking in a calm, reassuring manner that conveys respect and professionalism. By adopting respectful language, you create a positive and dignified care environment that values the individual's worth and autonomy.

Foster Independence:

Promoting independence is a key aspect of upholding dignity in personal care. Encourage the individual to participate in their care routine to the best of their abilities, even if it means completing small tasks or making minor decisions. This could involve letting them wash their face, brush their hair, or choose their clothing for the day.

By fostering independence, you reinforce the individual's sense of control and self-efficacy, enhancing their self-esteem and overall well-being. Offer assistance as needed but avoid taking over tasks that the individual can do themselves. Celebrate their achievements and progress, no matter how small, and positively reinforce their efforts.

Offer Emotional Support:

Personal care routines can be emotionally challenging for both the individual receiving care and the caregiver providing it. It is important to recognize and confirm any feelings of vulnerability, embarrassment, or anxiety that may arise during these intimate tasks. Offer reassurance and empathy, letting the individual know that their feelings are normal and understandable.

Be ready to listen actively and respond to any concerns or emotional needs with compassion and understanding. Create a supportive and non-judgmental space where the individual feels comfortable expressing their thoughts and emotions. By offering emotional support, you show genuine care and respect for their well-being, fostering a sense of dignity and trust in the caregiving relationship.

Professional Demeanor:

Maintaining a professional demeanor is essential in upholding dignity during personal care tasks. This includes being punctual, prepared, and focused on the individual's needs throughout the care routine. Make sure you have all necessary supplies and equipment readily available to reduce disruptions or delays.

Dress appropriately in clean, professional attire that reflects your role as a caregiver. Maintain good hygiene practices, such as washing your hands before and after each care task, to promote cleanliness and reduce the risk of infection. By approaching personal care with professionalism and attention to detail, you show respect for the individual and their dignity, creating a safe and trustworthy care environment.

Stay Adaptable:

Recognizing that personal care needs and preferences may change over time is important in providing dignified care. Regularly assess the individual's abilities, comfort level, and emotional state, and be ready to adapt your care practices. Encourage open communication and actively seek feedback from the individual and their loved ones regarding their care experiences.

Be receptive to suggestions for improvement and willing to make changes to make sure their dignity and comfort remain the top priorities. By staying adaptable and responsive to the individual's evolving needs, you create a personalized and respectful care approach that upholds their sense of self-worth and autonomy.

Chapter Summary:

Upholding dignity in personal care is a fundamental responsibility of every caregiver. By integrating principles of transparent communication, privacy, choice, personal space, confidentiality, respectful language, independence, emotional support, professionalism, and adaptability into your caregiving approach, you create a care environment that focuses on the individual's comfort, autonomy, and sense of self-worth.

Remember, personal care routines are not just about completing tasks; they are opportunities to foster connection, trust, and respect between the caregiver and the individual receiving care. By approaching these intimate moments with sensitivity, compassion, and a commitment to dignity, you have the power to enhance the overall well-being and quality of life of the person in your care.

As a caregiver, it is also important to focus on your own self-care and seek support when needed. Providing personal care can be emotionally and physically demanding, and it is essential to maintain your own well-being to provide the best care. Contact colleagues, supervisors, or support groups for guidance, resources, and emotional support as needed.

By embracing the principles outlined in this guide and making dignity the cornerstone of your caregiving approach, you can make a profound difference in the lives of those you care for, making sure they receive the respect, compassion, and dignity they deserve.

~

OPTIMIZING PERSONAL HYGIENE CARE: A GUIDE FOR CAREGIVERS

PROVIDING effective personal hygiene care is a critical part of caregiving that directly affects the health, comfort, and dignity of the individuals you care for. As a caregiver, it is essential to approach personal care and hygiene assistance with sensitivity, respect, and a focus on meeting the unique needs and preferences of each person.

This guide offers practical strategies and considerations to help you optimize personal hygiene care, making sure the individuals under your care receive the highest quality of support and maintain a sense of autonomy and self-worth throughout the process.

Personalize Hygiene Care:

Understanding the individual's specific needs, preferences, and challenges is the foundation of providing personalized hygiene care. Take the time to learn about their daily routines, favorite products, and any sensitivities or allergies they may have.

Observe and ask about any mobility constraints or physical limitations that might affect their ability to engage in personal care tasks independently. By tailoring your approach to their unique circumstances, you show respect for their individuality and create a more comfortable and dignified care experience.

Select Suitable Products:

Choosing the right hygiene products is important for promoting skin health and overall comfort. Pay attention to the individual's skin type and preferences when selecting soaps, shampoos, lotions, and other personal care items.

Choose gentle, hypoallergenic, and fragrance-free products designed for sensitive skin to reduce the risk of irritation or allergic reactions. Consider the individual's specific needs, such as dry skin, eczema, or incontinence, and choose products that address these concerns. Involve the individual in the choosing process respecting their choices and preferences.

Incorporate Assistive Tools:

Assistive devices can greatly enhance the comfort, safety, and independence of individuals during personal care routines. Assess the individual's mobility and dexterity to determine which assistive tools may be most beneficial.

Shower chairs or benches provide stability and support for those with balance or strength issues, letting them sit comfortably while bathing. Handheld showerheads with adjustable settings offer flexibility and control, making it easier to direct water flow and regulate temperature. Long-handled sponges, brushes, and combs enable individuals with limited reach to maintain their personal hygiene more independently.

By incorporating these tools, you empower the individual to participate in their care and promote a sense of autonomy.

Modify the Environment:

Creating a safe and accessible personal care environment is essential for ideal hygiene care. Assess the bathroom and other personal care areas to identify any potential hazards or barriers. Install grab bars near the toilet, shower, and bathtub to provide more support and stability. Use non-slip bathmats or textured floor surfaces to prevent falls and increase traction. Make sure the bathroom is well-lit, with easily accessible light switches or motion-activated lighting.

Arrange personal care items within easy reach and consider using labeled containers or organizers for individuals with cognitive impairments. By changing the environment, you create a space conducive to safe and comfortable personal hygiene routines.

Promote Autonomy:

Encouraging the individual to participate in their personal care to the best of their abilities is a key aspect of promoting autonomy and dignity. Assess the individual's capabilities and provide help only where necessary, letting them handle tasks they can manage independently. This may include washing their face, brushing their teeth, or applying lotion to accessible areas of their body.

Offer verbal cues, visual prompts, or step-by-step instructions to guide them through the process, but avoid taking over unless necessary. Celebrate their efforts and achievements, providing positive reinforcement and encouragement throughout the care routine. By fostering independence, you enhance the individual's self-esteem and sense of control over their personal hygiene.

Approach with Sensitivity:

Personal hygiene care involves intimate and potentially vulnerable moments, and it is important to approach these tasks with the utmost sensitivity and respect. Always communicate clearly and calmly, explaining each step of the process before beginning.

Seek the individual's consent and permission before touching or helping with any personal care tasks. Use respectful language and avoid any comments or actions that could be perceived as demeaning or embarrassing. Protect the individual's privacy by ensuring proper draping or covering during care routines and closing doors or curtains when appropriate.

By approaching personal hygiene care with sensitivity and respect, you create a safe and trusting environment that upholds the individual's dignity.

Maintain Equipment:

Regular maintenance of hygiene products and assistive devices is essential for ensuring their effectiveness and preventing the spread of infections. Establish a routine for cleaning and disinfecting items such as shower chairs, handheld showerheads, and combs or brushes. Follow manufacturer guidelines for proper cleaning methods and frequencies. Inspect assistive devices regularly for any signs of wear, damage, or malfunction, and replace them as needed to maintain safety and functionality.

Keep an inventory of hygiene supplies and restock items promptly to avoid running out. By maintaining equipment and supplies, you promote ideal hygiene standards and show a commitment to the individual's well-being.

Seek Expert Advice:

When faced with complex or unfamiliar personal hygiene situations, please seek guidance from healthcare professionals. Consult with the individual's primary care doctor, nurses, or occupational therapists for recommendations on specific hygiene products, techniques, or assistive devices that may be most appropriate for their health status and personal needs.

These experts can provide valuable insights into managing skin conditions, addressing mobility challenges, or adapting care routines to accommodate cognitive or sensory impairments. By collaborating with healthcare professionals, you make sure the individual receives evidence-based, personalized hygiene care that promotes their overall health and well-being.

Chapter Summary:

Optimizing personal hygiene care is an important responsibility of caregivers, as it directly affects the health, comfort, and dignity of the individuals they serve. By personalizing care routines, selecting suitable products, incorporating assistive tools, changing the environment, promoting autonomy, approaching with sensitivity, maintaining equipment, and seeking expert advice, you can provide the highest quality of personal hygiene support.

Remember, personal hygiene care goes beyond completing tasks; it is an opportunity to build trust, foster connection, and show respect for the individual's autonomy and self-worth. By focusing on their preferences, involving them in decision-making, and celebrating their abilities, you create a positive and empowering care experience.

As a caregiver, it is also essential to focus on your own well-being and seek support when needed. Providing personal hygiene care can be physically and emotionally demanding, and it is important to practice self-care, maintain proper ergonomics, and seek guidance from colleagues or supervisors when faced with challenges.

By embracing the strategies outlined in this guide and making personal hygiene optimization a central focus of your caregiving approach, you can significantly enhance the quality of life and overall well-being of the individuals under your care. Your dedication, compassion, and commitment to providing dignified and personalized hygiene support will have a lasting positive impact on their lives.

$\sim$

BEST PRACTICES IN PERSONAL CARE: ENSURING SAFETY AND UPHOLDING DIGNITY

PROVIDING personal care and hygiene assistance is a crucial part of caregiving that requires a thoughtful and respectful approach. Whether you are caring for someone due to age, illness, or disability, adhering to best practices is essential to ensure their safety, comfort, and dignity.

This guide outlines key principles and strategies to help you deliver high-quality personal care that focuses on the well-being and autonomy of the individuals you serve. By incorporating these guidelines into your caregiving routine, you can foster a positive and supportive care environment that enhances the quality of life for those under your care.

Effective Communication:

Clear and compassionate communication is the foundation of providing safe and dignified personal care. Before beginning any care task, take the time to explain what you will do and why. Use simple, non-technical language and make sure the individual understands and consents to the care being provided.

Actively listen to their concerns, preferences, and feedback, and adjust your approach. Maintain a calm and reassuring tone throughout the care process, offering encouragement and support. By engaging in open and respectful communication, you create a sense of trust and collaboration, empowering the individual to be an active participant in their own care.

Privacy Protection:

Respecting the individual's privacy is paramount in personal care. Always make sure doors, curtains, or privacy screens are used to create a secure and private environment during care tasks. Reduce unnecessary exposure of the individual's body, using towels or blankets for covering when appropriate.

Avoid discussing personal care matters in public spaces or with individuals not directly involved in the care process. Be mindful of the individual's personal boundaries and preferences and honor their right to privacy and modesty. By focusing on privacy protection, you show respect for the individual's dignity and create a safe and comfortable care environment.

Correct Body Mechanics:

Using proper body mechanics is crucial for preventing injuries to both the caregiver and the individual receiving care. When helping with transfers, lifting, or repositioning, maintain a straight back and engage your leg muscles, avoiding twisting or bending at the waist.

Use assistive devices, such as transfer belts or mechanical lifts, when necessary to reduce strain and ensure safe movements. Encourage the individual to participate in transfers to the best of their ability, promoting their independence and reducing the risk of injury.

Regularly assess the care environment for potential hazards, such as slippery surfaces or obstacles, and address them promptly. By practicing correct body mechanics, you focus on the physical safety and well-being of both yourself and the individual under your care.

Rigorous Infection Control:

Maintaining high standards of hygiene and infection control is essential in personal care. Always wash your hands thoroughly with soap and water before and after providing care and use hand sanitizer when soap and water are not readily available. Wear disposable gloves when handling bodily fluids or contaminated materials and change gloves between different care tasks. Make sure all equipment, such as bedpans, commodes, or shower chairs, is well cleaned and disinfected after each use. Follow established protocols for disposing of soiled materials and linens to prevent the spread of infection.

By adhering to rigorous infection control practices, you protect the health and safety of both the individual receiving care and yourself.

Safe Bathing Practices:

Assisting with bathing requires careful attention to safety and comfort. Before beginning, check the water temperature to ensure it is not too hot or cold, adjusting as needed. Use non-slip mats or textured surfaces in the bathtub or shower to prevent falls and make sure grab bars or handrails are securely installed and easily accessible.

Encourage the individual to participate in the bathing process to the extent they are able, promoting their independence and sense of control. Offer gentle help with washing and rinsing, being mindful of any physical limitations or sensitivities.

Monitor the individual's comfort level throughout the bathing process and be ready to adjust the water temperature or provide more support as needed. By implementing safe bathing practices, you focus on the individual's well-being and create a positive and comfortable care experience.

Dignified Toileting Assistance:

Providing toileting assistance requires the utmost respect for privacy and dignity. Approach the task with sensitivity and discretion, using privacy screens or closing doors when possible. Encourage the individual to handle as much of the process independently as they can, offering assistance only when necessary. Use protective hygiene practices, such as wearing gloves and properly disposing of soiled materials.

If the individual requires the use of incontinence products, ensure they are properly fitted and changed regularly to prevent skin irritation and infections. Consider making environmental changes, such as installing raised toilet seats or grab bars, to enhance safety and ease of use. By handling toileting assistance with dignity and respect, you promote the individual's self-esteem and overall well-being.

Assistance with Dressing:

Helping with dressing is an opportunity to promote the individual's independence and personal style. Encourage them to make choices about what they want to wear, offering options and respecting their preferences.

Provide help as needed, such as helping with buttons, zippers, or shoes, while letting them handle tasks they can manage independently. Consider adaptive clothing options, such as garments with Velcro closures or elastic waistbands, to simplify the dressing process for those with mobility challenges.

Be patient and allow ample time for the individual to dress at their own pace, offering encouragement and positive reinforcement along the way. By supporting independence and choice in dressing, you foster a sense of autonomy and self-expression.

Accident Prevention:

Minimizing the risk of accidents and falls is a critical part of personal care. Regularly assess the individual's mobility and balance, and provide appropriate assistive devices, such as walkers or canes, as needed. Make sure pathways are well-lit and free from clutter or tripping hazards. Install grab bars or handrails in key areas, such as near the bed, toilet, or shower, to provide more support and stability.

Encourage the use of non-slip footwear or socks to reduce the risk of slips and falls. Be vigilant about tracking for any changes in the individual's gait, strength, or balance, and report concerns to healthcare professionals promptly. By implementing effective accident prevention strategies, you create a safer care environment and promote the individual's overall well-being.

Providing Emotional Support:

Personal care tasks can be emotionally sensitive and potentially overwhelming for individuals receiving care. Recognize the vulnerability and intimacy involved in these activities, and approach them with empathy and understanding.

Offer reassurance and emotional support throughout the care process, acknowledging any fears, concerns, or discomfort the individual may express. Use a calm and soothing tone of voice and positively reinforce their efforts and progress. Listen actively to their needs and preferences and respond to their emotional state. By offering emotional support and validation, you create a caring and compassionate environment that promotes the individual's psychological well-being.

Continuous Learning and Self-Care:

Providing high-quality personal care requires ongoing learning and skill development. Seek training opportunities to enhance your knowledge and techniques in areas such as safe lifting, infection control, and emergency first aid. Stay up to date with best practices and evidence-based approaches to personal care, and be open to feedback and guidance from healthcare professionals and experienced caregivers.

Additionally, focus on your own self-care and well-being as a caregiver. Engage in stress-reduction activities, maintain a healthy work-life balance, and seek support from colleagues, supervisors, or caregiver support groups when needed. By investing in your own growth and well-being, you can provide the best care to those you serve.

Chapter Summary:

Providing personal care with a focus on safety and dignity is a fundamental responsibility of caregivers. By adhering to best practices, including effective communication, privacy protection, correct body mechanics, infection control, safe bathing, dignified toileting, assistance with dressing, accident prevention, emotional support, and continuous learning and self-care, you can make sure the individuals under your care receive the highest quality of support.

Remember, personal care is more than just a set of tasks; it is an opportunity to build trust, foster connection, and enhance the overall well-being of those you serve. By approaching each interaction with respect, compassion, and a commitment to upholding dignity, you can make a profound difference in the lives of the individuals you care for.

As a caregiver, it is also essential to focus on your own well-being and seek support when needed. Providing personal care can be physically and emotionally demanding, and it is important to maintain a healthy balance and engage in self-care practices to prevent burnout and maintain your ability to provide high-quality care.

By embracing the principles and strategies outlined in this guide, you can create a care environment that focuses on safety, respects individuality, and promotes the dignity and autonomy of those you serve. Your dedication and commitment to providing exceptional personal care will have a lasting positive impact on the lives of the individuals under your care and their families.

CARING WITH SENSITIVITY: A GUIDE TO PERSONAL CARE ASSISTANCE

PROVIDING personal care assistance is a profound responsibility that goes beyond the mere execution of physical tasks. It involves building a relationship rooted in trust, respect, and understanding, particularly when caring for individuals with dementia or other cognitive impairments. This guide aims to help caregivers navigate the sensitive parts of personal care with kindness, professionalism, and a deep commitment to preserving the dignity and well-being of those they serve. By embracing these principles and strategies, you can create a caring environment that nurtures both the physical and emotional needs of the individuals under your care.

Establish Trust and Respect:

The cornerstone of effective personal care is a strong, trusting relationship between the caregiver and the individual receiving care. Take the time to get to know the person you are caring for, engaging in open and honest communication about their preferences, fears, and concerns. Listen attentively to their stories, experiences, and opinions, showing genuine interest and respect for their individuality.

Consistently focus on their dignity and autonomy in every interaction, involving them in decision-making processes and honoring their choices. By cultivating a relationship built on trust and respect, you create a safe and supportive environment that fosters cooperation and enhances the overall care experience.

Maintain Privacy:

Respecting the privacy of the individual receiving care is essential to preserving their sense of dignity and security. When performing personal care tasks, such as bathing, dressing, or toileting, make sure doors are closed and privacy screens or curtains are used to create a protected space. Avoid unnecessary exposure of the individual's body, using towels or blankets for covering when appropriate.

Be mindful of the individual's comfort level and modesty preferences, and adjust your approach. Knock before entering their personal space and announce your presence to avoid startling them. By focusing on privacy, you show respect for the individual's personal boundaries and create an atmosphere of trust and safety.

Sensitivity to Cultural Differences:

Personal care practices can be deeply influenced by an individual's cultural background, values, and beliefs. As a caregiver, it is important to be aware of and sensitive to these cultural differences. Take the time to learn about the individual's cultural heritage, asking respectful questions and seeking guidance from family members or cultural liaisons when necessary.

Understand and respect any specific cultural norms, rituals, or taboos related to personal care, such as preferences for same-gender caregivers or the use of certain products or techniques. Adapt your approach to align with their cultural expectations, showing a commitment to providing culturally competent care. By honoring cultural diversity, you create a more inclusive and respectful care environment.

Communicate Clearly:

Clear and effective communication is important when discussing personal care needs and activities. Use plain, straightforward language to explain each step of the care process, avoiding medical jargon or euphemisms that may cause confusion or discomfort. Be patient and allow ample time for the individual to process the information and ask questions.

Encourage open dialogue about their concerns, fears, or preferences, and actively listen to their responses. Use nonverbal cues, such as gentle touch or eye contact, to convey empathy and support. If the individual has cognitive impairments, use simple, concise language and visual aids to help with understanding. By communicating clearly and openly, you foster a sense of trust and collaboration, empowering the individual to be an active participant in their own care.

Empathy and Compassion:

Providing personal care assistance requires a deep well of empathy and compassion. Recognize that the individual receiving care may be experiencing a range of emotions, including fear, vulnerability, frustration, or embarrassment. Put yourself in their shoes and approach each interaction with a gentle, understanding demeanor.

Offer reassurance and support throughout the care process, acknowledging their feelings and confirming their experiences. Use a calm, soothing tone of voice and positively reinforce their efforts and progress. Be patient and flexible, adapting to their changing needs and moods with grace and understanding. By extending empathy and compassion, you create a caring and supportive environment that promotes emotional well-being and resilience.

Incontinence Management:

Managing incontinence is a sensitive and often challenging part of personal care. Approach this task with the utmost discretion and respect for the individual's dignity. Use incontinence products, such as absorbent pads or adult briefs, that are properly fitted and changed regularly to prevent skin irritation and infections.

Establish a regular toileting schedule and help with prompt cleansing and changing to reduce discomfort and preserve skin integrity. Handle soiled materials discreetly and dispose of them properly to have a hygienic environment. Offer reassurance and emotional support throughout the process, acknowledging the potential embarrassment or distress the individual may experience. By handling incontinence management with sensitivity and professionalism, you help the individual maintain their self-esteem and quality of life.

Body Odor Management:

Maintaining personal hygiene and managing body odor is important for both physical health and emotional well-being. Encourage regular bathing, showering, or sponge baths, using gentle, fragrance-free cleansers suitable for the individual's skin type. Help with thorough cleansing of areas prone to odor, such as armpits, groin, and feet, while respecting the individual's privacy and comfort level.

Make sure the individual has access to fresh, clean clothing and undergarments, changing them regularly to prevent odor buildup. Use deodorants or antiperspirants considering any skin sensitivities or allergies. Maintain good oral hygiene, helping with brushing teeth, flossing, and using mouthwash as needed. By promoting regular hygiene habits and addressing body odor concerns with sensitivity, you help the individual maintain their self-esteem and social confidence.

Skin Conditions:

Caring for individuals with skin conditions requires special attention and gentle handling. Familiarize yourself with the specific skin condition and any prescribed treatment plans, following them closely to prevent complications or exacerbations. Apply creams, ointments, or medications as directed, using clean techniques to avoid contamination. Be mindful of the individual's comfort level and pain tolerance, adjusting your touch and pressure.

Monitor the skin regularly for signs of redness, irritation, or infection, reporting any concerns to healthcare professionals promptly. Use dressings or bandages as needed, changing them regularly to maintain a clean and protected environment. By providing attentive and gentle care for skin conditions, you promote healing, prevent further damage, and enhance the individual's overall comfort and well-being.

Seek Professional Guidance:

Providing personal care assistance can be complex and emotionally demanding, and sometimes, you feel overwhelmed or unsure of how to move forward. In these moments, it is essential to seek guidance and support from healthcare professionals, such as nurses, doctors, or occupational therapists. They can offer expert advice on managing specific care needs, addressing challenging behaviors, or adapting care techniques to the individual's unique circumstances.

Please reach out for help when needed, recognizing that collaboration with healthcare professionals is an important part of providing high-quality care. By seeking professional guidance, you expand your knowledge, skills, and confidence as a caregiver, ultimately benefiting the individual under your care.

Self-Care for Caregivers:

Caring for others can be physically and emotionally taxing, and caregivers must prioritize their own well-being. Engage in regular self-care practices, such as exercise, meditation, hobbies, or spending time with loved ones, to manage stress and maintain a healthy work-life balance. Seek support from family, friends, or caregiver support groups, sharing your experiences and challenges in a safe and understanding environment. Set realistic boundaries and learn to say no when necessary, recognizing that you cannot pour from an empty cup.

Take regular breaks throughout the day to rest and recharge and consider respite care options to allow for longer periods of self-care. By attending to your own physical, emotional, and mental health needs, you can provide more compassionate, patient, and effective care to those you serve.

Chapter Summary:

Providing personal care assistance with sensitivity and respect is a profound act of compassion with the power to transform lives. By establishing trust and respect, maintaining privacy, being sensitive to cultural differences, communicating, extending empathy and compassion, managing incontinence and body odor, caring for skin conditions, seeking professional guidance, and focusing on self-care, you create a nurturing and dignified care environment.

Remember, personal care is not just about completing tasks; it is about honoring the humanity and individuality of the person you are caring for. By approaching each interaction with kindness, patience, and understanding, you have the opportunity to make a meaningful difference in their lives, promoting their physical comfort, emotional well-being, and overall quality of life.

As a caregiver, your role is both challenging and rewarding, and it is essential to recognize the value and importance of your work. By embracing the principles and strategies outlined in this guide, you can navigate the sensitive parts of personal care with confidence, compassion, and a deep commitment to upholding the dignity of those you serve. Your dedication and empathy will have a profound impact on the lives of the individuals under your care, creating a positive and supportive environment that nurtures their physical, emotional, and social well-being.

Your role as a caregiver extends far beyond completing daily tasks; you are a source of comfort, security, and companionship for those you serve. Through your attentive and compassionate care, you help individuals maintain their sense of self-worth, autonomy, and connection to the world around them. Your patience, understanding, and unwavering commitment to their dignity serve as a beacon of hope and reassurance, even in the face of complex challenges.

As you start this journey of caregiving, remember to extend the same kindness and compassion to yourself. Recognize that your work is valuable and that your efforts make a significant difference in the lives of others. Seek support when needed, focus on your own self-care, and celebrate the small victories and moments of connection that make your role so rewarding.

By embracing the principles of sensitive and respectful personal care, you not only enhance the quality of life for those you serve but also contribute to a more compassionate and inclusive society. Your dedication to upholding the dignity and well-being of others is a testament to the power of empathy and the transformative potential of person-centered care.

~

NAVIGATING SENSITIVE PERSONAL CARE TOPICS: A COMPASSIONATE APPROACH

When you're providing personal care for someone, whether due to age, disability, or illness, there may be sensitive topics that come up. These can be related to hygiene, bodily functions, or cultural differences. As a caregiver, it's important to approach these subjects with understanding, respect, and a gentle touch.

Here's how you can navigate these delicate areas while maintaining the dignity of the person you're caring for:

Build Trust and Respect: The first step is to establish a strong bond of trust with the person you're caring for. Take the time to have open and honest conversations with them. Really listen to their concerns and preferences. Make sure that every interaction you have is based on mutual respect. This will create a solid foundation for addressing sensitive topics.

Uphold Privacy: Privacy is essential regarding personal care. Always make sure to close doors, use curtains, or provide coverings when needed. This helps protect the individual's dignity and makes them feel more secure. If you're in a shared living space, try to create a designated area for personal care activities that offers some privacy.

Cultural Sensitivity: It's important to remember that cultural backgrounds can influence personal care preferences. What may seem normal to you might not be comfortable for someone from a different culture. Take the time to learn about the individual's cultural needs and beliefs. Discuss their preferences and adjust your care practices. This shows respect for their heritage and helps build trust.

Clear Communication: When you need to discuss personal care topics, use language easy to understand. Avoid medical jargon or euphemisms that could cause confusion. Explain each step of the care process clearly, and encourage the person to ask questions. If they express any discomfort or concerns, listen carefully and address them with patience and understanding.

Empathetic Approach: Sensitive personal care issues can be emotionally challenging for the person you're caring for. They may feel embarrassed, anxious, or even ashamed. Approach these topics with empathy and compassion. Acknowledge their feelings and provide reassurance and support. Let them know that you're there to help them through this and that nothing is to be embarrassed about.

Dignified Incontinence Care: Incontinence can be a sensitive issue. When providing care, always focus on the individual's privacy and dignity. Use products and practices that are discreet and reduce any embarrassment. Be gentle and patient when helping to cleanse and change. Avoid any language or actions that could make the person feel ashamed or undignified.

Tactful Body Odor Management: Body odor can be another delicate topic. If you need to address this, do so with kindness and tact. Avoid any language that could cause embarrassment or shame. Instead, focus on encouraging regular hygiene practices, like bathing and changing clothes. Make sure the person has easy access to clean clothing, towels, and toiletries. If there are any underlying medical issues causing the odor, discuss this with a healthcare professional.

Gentle Skin Care: If the person you're caring for has any skin conditions, it's important to handle their skin with extra care. Follow any treatment plans from their healthcare team. When applying creams, ointments, or other products, do so gently to avoid causing any discomfort. Keep an eye out for any signs of skin irritation, infection, or distress, and report these to a medical professional if needed.

Professional Support: There may be times when you encounter a care situation that feels beyond your expertise. In these cases, don't hesitate to seek guidance from medical professionals, such as nurses or doctors. They can provide valuable advice and support on how to handle complex care needs. Remember, you need not figure everything out on your own.

Caregiver Self-Care: Providing care for others can be emotionally and physically demanding. It's important not to neglect your own well-being in the process. Prioritize self-care activities, like exercise, relaxation, and hobbies. Seek support from other caregivers or professionals when you need it. Take breaks when necessary to recharge your batteries. Remember, you can't pour from an empty cup.

By approaching sensitive personal care topics with compassion, respect, and a gentle touch, you can create a positive and dignified care experience. Always keep the individual's preferences and emotional needs at the forefront. With patience, understanding, and a commitment to their well-being, you can navigate even the most delicate situations with grace.

$\sim$

FREQUENTLY ASKED QUESTIONS:

1. How can I maintain my loved one's dignity while helping with personal hygiene? Dignity starts with respecting their privacy and preferences. Use a gentle, reassuring approach and involve them in the process letting them do what they can independently. For tasks that require more intimate assistance, ensure privacy by closing doors or using a screen, and explain what you are doing step by step to keep them informed. Always choose times that are best for them, respecting their routine and comfort levels.

2. What's the best way to approach sensitive topics, like incontinence? Approach sensitive topics with empathy and directness. Frame the conversation around their comfort and well-being, avoiding any language that might cause embarrassment. For example, when discussing incontinence, you might say, "I've noticed this might be uncomfortable for you. Let's find a way to make things easier and more comfortable." Offering solutions and involving them in decision-making can help maintain their sense of control and dignity.

3. My loved one is resistant to receiving help with bathing. How can I encourage them without causing distress? Resistance is often rooted in a loss of independence or embarrassment. Start by acknowledging their feelings and reassure them of their right to feel comfortable and respected. Offer choices where possible, such as the time of day for bathing or the type of bath they prefer. Emphasize the positive aspects, like how refreshed they will feel afterward. Showing patience and understanding can gradually reduce resistance.

4. How can I make the personal care process easier for both of us? Simplifying the personal care routine can make the process more manageable. Break down tasks into smaller, more achievable steps and communicate clearly what each step involves. Use adaptive equipment and clothing to reduce physical strain and maintain their independence. Establishing a predictable routine can also help them feel more secure and cooperative.

5. What should I do if I'm feeling overwhelmed by my caregiving responsibilities, especially concerning personal care? Feeling overwhelmed is natural. It's important to recognize when you need a break and to seek support. Contact family members, friends, or professional caregivers for help. Consider joining a caregiver support group to share experiences and strategies. Taking care of your own well-being is important to providing compassionate care. Consult healthcare professionals for advice on managing specific challenges you face.

Providing personal care with dignity is about respecting the individual's preferences, involving them in their care, and maintaining open, empathetic communication. By using these strategies, you can make sure personal care strengthens the trust and bond between you and your loved one.

∼

CASE STUDY: MARIA AND HER MOTHER, ROSA

MARIA, a 45-year-old bank manager, found herself in the role of a primary caregiver for her 76-year-old mother, Rosa, who was diagnosed with moderate Alzheimer's disease. One of the most challenging parts of her caregiving journey involved managing personal care tasks while ensuring her mother's dignity was maintained. This case study explores Maria's approach to navigating the sensitive parts of personal care and the lessons learned along the way.

Background: Rosa was a fiercely independent woman who had always taken pride in her appearance. As her Alzheimer's progressed, she began to struggle with basic personal care tasks, such as bathing, dressing, and grooming. Maria noticed her mother's increasing frustration and embarrassment, which often led to Rosa refusing help.

Approaching Personal Care with Dignity: Maria realized early on that maintaining her mother's dignity was paramount. She dedicated herself to learning how best to provide care while respecting Rosa's autonomy.

Strategies Implemented:

- **Establishing a Routine:** Maria set a regular schedule for personal care tasks, creating a sense of predictability and security for Rosa. This routine helped reduce Rosa's anxiety around personal care activities.
- **Open Communication:** Maria involved her mother in discussions about her care plan. She presented options and let Rosa make choices, whether it was about what outfit to wear or which shampoo to use.
- **Flexibility and Adaptability:** Understanding that some days were better than others, Maria remained flexible, adjusting the care plan according to her mother's mood and needs on any given day.
- **Simplifying Tasks:** Breaking down personal care activities into smaller, manageable steps helped Rosa participate in her own care, promoting her independence.
- **Visual Supports:** For tasks that Rosa found challenging, Maria used visual aids like picture schedules, which served as gentle reminders and support.
- **Encouraging Self-Care:** Maria gently encouraged her mother to do as much as she could on her own, providing help only when necessary. This approach boosted Rosa's self-esteem and contributed to a positive self-image.
- **Gentle Encouragement:** Maria found that offering kind reminders and encouragement helped maintain a daily routine without causing distress.

Lessons Learned by Maria:

- **Patience is Key:** Maria learned that patience was important in navigating personal care tasks. Rushing only increased Rosa's anxiety and resistance.
- **Communication Matters:** Effectively communicating in a clear, respectful manner was essential in making Rosa feel involved and respected in her care.
- **The Importance of Choices:** Allowing Rosa to make choices empowered her, giving her a sense of control over her life.

- **The Value of Flexibility:** Being adaptable to Rosa's needs and moods on any given day made sure personal care tasks were completed with minimal stress.
- **Empathy and Understanding:** Approaching care tasks with empathy and an effort to understand Rosa's perspective made a significant difference in their effectiveness and the overall caregiving experience.

Chapter Summary: Maria's journey with her mother taught her the delicate balance between providing necessary care and maintaining dignity. By implementing a structured yet flexible approach, communicating openly, and empowering Rosa through choices, Maria navigated personal care tasks with compassion and respect. This case study underscores the importance of dignity in caregiving and offers valuable insights for caregivers facing similar challenges.

~

PART NINE WRAP-UP:
ACTION ITEMS FOR THE CAREGIVER:

BASED ON MARIA'S experience in providing dignified personal care for her mother, Rosa, here are action items for caregivers to enhance the personal care experience while maintaining the dignity of their loved ones:

1. **Establish a Consistent Routine**: Create a predictable daily schedule for personal care tasks to help reduce anxiety and create a sense of security.
2. **Involve Your Loved One in Care Planning**: Engage them in conversations about their care preferences and decisions to respect their autonomy and make them feel valued.
3. **Be Flexible and Adaptable**: Recognize that their needs and moods may vary day by day. Be ready to adjust the care plan to ensure comfort.
4. **Break Down Tasks into Manageable Steps**: Simplify personal care activities to prevent feelings of overwhelm and promote a more manageable experience for both of you.
5. **Use Visual Aids**: For individuals with cognitive challenges, visual supports like checklists or picture schedules can be helpful reminders and support independence.

6. **Encourage Participation in Self-Care**: Motivate them to participate in their own care to the extent possible, which can significantly boost their self-worth and contribute to a positive self-image.

7. **Offer Gentle Encouragement and Reminders**: Use kind and encouraging words to guide them through their daily routines, reducing stress and confusion.

8. **Provide Choices**: Give options in personal care decisions, such as clothing or toiletry preferences, to respect personal tastes and engage them in the care process.

9. **Communicate Clearly and Calmly**: Use simple, reassuring language and maintain a calm demeanor to ease communication and reduce potential tension.

10. **Maintain Privacy**: Ensure privacy during personal care tasks using curtains or doors, reinforcing their dignity and comfort.

11. **Exercise Patience**: Recognize the importance of patience in helping with a positive care experience, allowing extra time for tasks without rushing.

12. **Seek Professional Advice When Needed**: Consult healthcare professionals for more strategies or support in managing personal care challenges effectively.

13. **Join Support Groups**: Connect with caregiver support communities for shared experiences, emotional support, and practical tips.

14. **Focus on Your Own Well-being**: Acknowledge the importance of self-care to maintain your ability to provide compassionate and effective care.

15. **Reflect on Each Day**: Take time to consider what worked well and what could be improved in your caregiving approach, adapting your strategies as necessary.

By following these action items, caregivers can provide personal care with respect, dignity, and compassion, enhancing the well-being and comfort of their loved ones.

∾

IN OUR NEXT PART...

IN OUR NEXT PART, we dig into the heart of creating enriching and
nurturing experiences through nutrition and meal planning for individuals living with dementia. This journey is not just about ensuring a
balanced diet; it's a pathway to enhancing the overall well-being and
happiness of your loved one. We'll explore practical strategies to navigate dietary challenges, turning mealtime into a positive, engaging,
and comforting experience for everyone involved. From understanding the importance of nutrient-rich foods to adapting meals to
meet changing needs and preferences, we'll give you a comprehensive
guide to make nutrition a cornerstone of dementia care. This Part is
designed to empower you with knowledge and tools to enrich your
caregiving journey, emphasizing the profound impact of thoughtful
meal planning on the health and enjoyment of individuals with
dementia.

We'll look closely at the significance of maintaining social connections
and engaging in meaningful activities. Dementia can often lead to feelings of isolation and disconnection, but we'll show you how to weave a
tapestry of social interactions that support and uplift your loved one.
From fostering family connections to leveraging technology for

enhanced interaction, we'll offer insights into creating a supportive and stimulating environment.

This Part aims to inspire you to embrace the power of social engagement and activity participation, showing how they can transform the day-to-day lives of individuals with dementia. Join us as we navigate these essential parts of dementia care, aiming to bring joy, comfort, and a sense of belonging to your loved one's life.

~

PART TEN
NUTRITION AND MEAL PLANNING FOR INDIVIDUALS WITH DEMENTIA

NOURISHING THE MIND AND BODY: A GUIDE TO NUTRITION AND MEAL PLANNING IN DEMENTIA CARE

WHEN CARING for someone with dementia, ensuring they get proper nutrition is an important part of supporting their overall well-being. What we eat not only affects our physical health but also our cognitive function and quality of life.

As dementia progresses, mealtime can become more challenging, but with some thoughtful planning and preparation, you can make sure your loved one is getting the nutrients they need while still enjoying their food. Here are strategies to help you navigate nutrition and meal planning in dementia care:

Focus on Nutrient-Rich Foods: When planning meals, aim to include a variety of fruits, vegetables, whole grains, lean proteins, and healthy fats. These nutrient-dense foods provide the essential vitamins, minerals, and other compounds that support brain health and overall well-being. For example, leafy greens, berries, fatty fish, and nuts are all great options to incorporate into the diet.

Diversify the Menu: Offering a range of different foods can help make sure your loved one is getting a comprehensive mix of nutrients. It can also make mealtimes more interesting and enjoyable. Try experimenting with different colors, textures, and flavors to keep things engaging. You might try a colorful salad, a comforting soup, or a fragrant curry. Variety is key to a well-rounded diet.

Adapt for Ease of Eating: As dementia progresses, some individuals may have difficulty chewing or swallowing. In these cases, it's important to adapt the food consistency to make eating easier and safer. Soft, well-cooked foods cut into small pieces or pureed can be much more manageable. Things like scrambled eggs, smoothies, or soft-cooked vegetables can be good options. Always be mindful of the individual's abilities and adjust.

Stay Hydrated: Dehydration can be a common issue for people with dementia, so make sure they're getting enough fluids. Offer water, herbal teas, and other non-caffeinated beverages throughout the day. You can also boost hydration through foods with high water content, like watermelon, cucumber, or soups. Aim for a minimum of 6-8 glasses of fluid per day, or more if recommended by a healthcare professional.

Reduce Processed Foods: While they may be convenient, processed and sugary foods often lack nutritional value and can contribute to health issues. Try to limit these foods and instead focus on whole, unprocessed options. Fresh fruits, vegetables, whole grains, and lean proteins are all good choices. When you use packaged foods, look for those with simple, recognizable ingredients.

Supplement Wisely: In some cases, dietary supplements may be necessary to address specific nutritional deficiencies. However, consult with a healthcare professional before adding any supplements to the diet. They can assess the individual's needs and recommend supplements that are safe and beneficial. Remember, supplements should be used to complement a healthy diet, not replace it.

Foster a Relaxing Mealtime Atmosphere: The dining environment can have a big impact on the enjoyment of meals. Try to create a calm, relaxing atmosphere free from distractions like loud noises or television. Soft, soothing background music can be a nice touch. Keep the table setting simple and uncluttered to reduce confusion. A peaceful environment can help your loved one focus on their meal and enjoy the experience.

Engage in Mealtime Activities Involve your loved one in meal planning and preparation. This could be something as simple as having them choose between two dinner options or stirring a bowl of ingredients. These activities can provide a sense of autonomy and routine, which can be comforting for individuals with dementia. It's also a nice way to spend quality time together.

Professional Nutrition Advice: For personalized dietary guidance, especially if your loved one has specific health issues or dietary restrictions, consider consulting with a registered dietitian with experience in dementia care. They can provide expert advice on meal planning, dietary changes, and strategies to ensure ideal nutrition. They can also monitor your loved one's nutritional status over time and make changes as needed.

Putting these nutrition and meal planning strategies into practice can have a profound effect on the well-being of individuals with dementia. By providing the nutrients they need in an enjoyable, stress-free way, you can support their physical health, cognitive function, and overall quality of life. Mealtimes can become a source of comfort and connection, rather than a challenge. With a thoughtful, compassionate approach to nutrition, you can nourish both the mind and body of your loved one living with dementia.

～

CRAFTING NUTRITIOUS AND APPEALING MEAL PLANS FOR DEMENTIA CARE

WHEN CARING for someone with dementia, mealtimes are about more than just providing sustenance. It's an opportunity to create a positive, engaging experience that nourishes both the body and the soul. By focusing on nutrient-dense foods, adapting to individual needs, and fostering a pleasant dining environment, you can make sure the meals you prepare are both healthy and enjoyable.

Here are strategies to help you craft nutritious and appealing meal plans for your loved one with dementia:

Focus on Nutrient-Dense Choices: Every meal is an opportunity to provide essential nutrients that support overall health and cognitive function. When planning meals, focus on colorful fruits and vegetables, whole grains, lean proteins, and healthy fats. These nutrient-dense foods are packed with vitamins, minerals, antioxidants, and other beneficial compounds that can help protect brain health and promote overall well-being.

Adapt to Smaller Appetites: As dementia progresses, some individuals may experience a decrease in appetite. Large meals may feel overwhelming, leading to reduced food intake. To counteract this, try offering smaller, more frequent meals throughout the day. This approach can help maintain energy levels and make sure nutritional needs are met without overwhelming the individual. Aim for five to six small meals or snacks, rather than three large ones.

Stay Hydrated: Proper hydration is important for overall health, but it can be a challenge for individuals with dementia. Encourage your loved one to drink water and other hydrating fluids regularly throughout the day. You can also boost hydration by offering foods with high water content, such as fruits, vegetables, and soups. If plain water isn't appealing, try infusing it with fresh fruit or herbs for a subtle flavor.

Simplify Eating and Drinking: For individuals who may struggle with utensils or have difficulty grasping cups, there are ways to make eating and drinking easier. Choose finger foods that can be easily picked up and consumed, such as sliced fruits, vegetables, sandwiches, or bite-sized portions. You can also use adaptive dishes and cutlery designed for easier handling, such as plates with raised edges or utensils with larger grips. Making food easier to consume can enhance independence and reduce frustration at mealtimes.

Keep Recipes Simple: When preparing meals, choose recipes that are straightforward and quick to make. Complex, time-consuming dishes can add unnecessary stress to your caregiving responsibilities. Look for recipes with fewer ingredients and simple preparation methods. One-pot meals, slow cooker recipes, or sheet pan dinners can be great options. By keeping recipes simple, you can provide nutritious meals without adding extra burden to your daily routine.

Incorporate Familiar Favorites: Familiarity can be comforting for individuals with dementia, and this extends to food preferences. When planning meals, try to incorporate dishes that your loved one has enjoyed throughout their life. This could be a favorite childhood meal, a traditional family recipe, or a dish from their cultural background. Familiar flavors and aromas can stimulate appetite and provide a sense of comfort and connection to the past.

Promote Social Interaction: Mealtimes are a great opportunity for social engagement, which is important for individuals with dementia.

Try to make dining a social event. Sit down and share meals, engaging in conversation and creating a positive atmosphere. If your loved one is in a care facility, encourage them to dine with others in a communal setting. Social interaction during meals can stimulate appetite, reduce feelings of isolation, and provide valuable cognitive stimulation.

Regularly Review Nutritional Needs: As dementia progresses, nutritional requirements may change. Regularly assess your loved one's dietary needs in consultation with healthcare professionals, such as a registered dietitian or doctor. They can help you make sure the meal plan remains appropriate and effective, providing guidance on any necessary changes or interventions. This may include adding nutritional supplements, changing food textures, or addressing specific health concerns.

Customize for Dietary Restrictions: If your loved one has any dietary restrictions or health conditions that require a special diet, it's important to tailor their meals. This may include low-sodium, low-sugar, or gluten-free diets, among others. Work with a healthcare professional to understand the specific requirements and how to incorporate them into the meal plan. By customizing meals to accommodate these needs, you can support your loved one's overall health and well-being.

Create a Pleasant Dining Environment: The dining atmosphere can greatly influence the enjoyment of meals. Aim to create a calm, inviting environment that encourages relaxation and appetite. Use simple table settings with minimal distractions, such as soothing background music or a vase of fresh flowers.

Make sure the eating area is comfortable, well-lit, and free from clutter. A pleasant dining environment can make mealtimes more enjoyable and reduce stress for both the individual with dementia and their caregivers.

By putting these strategies into practice, you can craft nutritious and appealing meal plans that support the health and happiness of your loved one with dementia.

Remember, mealtimes are an opportunity for nourishment, enjoyment, and connection. By focusing on nutrient-dense foods, adapting to individual needs, and creating a positive dining experience, you can make a significant difference in your loved one's quality of life. Don't hesitate to seek guidance from healthcare professionals to make sure you're providing the best nutrition and care.

～

NAVIGATING MEALTIME CHALLENGES IN DEMENTIA CARE: STRATEGIES FOR SUCCESS

MEALTIMES CAN BE a challenging part of caring for someone with dementia. From forgetfulness to changes in appetite or difficulty swallowing, several issues may arise. However, by addressing these challenges proactively and with compassion, you can make sure mealtimes remain a positive, nourishing experience for your loved one. Here are strategies to help you navigate common mealtime challenges in dementia care:

Establish a Consistent Routine: Familiarity and routine can be comforting for individuals with dementia. Try to serve meals at the same time each day to create a predictable structure. This can help reduce anxiety and confusion around mealtimes. It can also help regulate appetite and digestion. In addition to consistent timing, try to create a familiar setting by using the same dishes, utensils, and seating arrangements.

Opt for Nutrient-Dense Choices: As appetite and food intake may go down, it's important to make every bite count. Focus on incorporating nutrient-dense foods into the diet to make sure your loved one is getting the vitamins, minerals, and other essential nutrients they need. Focus on colorful fruits and vegetables, lean proteins, whole grains, and healthy fats. These foods provide a powerful mix of nutrients that can support overall health and cognitive function.

Adapt Food Textures: Dementia can affect chewing and swallowing abilities, making certain food textures difficult or even dangerous to consume. If you notice your loved one struggling with certain foods, consider adapting the texture. Pureed, soft-cooked, or mashed foods can be much easier to manage. You can also try moistening dry foods with sauces or gravies. If swallowing issues persist, talk to a healthcare professional about the possibility of a texture-modified diet.

Introduce Finger Foods: For individuals with difficulty using utensils, finger foods can be a great solution. They allow for greater independence and can make mealtimes feel less frustrating. Choose foods easy to pick up and hold, such as bite-sized fruits, vegetable sticks, cheese cubes, or small sandwiches. Finger foods can also be a good option for those who usually wander during meals, as they can be eaten on the go.

Implement Smaller, Frequent Meals: Large meals can be overwhelming for some individuals with dementia, leading to lower appetite or disinterest in eating. Instead of three large meals, try offering smaller, more frequent meals and snacks throughout the day. This can help maintain energy levels and make sure nutritional needs are met. It can also be less daunting for those with diminished appetites.

Create a Distraction-Free Environment: Distractions can make it difficult for individuals with dementia to focus on eating. To create a more conducive dining environment, try to reduce background noise and activity. Turn off the TV or radio and avoid having conversations unrelated to the meal. Use simple table settings and remove any clutter that could be distracting. A calm, quiet atmosphere can help your loved one concentrate on the task at hand.

Promote Hydration: Dehydration is a common concern for individuals with dementia, as they may forget to drink or not recognize thirst cues. Make a conscious effort to offer fluids regularly throughout the day. Water is always a good choice, but you can also offer other hydrating options like herbal teas, broths, or foods with high water content, such as fruits and soups. Aim for at least 6-8 glasses of fluid per day, or more if recommended by a healthcare professional.

Engage in Meal Preparation: Involving your loved one in meal preparation can help stimulate appetite and provide a sense of purpose. Even simple tasks like stirring a bowl, tossing a salad, or setting the table can be engaging. Focus on tasks that are safe and manageable for their current abilities. The process can make them feel more connected to the meal and more interested in eating.

Be Attentive to Preferences: As dementia progresses, food preferences and aversions may change. What was once a favorite dish may no longer be appealing. Be attentive to these changes and try to offer many options. Keep track of what your loved one seems to enjoy and what they avoid. Respecting individual preferences can make mealtimes more pleasant and reduce the likelihood of mealtime battles.

Consult a Dietitian: For personalized guidance on navigating mealtime challenges, consider consulting with a registered dietitian with experience in dementia care. They can provide expert advice on nutrition, meal planning, and strategies to address specific issues like weight loss, chewing and swallowing difficulties, or medication side effects. They can also help you make sure your loved one's diet meets their unique needs.

Remember, the goal of mealtimes is not just to provide nourishment, but also to create a positive, enjoyable experience. By approaching challenges with patience, creativity, and a focus on your loved one's individual needs, you can make mealtimes a highlight of the day.

Please reach out for support and guidance from healthcare professionals when needed. With the right strategies and a compassionate approach, you can make sure your loved one receives the nutrition they need while still finding joy and comfort in the dining experience.

～

EMPOWERING HEALTHY EATING IN DEMENTIA CARE: THE VITAL ROLE OF CAREGIVERS

As a caregiver for someone with dementia, you play an important role in supporting their overall well-being, and nutrition is a key aspect of this care. What your loved one eats can have a profound impact on their physical health, cognitive function, and quality of life.

However, as dementia progresses, many challenges can arise that make maintaining healthy eating habits more difficult. Memory loss, decreased appetite, and changes in taste and smell are a few issues that may come into play. This is where you, as a caregiver, can make a significant difference. By creating a supportive and nurturing dietary environment, you can help your loved one get the nutrition they need to thrive.

Here are ways you can actively promote healthy eating habits:

Establish a Routine: Consistency and familiarity can be comforting for individuals with dementia. By setting regular times for meals and snacks, you create a predictable structure that can reduce confusion and anxiety. This routine can also help regulate appetite and make sure your loved one is eating at regular intervals throughout the day. Try to serve meals at the same time each day and consider using visual cues like a clock or a daily schedule to reinforce the routine.

Focus on Nutrient-Rich Foods: A diet rich in essential nutrients is important for maintaining overall health and potentially mitigating symptoms of dementia. When planning meals, focus on incorporating many colorful fruits and vegetables, whole grains, lean proteins, and healthy fats. These foods are packed with vitamins, minerals, and antioxidants that can support brain health and overall well-being. Aim to create balanced, visually appealing plates that offer a range of nutrients.

Create a Calm Dining Environment: The atmosphere in which meals are eaten can greatly influence the dining experience. A serene, distraction-free environment can help your loved one focus on eating and enjoy their food more. Try to reduce background noise, such as turning off the TV or radio. Use simple table settings and remove any clutter that could be distracting. Make sure the eating area is well-lit and comfortable. A calm, inviting space can make mealtimes more pleasant and less stressful.

Promote Autonomy and Engagement: Encouraging your loved one to be involved in meal preparation and dining can help maintain a sense of independence and engagement. Even simple tasks, like washing vegetables, stirring a bowl, or setting the table, can be empowering. Focus on activities that are safe and manageable for their current abilities. The process can boost their interest in the meal and provide a sense of accomplishment. It's also an opportunity for meaningful interaction and connection.

Simplify Meal Consumption: As dementia progresses, using utensils and managing certain food textures can become challenging. To make eating easier and more enjoyable, consider offering finger foods or items that can be easily consumed without utensils. Soft, bite-sized portions of fruits, vegetables, sandwiches, or cheese can be good options. This approach allows for greater independence in self-feeding and can reduce frustration at mealtimes. Adaptive utensils and dishes can also be helpful for those with grip or coordination difficulties.

Focus on Hydration: Dehydration is a common concern for individuals with dementia, as they may forget to drink or not recognize thirst cues. As a caregiver, you can help by regularly offering and encouraging fluid intake. Water is always a good choice, but you can also offer other hydrating options like herbal teas, broths, or foods with high water content. Make drinks easily accessible and consider using brightly colored cups or straws to draw attention to them. Aim for at least 6-8 glasses of fluid per day, or more if recommended by a healthcare professional.

Foster a Collaborative Care Approach: Caring for someone with dementia is a team effort, and this extends to managing dietary needs. Involve other family members, friends, or professional caregivers in meal planning, preparation, and encouragement. A supportive network can help make sure your loved one's nutritional needs are consistently met. It can also give you much-needed respite and support. Please ask for help when needed and communicate openly with your care team.

Remember, as a caregiver, you are not just a passive observer but an active participant in your loved one's nutritional journey. By putting thoughtful strategies into practice, showing empathy and patience, and creating a nurturing environment, you can make a significant difference in their dietary well-being. Each meal becomes an opportunity for nourishment, enjoyment, and connection. Your efforts, no matter how small they may seem, can have a profound impact on your loved one's quality of life. Take pride in the important role you play and the love and care you provide.

$\sim$

DIVERSE AND ADAPTABLE MEAL PLANNING FOR DEMENTIA CARE: STRATEGIES FOR NUTRITION AND ENJOYMENT

When planning meals for someone with dementia, it's important to consider not just their nutritional needs, but also their overall enjoyment of food. Eating should be a pleasurable experience that brings comfort and satisfaction, even as abilities and preferences may change. By incorporating variety, flexibility, and a focus on nutrient-dense options, you can create meal plans that support both physical health and quality of life.

Here are strategies to help you infuse diversity and adaptability into your approach:

Embrace Food Variety: One of the keys to a well-rounded diet is variety. Aim to include a wide range of fruits, vegetables, proteins, and whole grains in your meal plans. This not only ensures a comprehensive intake of essential nutrients but also adds visual appeal and flavor diversity to meals. Variety can help keep things interesting and prevent boredom with repetitive food choices. Experiment with different cuisines, herbs, and spices to introduce new tastes and textures.

Focus on Nutrient-Dense Choices: While variety is important, it's also important to focus on nutrient-dense foods. These are options that pack a lot of essential nutrients into relatively few calories. Leafy greens, colorful fruits and vegetables, fatty fish, lean proteins, and whole grains are all excellent examples. These foods provide vitamins, minerals, antioxidants, and other beneficial compounds that support overall health and cognitive function. Try to incorporate these nutrient powerhouses into meals and snacks.

Adapt to Changing Preferences: As dementia progresses, an individual's food preferences and appetite may change. What they once loved may no longer be appealing, or they may develop new taste preferences. Be attentive to these changes and be willing to adapt meal plans. Keep a record of what foods are well-received and which ones are consistently left uneaten. This flexibility in planning can help make sure meals remain enjoyable and nutritionally adequate.

Offer Smaller, More Frequent Meals: For some individuals with dementia, large meals may be overwhelming or difficult to manage. They may have reduced appetites or get easily distracted during long meals. In these cases, offering smaller, more frequent meals and snacks throughout the day can be a helpful strategy. This approach can help maintain energy levels and make sure nutritional needs are met without the pressure of consuming large portions. Aim for five to six small meals or snacks, rather than three large ones.

Simplify Meal Consumption: As dementia advances, some individuals may experience difficulties with chewing, swallowing, or using utensils. To make eating easier and more enjoyable, focus on preparing foods simple to consume. Soft-cooked vegetables, ground meats, and smooth purees can be much gentler on the mouth and throat. Finger foods like bite-sized fruits, cheese cubes, or small sandwiches can also be a good option for those who struggle with utensils. The goal is to make eating as comfortable and stress-free as possible.

Keep Hydration in Focus: Adequate hydration is essential for overall health, but it can be a challenge for individuals with dementia. They may forget to drink, not recognize thirst cues, or have difficulty swallowing fluids. Make a concerted effort to encourage fluid intake throughout the day. Offer a variety of beverages like water, herbal teas, or diluted juices. You can also boost hydration through foods with high water content, such as soups, fruits, and vegetables. Make drinks easily accessible and offer them regularly.

Customize Food Textures: In some cases, modifying food textures may be necessary to ensure safe and comfortable eating. This may involve pureeing, mashing, or finely chopping foods to make them easier to chew and swallow. Work with a healthcare professional, such as a speech therapist or dietitian, to determine the most appropriate texture modifications for your loved one's needs. Be creative in presenting these modified foods in an appealing way, using molds or attractive garnishes.

Consult with Nutrition Experts: If you're unsure about how to meet your loved one's nutritional needs through meal planning, don't hesitate to seek guidance from a registered dietitian. They can provide personalized recommendations based on individual health status, dietary restrictions, and food preferences.

They can also offer creative ideas for meals and snacks that are both nutritious and appealing. Their knowledge can be invaluable in navigating the challenges of dementia-related changes in eating habits.

Remember, the ultimate goal of meal planning in dementia care is to nourish both the body and the soul.

By embracing variety, focusing on nutrient-dense options, and remaining flexible in your approach, you can create a dining experience that is both nutritionally sound and deeply satisfying. Be patient, be creative, and focus on your loved one's enjoyment of food. Your efforts in crafting diverse and adaptable meal plans can have a profound impact on their overall well-being and quality of life.

~

RESOURCES AND TOOLS FOR FURTHER GUIDANCE ON NUTRITION AND MEAL PLANNING FOR INDIVIDUALS WITH DEMENTIA

HERE ARE key resources and tools that can help guide nutrition and meal planning for individuals with dementia:

Alzheimer's Association (alz.org): The Alzheimer's Association is a leading resource that provides comprehensive information on dementia care, including tips on nutrition and how diet affects cognitive health. Their website offers guidelines for creating dementia-friendly meals that cater to the specific needs of those with cognitive impairment.

Academy of Nutrition and Dietetics (eatright.org): The Academy's website lets you find and connect with registered dietitian nutritionists who specialize in various areas, including nutrition for older adults. An RDN can provide personalized nutrition advice and strategies for meal planning tailored to the unique needs of an individual with dementia.

The MIND Diet: While not designed exclusively for dementia, the MIND diet focuses on foods that have been shown to support brain health and cognitive function. The diet's principles can be adapted to help guide food choices for those with dementia. Various health and wellness websites provide resources and information on following the MIND diet.

Meal Delivery Services: Services like Meals on Wheels or other local meal providers can be helpful for caregivers who may not have the time to prepare nutritious meals. These services often cater to the dietary needs of seniors, including those with cognitive impairment.

Dementia-Specific Cookbooks and Online Recipes: There are several cookbooks and websites dedicated to recipes and meal ideas suitable for individuals with dementia. These focus on nutrient-dense foods that are easy to eat, and often include tips for making mealtimes less stressful.

Memory Cafés and Support Groups: Many communities have Memory Cafés or support groups for people with dementia and their caregivers. These can provide a space to share meal planning tips and recipes with others who understand the challenges.

Adaptive Dining Equipment: Companies make dining tools specially designed for people with cognitive and physical impairments. Things like plate guards, adaptive utensils, and no-spill cups can help make meals easier and more enjoyable.

Educational Workshops: Dementia care organizations often host workshops and webinars on a range of topics, which may include information on nutrition and practical tips for meal planning. These can provide helpful foundational knowledge.

The key is finding strategies and resources that work well for each individual's unique preferences and challenges. A mix of nutritional guidance from experts, practical tools and tips, support from other caregivers, and some trial and error can help establish a healthy and enjoyable meal planning routine.

The Alzheimer's Association and Academy of Nutrition and Dietetics websites are great starting points for accessing reliable information and connecting with knowledgeable professionals.

∼

KEEPING YOUR LOVED ONE WITH DEMENTIA CONNECTED AND ENGAGED

As a caregiver, you play an important role in supporting your loved one with dementia. One of the most important parts of this care is helping them maintain social connections and participate in meaningful activities. Engaging with others and staying active can have a profound impact on their overall well-being, including their cognitive function, emotional health, and sense of belonging.

Let's explore practical ways you can foster social engagement in your loved one's life.

Encourage Regular Social Interactions: Staying in touch with friends, family, and community members is important for combating feelings of isolation. Encourage loved ones to visit, schedule regular phone calls, or set up video chats to keep your family member involved in their social circle. Even brief interactions can make a big difference in their day.

Participate in Group Activities: Look for group activities in your community tailored to individuals with dementia. These might include music therapy sessions, art classes, or exercise groups designed to meet their specific needs and abilities. These activities can provide a sense of camaraderie and support.

Promote Hobbies and Interests: Engage your loved one in activities they've always enjoyed, whether it's gardening, painting, or listening to their favorite music. These familiar pastimes can bring them joy and a sense of accomplishment. You can also explore new hobbies together, focusing on themes they find interesting.

Explore Volunteer Opportunities: If your loved one is able, consider exploring volunteer opportunities that match their skills and interests. Contributing to community projects, even in small ways, can provide a sense of purpose and fulfillment. Look for dementia-friendly opportunities that provide a supportive environment.

Use Technology: Technology offers innovative ways to keep your loved one connected. Look for apps and platforms designed specifically for seniors, which can help them communicate with friends and family more easily. They may also enjoy virtual events or activities tailored to their interests.

Create a Memory Café: Memory Cafés are welcoming spaces where individuals with dementia and their caregivers can socialize and share experiences. Consider starting one in your community or seeking existing gatherings. These can provide a sense of belonging and support for both you and your loved one.

Develop a Routine: Creating a consistent routine that incorporates social activities can provide structure and reduce anxiety for your loved one. Tailor the schedule to include manageable social interactions that won't overwhelm them. Regular social engagements, even brief ones, can give them something to look forward to.

Encourage Physical Activity: Staying physically active is important for overall health and can provide opportunities for social engagement. Consider group walks, gentle exercise classes, or dance activities designed for individuals with dementia. Joining others for movement can boost both physical and emotional well-being.

Seek Support Groups: Support groups for individuals with dementia and their caregivers can provide a valuable space to share experiences, tips, and companionship. Connecting with others who understand the challenges you face can foster a sense of community and provide much-needed support for both you and your loved one.

Tailor Activities to Individual Needs: Always consider your loved one's current abilities and preferences when planning social activities. What works for one person may not work for another. Tailoring engagements to fit their specific needs can make sure activities are both enjoyable and meaningful for them.

Remember, maintaining social connections and engaging in activities can have a significant impact on your loved one's overall well-being. By focusing on these aspects of care, you can support them in leading a more fulfilling and connected life, despite the challenges of dementia. Your efforts to nurture these social connections can make all the difference in their happiness and quality of life.

~

NURTURING ENGAGEMENT AND SOCIAL CONNECTION IN DEMENTIA CARE

As a caregiver, one of your primary goals is to make sure your loved one with dementia remains engaged and socially connected. Participating in meaningful activities and maintaining relationships can significantly improve their overall quality of life, including their emotional well-being, cognitive function, and sense of belonging.

Let's explore practical ways you can foster engagement and social interaction in both individual and group settings.

Revisit Past Interests and Hobbies: Begin by thinking about the activities your loved one enjoyed before the onset of dementia. Consider how you can adapt these hobbies to match their current abilities. Reengaging with familiar pastimes can spark their interest and provide a comforting sense of continuity.

Help with Social Connections: Regular interaction with friends, family, and community members is essential for combating feelings of loneliness and isolation. Consider organizing small, intimate gatherings or encouraging video calls with loved ones. Look for local community events tailored to seniors or individuals with dementia and offer support to help them participate.

Incorporate Physical Activity: Engaging in simple physical activities, such as going for walks, doing light gardening, or participating in seated exercises, can provide many benefits for both physical and mental health. These activities also offer natural opportunities for social interaction. Consider joining a group exercise class designed specifically for older adults to foster a sense of camaraderie and support.

Explore New Experiences: While familiarity is comforting, introducing new experiences can stimulate the brain and add excitement to daily life. Explore new hobbies together, visit local attractions, or go to cultural events that are accessible and enjoyable for your loved one. Be open to trying new things and see what resonates with them.

Use Technology for Connection: Digital platforms offer innovative ways to keep your loved one engaged and connected. Introduce them to senior-friendly apps that align with their interests, such as music apps, brain-stimulating games, or virtual reality experiences. Online forums and social media groups can also help them connect with broader communities who share similar interests.

Be Flexible and Adaptable: It's important to remember that your loved one's interests and abilities may change. Be willing to adjust activities based on their daily mood and energy levels. If an activity becomes frustrating or unenjoyable, please try something different. The goal is to make sure engagement remains pleasant and rewarding.

Encourage Creative Expression: Art, music, and storytelling can be powerful outlets for expression and communication, particularly for individuals who may have difficulty with traditional conversation. Engage in creative arts programs together or enjoy simple arts and crafts projects at home. These activities provide opportunities for self-expression and can evoke positive emotions.

Focus on Engagement Over Perfection: Remember, the primary goal is to enjoy the process and the engagement itself, rather than focusing on achieving a specific outcome. Celebrate your loved one's participation and effort, making sure activities remain pressure-free and enjoyable. The joy is in the journey, not the destination.

Leverage Community Resources: Many communities offer programs and services designed specifically for individuals with dementia, such as day programs, support groups, and recreational activities. These resources can provide valuable opportunities for socialization and engagement in a supportive environment. Please reach out and explore what's available in your area.

Involve Them in Daily Tasks: Encouraging your loved one to participate in simple, everyday tasks like setting the table or folding laundry can provide a sense of purpose and accomplishment. Tailor these tasks to their current ability level to ensure success and positive reinforcement. Celebrating their contributions, no matter how small, can boost their self-esteem and sense of belonging.

By putting these strategies into practice, you can significantly enhance the social and emotional well-being of your loved one with dementia. The key is to provide supportive, enjoyable, and meaningful opportunities for engagement that respect their unique preferences and capabilities. Remember, your efforts to nurture these connections and experiences can make a profound difference in their overall happiness and quality of life.

∽

CULTIVATING A SUPPORTIVE SOCIAL CIRCLE FOR YOUR LOVED ONE WITH DEMENTIA

As a caregiver, one of the most impactful things you can do for your loved one with dementia is to help them maintain a strong social support network. A nurturing social circle can provide emotional comfort, cognitive stimulation, and a profound sense of belonging, which contribute to a better quality of life.

Let's explore practical ways you can cultivate a supportive community around your loved one.

Strengthen Family Ties: Encourage family members to actively engage in your loved one's life. Regular visits, phone calls, and video chats can provide a consistent source of love and connection. Consider organizing family gatherings that are inclusive and mindful of your loved one's needs, creating joyful and memorable moments together.

Maintain Existing Friendships and Encourage New Ones: Help your loved one sustain their long-standing friendships by helping with social gatherings or encouraging regular communication. You can also help to form new friendships by connecting your loved one with peers who share similar interests or experiences. Look for community groups, hobby clubs, or support networks that can provide opportunities for meaningful social interactions.

Use Community Resources: Research local senior centers, libraries, or community organizations that offer programs specifically designed for older adults or individuals with cognitive impairments. These resources can provide a range of engaging activities, from social gatherings to educational workshops, allowing your loved one to connect with others while enjoying enriching experiences.

Embrace Technology for Connection: Introduce your loved one to user-friendly technology that can help them stay connected with friends and family who may live far away. Social media platforms, video call applications, and online community forums can offer valuable opportunities for engagement and communication. Help them to learn how to use these tools and provide ongoing support as needed.

Promote Physical Activity and Social Interaction: Look for group activities that combine physical movement with social engagement, such as senior fitness classes, walking clubs, or gentle yoga sessions. These activities can help maintain physical health while also fostering social connections with others who share similar interests and abilities.

Encourage Cognitive Stimulation: Engage your loved one in mentally stimulating group activities that provide opportunities for social interaction, such as board game clubs, book discussion groups, or art classes tailored to their cognitive abilities. These activities not only offer intellectual stimulation but also help with meaningful conversations and social bonds.

Plan Regular Outings: Organize outings that align with your loved one's interests and preferences, such as visits to museums, attending concerts, or enjoying nature walks. These excursions provide fresh experiences and opportunities to interact with others in a social setting, promoting a sense of adventure and connection to the wider world.

Building and maintaining a supportive social network for your loved one with dementia requires ongoing effort, creativity, and patience. However, the positive impact on their emotional well-being and cognitive health is immeasurable. By thoughtfully weaving together a network of family, friends, and community resources, you can make sure your loved one feels valued, understood, and deeply connected to the people and experiences that matter most to them.

Remember, every small gesture of love and inclusion makes a difference. Your dedication to fostering a nurturing social environment will not only enhance your loved one's quality of life but also give you the support and encouragement you need as a caregiver. Embrace the power of community and watch as it transforms your loved one's journey with dementia into one filled with joy, purpose, and meaningful connections.

~

HARNESSING TECHNOLOGY TO ENHANCE SOCIAL CONNECTION AND MENTAL STIMULATION IN ELDER CARE

TODAY, technology can be a powerful tool for enhancing the quality of life for older adults, especially those facing cognitive challenges like dementia. By thoughtfully integrating technology into their daily routines, you can help your loved one stay connected with others, engage in mentally stimulating activities, and enjoy a greater sense of fulfillment.

Let's explore some practical ways to leverage technology for social engagement and cognitive enrichment.

Video Calling Platforms: Applications like Skype, Zoom, or FaceTime provide a wonderful opportunity for face-to-face interaction with family and friends, even when physical distance separates them. These video calls can help combat feelings of isolation by allowing your loved one to see and connect with familiar faces, making the experience more personal and meaningful.

Social Media Engagement: Encouraging your loved one to engage with social media can help them stay connected to their community and the broader world. Platforms like Facebook let them stay updated on family news, reconnect with old friends, and join groups centered on their interests. This sense of belonging and participation can be fulfilling.

Online Communities and Forums: Introduce your loved one to websites and forums related to their hobbies or areas of interest, such as gardening, literature, or history. Participating in these online communities can provide mental stimulation and a platform for sharing knowledge and experiences with like-minded individuals.

Virtual Experiences and Tours: Many museums, historical sites, and cultural institutions now offer virtual tours and immersive experiences. These digital adventures can provide mental stimulation and a sense of exploration without the need for physical travel. Enjoy these virtual journeys together, fostering conversation and curiosity.

Educational Platforms: Websites like Coursera or Khan Academy offer a wide range of online courses on various subjects. Encourage your loved one to pursue a topic they've always been curious about or revisit a subject they enjoyed in the past. Continuous learning provides mental stimulation and a rewarding sense of personal growth.

Interactive Games and Brain-Training Apps: Digital games and applications designed to enhance cognitive skills can be both entertaining and beneficial for mental acuity. Look for games that involve strategy, puzzle-solving, or memory exercises to keep the mind engaged and challenged. Many of these apps adapt to the user's skill level, ensuring a satisfying experience.

Assistive Technology Devices: Consider introducing devices specifically designed for seniors, such as simplified smartphones or tablets with user-friendly interfaces. Features like voice commands or enlarged text can make navigating technology more accessible and less frustrating for your loved one.

Digital Photo Sharing: Sharing digital photos through cloud-based albums or digital picture frames can help your loved one feel connected to cherished memories and family moments. Revisiting these images together can prompt meaningful conversations and encourage reminiscence, which is valuable for those with memory challenges.

Safety and Health Monitoring Technology: In addition to social and cognitive benefits, technology can also support the health and safety of your loved one. Wearable devices can track important health indicators and alert caregivers to potential concerns, while GPS tracking technology can provide peace of mind for those prone to wandering or disorientation.

When introducing new technologies to your loved one, it's essential to do so gradually and with patience. Provide clear, step-by-step guidance and be available to offer support as they learn to navigate these digital tools. Celebrate their successes and encourage them to explore the features that resonate with their interests and abilities.

By thoughtfully incorporating technology into the care plan for your elderly loved one, you can open up new avenues for social connection, mental engagement, and overall well-being. These digital tools have the power to enrich their daily lives, foster a sense of purpose, and help them feel more connected to the world around them. Embrace the potential of technology and witness the positive impact it can have on your loved one's journey through their golden years.

~

EMPOWERING INDIVIDUALS WITH DEMENTIA THROUGH COMMUNITY ENGAGEMENT AND VOLUNTEERING

Encouraging your loved one with dementia to participate in community service and volunteering activities can offer a wide range of benefits that significantly enhance their overall quality of life.

Let's explore the compelling reasons fostering community engagement is so valuable and discuss practical ways to support your loved one in finding fulfilling volunteer opportunities.

Strengthening Social Connections: Volunteering provides a natural platform for meeting new people and expanding social networks. These social interactions can be powerful in combating feelings of loneliness and isolation, which are common challenges faced by individuals with dementia. By engaging with others in a purposeful context, your loved one can develop a strong sense of belonging and connection to their community.

Rekindling a Sense of Purpose: Contributing to the community or a meaningful cause can instill a profound sense of purpose and accomplishment in individuals with dementia. Volunteer work allows them to feel valued and needed, boosting their self-esteem and counteracting feelings of loss or uselessness that may go along with the progression of dementia. Knowing that their efforts make a difference can be empowering and emotionally uplifting.

Promoting Cognitive and Physical Stimulation: Volunteering often involves many tasks that stimulate both the mind and body. From organizing events to interacting with others or even engaging in light physical work, these activities can help maintain cognitive function and physical health. Engaging in mentally stimulating tasks and staying physically active, within their abilities, can slow down cognitive decline and improve overall well-being.

Building Confidence and Self-Esteem: Successfully participating in volunteer activities can reinforce an individual's existing abilities and strengths, helping to build confidence and foster a positive self-image. Accomplishing tasks and receiving appreciation for their contributions can be validating, reminding them of their capabilities and value within the community.

Fostering Community Ties and Identity: Being an active member of the community helps individuals with dementia maintain a sense of identity and continuity in their lives. Volunteer work allows them to feel connected to something larger than themselves, providing a sense of belonging and purpose. These community ties can be grounding and emotionally supportive.

To support your loved one in starting a fulfilling volunteer journey, consider these steps:

1. **Identify Suitable Opportunities**: Research volunteer roles that align with your loved one's interests, skills, and abilities. Many organizations welcome volunteers with dementia and offer accommodating roles that provide meaningful engagement without being overwhelming. Consider your loved one's passions and look for opportunities that match their strengths and limitations.
2. **Start with Manageable Commitments**: Begin by exploring volunteer activities or community events that don't require a long-term commitment. This allows your loved one to test the

waters and gauge their interest and capacity for volunteering without feeling pressured. Short-term or one-time events can be a great starting point.

3. **Provide Support and Encouragement**: Offer to go along with your loved one to volunteer activities or community events, providing a familiar presence and emotional support. As they grow more comfortable and confident, they may wish to participate independently or with peers who share similar experiences. Be there to cheer them on and celebrate their involvement.

4. **Celebrate Their Contributions**: Recognize and celebrate the contributions your loved one makes, no matter how small they may seem. Acknowledging their efforts and expressing appreciation for their dedication can reinforce the value of their participation. Celebrate their successes and let them know the positive impact they are making.

5. **Monitor and Adapt as Needed**: Keep a close eye on how volunteering affects your loved one's mood, energy levels, and overall well-being. If the activities become stressful or overwhelming, be open to adjusting the type or duration of involvement to better suit their needs. Regularly check in with them and be flexible in adapting their volunteer commitments as their abilities or preferences change.

By promoting and supporting community engagement and volunteering, you can help your loved one with dementia lead a more fulfilling and purposeful life. These activities provide a unique avenue for meaningful social connections, cognitive stimulation, and a profound sense of belonging.

Embracing the power of community involvement can significantly enhance their emotional, mental, and social well-being, letting them thrive despite the challenges posed by dementia.

Remember, every individual's journey with dementia is unique, so it's essential to approach volunteering and community engagement with patience, understanding, and flexibility. Celebrate the small victories and cherish the moments of joy and connection that these activities bring. By empowering your loved one to make a difference in their community, you are not only enriching their life but also creating a more inclusive and supportive society for all individuals living with dementia.

~

DESIGNING A STRUCTURED AND STIMULATING ENVIRONMENT FOR INDIVIDUALS WITH DEMENTIA

CREATING a structured routine and incorporating engaging activities can significantly enhance the quality of life for individuals living with dementia. By providing a predictable and stimulating environment, you can help reduce confusion, alleviate anxiety, and promote a sense of purpose and joy in your loved one's daily life.

Let's explore practical ways to integrate these elements effectively.

Establish a Consistent Daily Routine: Implementing a predictable daily routine can greatly help individuals with dementia by providing a sense of stability and comfort. Structure their day around regular mealtimes, personal care activities, and scheduled engagements. This consistency helps to reduce confusion and anxiety, as your loved one knows what to expect and can feel more in control of their day.

Focus on Regular Social Interactions: Facilitate regular social activities that allow your loved one to connect and interact with others. This can be achieved through participation in local clubs, community centers, or family gatherings. Encourage involvement in group activities that align with their interests, such as book clubs, art classes, or music groups. Regular social interaction can improve mood, maintain social skills, and combat feelings of isolation and loneliness.

Leverage Technology for Connection: In the digital age, technology can be a powerful tool for keeping your loved one connected with friends and family, both near and far. Set up regular video calls using user-friendly platforms, introduce them to social media sites tailored to their interests, or explore online communities together. These digital connections can provide a sense of belonging and help have important relationships.

Plan Engaging Outings: Regular outings to places of interest, such as parks, museums, or community events, can provide mental stimulation and a refreshing change of scenery. When planning these outings, consider your loved one's interests, abilities, and comfort level. Aim for experiences that are enjoyable, manageable, and aligned with their current capabilities. These outings can spark conversations, evoke pleasant memories, and create new, positive associations.

Nurture Hobbies and Personal Interests: Encourage activities that resonate with your loved one's hobbies and passions. Whether it's gardening, painting, listening to music, or engaging in crafts, participating in familiar and enjoyable activities can provide a sense of accomplishment, purpose, and pleasure. Adapt these activities as needed to match their current abilities, making sure they remain stimulating without being overwhelming.

Incorporate Physical Activity: Regular physical activity is essential for maintaining physical health and promoting mental well-being. Incorporate light physical activities into your loved one's daily routine, tailored to their individual abilities. This can include walks in nature, gentle stretching exercises, or simple chair-based movements. Physical activity can improve mobility, boost mood, and provide a sense of accomplishment.

Foster Meaningful Relationships: Support your loved one in nurturing and maintaining meaningful relationships with family, friends, and peers. Encourage regular communication, shared activities, and opportunities for emotional connection. Strong social ties can offer invaluable support, reduce feelings of isolation, and decrease the risk of depression. Facilitate these connections and creating opportunities for social engagement.

Adapt to Changing Needs: As dementia progresses, your loved one's abilities, interests, and needs may evolve. Continuously assess and adapt their daily routine and activities to align with their current stage and capabilities. Be flexible in adjusting schedules, changing activities, and introducing new elements that keep them engaged and stimulated without causing undue stress or frustration.

Remember, creating a structured and engaging environment for your loved one with dementia is an ongoing process that requires patience, creativity, and attentiveness to their unique needs. By providing a predictable routine, fostering social connections, and incorporating stimulating activities, you can significantly enhance their sense of well-being, purpose, and happiness.

Celebrate the small joys and cherish the moments of connection and engagement that these efforts bring. Your dedication to a nurturing and supportive environment can make a profound difference in your loved one's quality of life, helping them navigate the challenges of dementia with greater comfort, dignity, and fulfillment.

$\sim$

ENHANCING SOCIAL ENGAGEMENT THROUGH PROFESSIONAL SUPPORT IN DEMENTIA CARE

PROVIDING A SOCIALLY engaging and fulfilling life for your loved one with dementia can be a complex and challenging task. Seeking the guidance and support of professionals who specialize in dementia care can be a game-changer in making sure your loved one's social needs are met in a meaningful and personalized way.

Let's explore how leveraging expertise can make a significant difference in enhancing social engagement and activity participation.

Comprehensive Needs Assessment: Engaging professionals, such as social workers and occupational therapists, to thoroughly assess your loved one's social interests, abilities, and needs is an important first step. This personalized approach makes sure the social activities and connections recommended align with their preferences and capabilities, making the experiences more enjoyable and rewarding.

Therapeutic Interventions: Psychologists or therapists who specialize in geriatric care can provide targeted interventions designed to boost confidence in social situations, address feelings of isolation, and help your loved one cope with the emotional challenges that often go along with dementia. These professionals may use cognitive-behavioral strategies to enhance social interaction skills, improve communication, and promote overall emotional well-being.

Access to Community Resources: Social workers are invaluable allies in connecting families with community resources tailored to the needs of individuals with cognitive impairments. They can help navigate the many available services, such as senior centers, social clubs, and volunteer opportunities, making it easier for families to find appropriate and engaging social activities. Their knowledge in identifying suitable resources can save caregivers time and effort while making sure their loved one has access to many stimulating social experiences.

Family Support and Education: Caring for a loved one with dementia can be emotionally and mentally demanding. Professionals can offer valuable education and support to family members, equipping them with effective communication strategies, a deeper understanding of dementia-related challenges, and practical ways to encourage social participation. Additionally, support groups facilitated by professionals provide a platform for caregivers to share experiences, learn from one another, and find emotional support within a community of individuals facing similar challenges.

Individualized Activity Planning: Occupational therapists can work closely with your loved one to identify hobbies and activities that are not only enjoyable but also adapted to their specific cognitive and physical abilities. These professionals can suggest changes to activities, making sure they remain engaging and accessible as dementia progresses. By tailoring activities to your loved one's changing needs, occupational therapists help maintain a sense of purpose, accomplishment, and joy through meaningful participation.

Navigating Social Challenges: For individuals with dementia who experience difficulties in social situations due to cognitive impairments, speech-language pathologists and therapists can provide targeted interventions to improve communication skills and enhance social confidence. These professionals can teach strategies for starting and maintaining conversations, understanding nonverbal cues, and expressing thoughts and feelings effectively, thus promoting more successful and fulfilling social interactions.

Monitoring and Adjusting Care Plans: As dementia progresses, your loved one's social needs and abilities may change. Professionals can continuously evaluate and adjust care plans to reflect these changes, making sure social engagement remains a central focus of the overall care strategy. By regularly reassessing and adapting to your loved one's evolving needs, professionals help maintain a consistent quality of life and social connectedness throughout the dementia journey.

Seeking the knowledge of professionals in dementia care is a proactive and empowering step toward making sure your loved one enjoys a socially rich and fulfilling life. By collaborating with a team of skilled professionals, you can access personalized support, tailored resources, and evidence-based strategies designed to maintain and enhance your loved one's social connections and engagement in meaningful activities.

This holistic approach not only enriches the life of your loved one with dementia but also provides invaluable support to you as a caregiver. With the guidance and knowledge of professionals, you can navigate the complexities of dementia care with greater confidence, knowing you are providing the best care and opportunities for social engagement.

Remember, enhancing social engagement is an ongoing process that requires patience, flexibility, and a willingness to adapt to changing needs. By leveraging the knowledge and skills of professionals, you can create a supportive and stimulating environment that promotes your loved one's overall well-being and quality of life, making sure they continue to find joy, purpose, and connection in their social interactions.

∿

FREQUENTLY ASKED QUESTIONS:

1. How can I ensure my loved one with dementia receives proper nutrition when they have a diminished appetite?

Answer: Start by offering smaller, more frequent meals throughout the day instead of three large ones. Focus on nutrient-dense foods that provide essential vitamins, minerals, and energy in smaller servings. Enhancing the flavor and aroma of meals can also stimulate appetite. If chewing or swallowing is an issue, try serving soft foods or smoothies that are easier to consume. Always ensure a comfortable, distraction-free meal setting to encourage eating.

2. My family member with dementia is becoming increasingly selective with their food. How can I manage this?

Answer: It's common for individuals with dementia to develop specific food preferences or aversions. Offer a variety of healthy options to choose from and pay attention to which foods are consistently accepted or rejected. Incorporating their favorite foods into meals can increase intake but try to balance this with nutritional needs. Experiment with different textures and flavors and involve them in meal choices to provide a sense of control and engagement.

3. What strategies can I use to handle difficulties with chewing and swallowing?

Answer: Modify the texture of foods to make them easier to chew and swallow. This might involve pureeing, mashing, or chopping foods into small, manageable pieces. Ensure foods are cooked until soft, and consider adding sauces or gravies to moisten dry meals. Always monitor your loved one while they eat to reduce the risk of choking and consult with a healthcare professional for personalized advice and swallowing exercises that may help.

4. How do I keep my loved one with dementia hydrated, especially if they forget to drink water?

Answer: Regular reminders and having a glass of water within easy reach can help. Offer fluids in small amounts throughout the day rather than large volumes at once. You can also increase fluid intake through foods with high water content, such as fruits, vegetables, soups, and smoothies. Consider offering a variety of beverages, like herbal teas or flavored waters, to make hydration more appealing.

5. Mealtime is becoming increasingly stressful for both of us. How can I make it a more positive experience?

Answer: Establishing a routine can provide comfort and predictability. Keep the dining environment calm and free of distractions, and maintain a positive, patient demeanor. Engage your loved one in simple meal preparation tasks to foster participation and a sense of achievement. If confusion or agitation arises, take a gentle approach, offering reassurance and redirecting attention if necessary. Remember, the goal is to make mealtime enjoyable and stress-free, focusing on the quality of the experience rather than just nutritional intake.

By addressing these common concerns with empathy, patience, and creativity, caregivers can significantly improve the dietary health and overall well-being of individuals with dementia.

~

CASE STUDY: MARY AND HER MOTHER, JUNE

MARY, a dedicated caregiver, faced a challenge familiar to many in her situation: ensuring her mother, June, who lives with dementia, receives proper nutrition and stays engaged and connected. June, a 78-year-old widow with a love for gardening and a lifetime of active community involvement, had seen her world shrink significantly since her dementia diagnosis. Mary noticed changes in June's eating habits and social interactions, which prompted her to seek solutions that respected her mother's dignity and independence.

Nutrition and Meal Planning:

June had always been a healthy eater, but dementia made mealtimes difficult. She would often forget to eat or lose interest in food altogether. Mary recognized the importance of a balanced diet in managing her mother's condition and sought to make meals more appealing and nutritious. She focused on incorporating June's favorite foods, ensuring many colors and textures to stimulate her appetite. Mary also adjusted meal sizes to smaller, more frequent portions, which seemed to suit June better.

One successful strategy was involving June in meal preparation, making it a daily activity they could enjoy together. This not only gave

June a sense of accomplishment but also made her more interested in eating what she had helped prepare. Mary learned the value of patience and flexibility, understanding that her mother's preferences could change from one day to the next.

Social Engagement:

Mary knew her mother missed her gardening and community volunteer work, so she looked for ways to adapt these activities to her current abilities. She created a small garden where June could tend to plants without the risk of wandering off. For community involvement, Mary found a local memory café where they could meet others facing similar challenges. These outings became a highlight for June, offering her the social interaction she craved in a safe and understanding environment.

Technology also played a role in keeping June connected. Mary set up video calls with family and introduced her to simple online games and virtual garden tours, which June could navigate with minimal assistance. These activities provided stimulation and a sense of connection to the wider world.

Lessons Learned:

Through this journey, Mary learned the importance of adaptability and creativity in dementia care. She realized that maintaining her mother's nutrition and social engagement required ongoing effort and change. Mary also saw the value in seeking support, whether from healthcare professionals, community resources, or technology solutions.

Mary understood that her mother's dignity and sense of self were paramount. By involving June in decisions, respecting her preferences, and finding joy in shared activities, Mary made sure her mother's life with dementia was fulfilling and dignified.

This case study exemplifies the challenges and rewards of caregiving for someone with dementia. It highlights the important role of nutrition and social engagement in enhancing the quality of life for individuals with dementia and underscores the lessons of patience,

adaptability, and the importance of maintaining dignity and independence.

~

PART TEN WRAP-UP:
ACTION ITEMS FOR THE CAREGIVER:

Personalize Meal Planning:

- Incorporate the care recipient's favorite foods into their diet.
- Ensure meals are colorful and varied to stimulate appetite.
- Adapt portion sizes to smaller, more frequent meals to suit changing appetites.

Involve in Meal Preparation:

- Engage the care recipient in simple meal preparation tasks.
- Use this as an opportunity to stimulate interest in food and eating.

Adjust Food Textures and Sizes:

- Modify foods to make them easier to eat, considering any chewing or swallowing difficulties.
- Offer pureed, soft-cooked, or finely chopped foods as necessary.

Optimize Hydration:

- Regularly encourage the drinking of water and other hydrating fluids.
- Include foods with high water content in meals.

Foster Social Connections:

- Schedule regular video calls with family and friends.
- Introduce simple online games or activities that can be shared remotely.

Incorporate Technology:

- Use tablets or simple-to-use computers for social interaction and entertainment.
- Explore virtual tours or online communities related to interests like gardening.

Engage in Physical and Social Activities:

- Create a safe, accessible garden space for interaction with nature.
- Find and participate in local community activities suitable for individuals with dementia, such as memory cafés.

Seek Support and Resources:

- Consult with dietitians for personalized nutritional advice.
- Explore community resources and programs designed for individuals with dementia and their caregivers.

Promote Independence and Participation:

- Encourage the care recipient to participate in their own care and decision-making as much as possible.

- Recognize and celebrate their contributions and efforts.

Adapt to Changing Needs:

- Be ready to adjust strategies and activities based on the care recipient's evolving preferences and abilities.
- Track and reassess nutritional needs and social activities regularly.

Maintain a Positive and Patient Approach:

- Focus on the process and enjoyment of activities rather than outcomes.
- Practice patience and flexibility in daily care and activities.

Focus on Caregiver Self-Care:

- Acknowledge the importance of the caregiver's own well-being.
- Seek emotional and practical support from support groups, friends, and family.
- These action items can help caregivers provide comprehensive, compassionate care that supports the nutritional and social well-being of individuals with dementia, enhancing their quality of life and maintaining dignity.

IN OUR NEXT PART...

IN OUR NEXT PART, "Empowering Through Nutrition and Movement," we dig into the critical aspects of maintaining and enhancing the physical health of individuals with dementia. A balanced diet and regular physical activity are not just foundational for general well-being; they play a pivotal role in managing dementia symptoms and improving quality of life. We'll explore practical, tailored strategies for integrating nutritious meals and enjoyable physical activities into daily routines, emphasizing the importance of hydration, the benefits of a diverse diet, and the joy of movement. This guide aims to equip caregivers with the knowledge and tools to create a supportive environment that fosters both physical vitality and joy in their loved ones.

We'll address the common challenges caregivers face in encouraging physical activity and maintaining a nutritious diet, offering solutions that cater to varying abilities and preferences. From creating engaging meal plans that accommodate dietary needs and preferences to selecting activities that improve balance, flexibility, and strength, this Part is designed to inspire caregivers to embrace a holistic approach to care. By the end of this journey, caregivers will feel more confident in their ability to make informed decisions that enrich the lives of those they care for, making sure every day is lived to its fullest potential with dignity, comfort, and happiness.

~

PART ELEVEN
PROMOTING PHYSICAL HEALTH AND WELLNESS IN DEMENTIA CARE

Maintaining physical health and wellness is a crucial part of providing comprehensive care for individuals with dementia. Engaging in regular physical activities and adopting a healthy lifestyle can have a profound impact on their overall quality of life and well-being.

Let's explore practical ways to promote physical health for your loved one with dementia.

Tailored Physical Activity: Encourage regular physical activity by tailoring exercise routines to match your loved one's abilities, interests, and preferences. Activities such as walking, gentle stretching, or chair exercises can help improve mobility, balance, and overall physical health. Focus on activities that are enjoyable and safe to encourage consistent participation and make exercise a positive experience.

Nutritious Diet: Ensure that your loved one receives a well-balanced and nutritious diet. Focus on meals rich in fruits, vegetables, whole grains, lean proteins, and healthy fats. Proper nutrition plays an important role in supporting cognitive function and overall physical health. Pay attention to hydration too, encouraging your loved one to drink water regularly throughout the day to prevent dehydration.

Adequate Sleep: Establish a consistent sleep schedule to promote better sleep quality. Create a comfortable and distraction-free sleeping environment that encourages relaxation. Consider implementing bedtime routines that promote calmness, such as reading a book, listening to soothing music, or engaging in gentle stretching exercises. Adequate sleep is essential for physical and mental rejuvenation.

Stress Reduction: Incorporate activities and techniques that help reduce stress and promote relaxation. This can include mindfulness practices, such as deep breathing exercises or guided meditation, listening to calming music, or spending time in nature. Be attentive to signs of stress or agitation in your loved one and adopt strategies to alleviate these feelings, creating a more peaceful and supportive environment.

Regular Health Monitoring: Schedule regular check-ups with healthcare professionals to track your loved one's overall health status and manage any existing medical conditions. Keep a close eye on signs of discomfort, pain, or illness, as individuals with dementia may have difficulty communicating their needs. Prompt attention to health concerns can prevent complications and ensure timely interventions.

Hydration and Oral Health: Encourage regular fluid intake to prevent dehydration, which can harm physical and cognitive health. Additionally, focus on oral health by scheduling regular dental check-ups and helping with daily dental hygiene routines as needed. Good oral health can prevent infections, discomfort, and other health complications.

Social Engagement and Physical Activity: Encourage participation in social activities that incorporate gentle physical movement and promote emotional well-being. This can include group exercise classes, community walks, or engaging in hobbies that involve physical activity. Social interactions combined with physical movement can provide a sense of purpose, connection, and enjoyment.

Safe Environment: Assess and modify the living environment to reduce the risk of falls and injuries. Install grab bars in bathrooms and other areas where support may be needed, remove trip hazards such as loose rugs or clutter, and ensure adequate lighting throughout the living space. A safe environment allows for more confident and independent movement.

Encouraging Independence: Support your loved one in maintaining physical independence. Encourage them to participate in activities of daily living, such as walking, performing simple household tasks, or engaging in hobbies that involve physical movement. Providing opportunities for self-directed physical activity can boost self-esteem and a sense of accomplishment.

Professional Guidance: Consult with physical therapists or exercise specialists with experience working with individuals with dementia. These professionals can provide personalized recommendations for safe and beneficial exercises and activities tailored to your loved one's specific needs and abilities. They can also guide proper form and technique to prevent injuries and optimize the benefits of physical activity.

Remember, promoting physical health and wellness in dementia care is an ongoing process that requires patience, adaptability, and a supportive approach. By focusing on these key areas, you can help your loved one maintain their physical well-being, improve their quality of life, and experience the many benefits that come with an active and healthy lifestyle.

It's essential to celebrate the small victories and appreciate the efforts your loved one puts forth in maintaining their physical health. Offer encouragement, praise, and support throughout their journey, recognizing that every step toward better physical wellness is a significant accomplishment.

By focusing on physical health and wellness, you are not only enhancing your loved one's overall well-being but also creating opportunities for meaningful connections, shared experiences, and cherished moments. Your dedication to a healthy lifestyle can make a profound difference in their life, enabling them to navigate the challenges of dementia with greater resilience, comfort, and vitality.

~

THE POWER OF MOVEMENT: EMBRACING EXERCISE FOR BETTER HEALTH AND WELL-BEING

As a caregiver, it's important to understand the significant role that physical activity plays in maintaining overall health and well-being, not just for yourself but also for the person you're caring for, especially if they have dementia. Regular exercise offers a wide range of benefits that go beyond keeping fit. It's an important part of a healthy lifestyle that contributes to both physical and mental well-being. Let's explore how incorporating exercise into daily routines can make a positive difference.

Strengthening the Heart: Cardiovascular Benefits

One of the most important benefits of regular exercise is its positive impact on heart health. When you engage in physical activity, your heart muscle becomes stronger, letting it pump blood more efficiently throughout the body. This improved circulation helps deliver oxygen to organs and tissues more effectively and lowers the risk of developing heart diseases. Exercise also helps manage blood pressure and maintain healthy cholesterol levels, further supporting a healthy cardiovascular system.

Lifting the Mood: Emotional Benefits

Exercise doesn't just benefit the body; it also has a significant impact on mental well-being. You may have experienced a feeling of happiness or satisfaction after a workout. This is because exercise triggers the release of endorphins, which are natural mood boosters. Regular physical activity can help reduce symptoms of anxiety and depression, promoting a more balanced and positive emotional state. It also provides a healthy outlet for stress relief, letting you channel energy constructively and develop greater emotional resilience.

Boosting Energy Levels: Increasing Vitality

It may seem counterintuitive, but expending energy through exercise actually leads to increased vitality. When you engage in physical activity, your body experiences improved blood flow and oxygen delivery, resulting in a natural energy boost. Regular exercise helps fight off feelings of fatigue and sluggishness, leaving you feeling more alert, focused, and ready to take on daily challenges. By making exercise a part of your routine, you can tap into a renewable source of energy that benefits both the body and mind.

Managing Weight: A Balanced Approach

Exercise is an effective tool for maintaining a healthy weight. When you engage in physical activity, your body burns calories, contributing to weight management. However, the benefits go beyond burning calories. Regular exercise helps build and maintain lean muscle mass, which has a higher metabolic rate than fat tissue. This means that even when you're resting, your body continues to burn calories more efficiently, supporting your weight management goals.

Boosting the Immune System: Strengthening Defenses

Regular physical activity acts as a powerful ally in strengthening the immune system. During exercise, the body experiences a temporary increase in the production of immune cells and antibodies, enhancing its ability to fight off infections and diseases. Consistent moderate exercise helps the immune system function optimally, enabling better defense against illnesses and faster recovery when sickness occurs.

Improving Sleep Quality: Promoting Restful Slumber

If getting a good night's sleep is a challenge, exercise may be the solution. Regular physical activity helps regulate the body's sleep-wake cycle, making it easier to fall asleep and promoting deeper, more restorative stages of sleep. By incorporating exercise into daily routines, you can establish healthier sleep patterns, leading to improved energy levels and overall well-being.

Developing Flexibility and Strength: Building a Resilient Body

Engaging in many physical activities, such as strength training, stretching, and balance exercises, contributes to the development of a strong and resilient body. Regular exercise helps maintain and improve flexibility, reducing the risk of injuries and enhancing overall mobility. By challenging muscles through resistance training, you can build lean muscle mass, increase bone density, and improve overall strength and stability. A well-rounded exercise routine that includes different activities promotes a balanced and capable physique.

Embracing exercise as a regular part of daily life is a powerful step toward achieving better health and well-being, not just for caregivers but also for those they care for, particularly individuals with dementia. By focusing on physical activity, you unlock many benefits that extend beyond just fitness. From strengthening the heart and boosting mood to increasing energy levels and enhancing sleep quality, exercise is a transformative tool that can greatly improve overall well-being.

As you start a more active lifestyle, remember to approach exercise with enjoyment and self-compassion. Find activities you and the person you're caring for can enjoy together, whether it's a gentle walk in the park, a simple stretching routine, or a fun dance session. Always consult with a healthcare provider to make sure the chosen activities are appropriate and align with individual needs and any existing health conditions.

By making exercise a consistent part of your daily routine, you invest in both your own well-being and that of the person you're caring for.

Embrace the power of movement and unlock the potential for a healthier, happier, and more vibrant life. Let your commitment to physical activity be a driving force for positive change, guiding you toward a path of improved wellness and endless possibilities.

~

HELPING YOUR LOVED ONE WITH DEMENTIA EAT WELL: MAKING HEALTHY CHOICES FOR BETTER NUTRITION

As a caregiver, you play an important role in supporting the overall health and well-being of your loved one with dementia. An important aspect of their care ensures that they maintain a well-balanced diet. Making smart food choices and adopting healthy eating habits can have a significant impact on their physical wellness and quality of life. Let's explore key aspects of eating well and how you can help your loved one incorporate them into their daily routine.

Embracing Variety: The Importance of a Colorful Plate

Encourage your loved one to eat a variety of foods by presenting them with a colorful plate filled with a diverse array of fruits, vegetables, whole grains, lean proteins, and healthy fats. Each color in the rainbow of foods represents different vitamins, minerals, and beneficial compounds that work together to support overall health. By offering a range of nutritious options, you make sure your loved one receives the diverse range of nutrients their body needs to thrive.

Mindful Portion Sizes: Eating in Moderation

Help your loved one in practicing portion control by serving them appropriate serving sizes. Be mindful of the amounts they consume and encourage them to listen to their body's signals of fullness. If they express hunger after finishing a meal, offer them additional small portions of nutritious foods. Remember, it's easier to start with smaller portions and provide more if needed, rather than overwhelming them with large quantities of food.

Staying Hydrated: The Importance of Water

Ensure that your loved one stays properly hydrated by encouraging regular water intake throughout the day. Aim for at least eight glasses or more, depending on their individual needs. If plain water doesn't appeal to them, try infusing it with slices of lemon, cucumber, or fresh berries to add a refreshing twist. Keep a water bottle nearby and offer it to them often as a gentle reminder to stay hydrated.

Planning Ahead: Preparing Nutritious Meals

Take the time to plan and prepare meals in advance for your loved one with dementia. By having wholesome meals and snacks readily available, you can make sure they consistently have access to nutritious options. Consider prepping ingredients, cooking in batches, or portioning out meals for the week ahead. This proactive approach not only saves time but also guarantees that nourishing choices are easily accessible when your loved one needs them.

Mindful Eating: Savoring Each Bite

Encourage your loved one to practice mindful eating by creating a calm and pleasant dining environment. Sit with them during meals and engage them in conversation about the flavors, textures, and aromas of the food. Encourage them to take their time, savoring each bite and being present in the moment. Mindful eating can help them tune into their body's hunger and fullness signals, letting them eat until comfortably satisfied rather than overeating.

Adapting to Changing Needs: Flexibility and Patience

As your loved one's dementia progresses, their eating habits and preferences may change. Be patient and flexible, adapting meals and routines as needed. If they experience difficulty with utensils, offer finger foods or provide help during mealtimes. If their appetite goes down, offer smaller, more frequent meals throughout the day. Continuously monitor their eating habits and make adjustments to ensure they receive the necessary nutrition.

Helping your loved one with dementia adopt smart eating habits is an essential part of their care. By encouraging variety, practicing portion control, ensuring hydration, planning ahead, promoting mindful eating, and adapting to their changing needs, you can support their overall physical wellness and quality of life.

Remember that making dietary changes is a gradual process, and small, consistent steps can lead to significant improvements. Be patient, celebrate progress, and find joy in the journey of nourishing your loved one with wholesome, delicious foods.

As you support your loved one on this path of mindful eating, remember that every healthy choice you help them make is an investment in their long-term well-being. By helping them to fuel their body with the right nutrients, you empower them to live life to the fullest, with the energy, vitality, and resilience to tackle the challenges that come with dementia. Embrace the power of smart eating habits and discover the transformative impact they can have on your loved one's physical wellness and overall quality of life.

∼

HELPING YOUR LOVED ONE WITH DEMENTIA GET RESTORATIVE SLEEP: UNLOCKING THE FOUNDATION OF HEALTH AND VITALITY

As a caregiver, making sure your loved one with dementia gets sufficient and restorative sleep is a crucial part of supporting their overall health and well-being. While managing dementia can present unique challenges, focusing on sleep is essential for their physical and mental wellness. In this comprehensive guide, we will explore why quality sleep is important for individuals with dementia and how you can help them cultivate healthy sleep habits to unlock their full potential.

The Vital Functions of Sleep for Individuals with Dementia:

Sleep is not merely a passive state of rest; it is an active process during which the body undergoes essential repairs, rejuvenation, and restoration. For individuals with dementia, quality sleep is especially important for these reasons:

Cognitive Function and Memory: Sleep plays an important role in cognitive function, including memory consolidation and mental clarity. Helping your loved one achieve restorative sleep can support their cognitive abilities and potentially slow down the progression of dementia symptoms.

Emotional Well-being and Behavioral Management: Quality sleep patterns are closely linked to improved mood, emotional regulation, and overall well-being. Enough rest can help reduce agitation, anxiety, and other behavioral challenges often associated with dementia.

Physical Health and Resilience: During sleep, the body releases growth hormones that stimulate muscle repair, tissue growth, and protein synthesis. Ensuring your loved one gets enough restorative sleep supports their physical health, boosts their immune system, and enhances their overall resilience.

Strategies for Enhancing Sleep Quality for Your Loved One with Dementia:

As a caregiver, you can play an active role in helping your loved one with dementia achieve better sleep quality. Here are effective strategies to implement:

Establish a Consistent Sleep Schedule: Maintain a regular sleep schedule for your loved one, aiming for consistent bedtimes and wake times. This consistency helps regulate their body's internal clock, known as the circadian rhythm, promoting more restful and rejuvenating sleep.

Create a Calming Bedtime Routine: Develop a soothing pre-sleep ritual for your loved one that signals to their body and mind that it's time to wind down. This can include activities such as reading together, playing soft music, or engaging in gentle stretching or relaxation techniques. Consistently following this routine helps create a sense of familiarity and comfort.

Optimize the Sleep Environment: Transform your loved one's bedroom into a sleep sanctuary that promotes relaxation and comfort. Keep the room cool, dark, and quiet, using blackout curtains, earplugs, or a white noise machine if needed. Ensure their bed is comfortable and supportive, with pillows and bedding that align with their preferences.

Manage Diet and Lifestyle Habits: Be mindful of your loved one's eating habits and their impact on sleep. Avoid serving heavy or large meals close to bedtime, as the digestive process can interfere with sleep. Limit caffeine and alcohol intake, especially in the late afternoon and evening, as they can disrupt sleep patterns.

Engage in Regular Physical Activity: Encourage your loved one to participate in regular physical activity, as it can promote better sleep quality. Engage them in gentle exercises, such as walking or stretching, during the day to help them expend energy and prepare their body for restful sleep at night.

Consult with Healthcare Professionals: Work closely with your loved one's healthcare team, including their primary care doctor and any specialists involved in their dementia care. They can provide personalized recommendations and guidance on managing sleep issues specific to your loved one's needs.

Chapter Summary:

As a caregiver, focusing on your loved one's sleep quality is an important investment in their overall health and well-being. By understanding the critical role that sleep plays in cognitive function, emotional well-being, and physical resilience, you can appreciate the transformative power of restorative rest for individuals with dementia.

Incorporating sleep-enhancing strategies into your loved one's daily routine, such as maintaining a consistent sleep schedule, creating a calming bedtime ritual, optimizing their sleep environment, managing their diet and lifestyle habits, and engaging them in regular physical activity, can significantly improve the quality and duration of their sleep.

Remember, supporting your loved one's sleep is an essential part of their dementia care. By making sleep a non-negotiable priority, you empower them to unlock their full potential, fostering resilience, vitality, and ideal health.

Embrace the restorative power of sleep for your loved one with dementia and witness the profound impact it can have on their physical, mental, and emotional well-being. As you start this journey toward better sleep, be patient, consistent, and compassionate in your efforts, knowing that each night of quality rest is a step toward a healthier, more comfortable life for your loved one.

～

HELPING YOUR LOVED ONE WITH DEMENTIA MANAGE STRESS: THE VITAL ROLE OF STRESS MANAGEMENT IN PHYSICAL WELLNESS

As a caregiver, supporting your loved one with dementia in managing stress is a crucial part of promoting their overall physical health and well-being. While providing a nurturing environment and ensuring their basic needs are met is essential, the impact of stress on their physical well-being cannot be understated. Stress can gradually erode their health from within, affecting nearly every system in their body.

In this comprehensive guide, we will explore the interconnectedness of stress management and physical wellness for individuals with dementia, providing actionable strategies to help you fortify their body against the harmful effects of chronic stress.

The Physiological Impact of Stress on Individuals with Dementia:

Stress is not merely a mental or emotional burden; it manifests itself in real physical ways. When your loved one with dementia experiences stress, their body enters a state of heightened alertness, triggering a cascade of physiological changes. The "fight or flight" response, mediated by the release of stress hormones such as cortisol and adrenaline, can be pronounced in individuals with dementia.

Prolonged exposure to stress can disrupt various bodily systems, leading to a range of health issues. Chronic stress has been linked to high blood pressure, cardiovascular disease, obesity, diabetes, and a weakened immune system. It can also exacerbate existing health conditions and impair their ability to recover from illness or injury. By understanding the profound impact of stress on your loved one's physical well-being, you can take proactive steps to help them manage it effectively.

Strategies for Effective Stress Management for Your Loved One with Dementia:

To shield your loved one's body against the harmful effects of stress and promote their overall physical wellness, consider integrating these practices into their daily routine:

Creating a Calming Environment: Establish a calm and soothing environment for your loved one. Reduce clutter, noise, and distractions, and incorporate elements that promote relaxation, such as soft lighting, comfortable seating, and gentle music or nature sounds.

Encouraging Physical Activity: Engage your loved one in regular physical activity, tailored to their abilities and preferences. Even gentle exercises like walking, stretching, or chair yoga can help alleviate stress, improve cardiovascular health, and boost overall well-being.

Providing a Balanced Diet: Ensure that your loved one receives a balanced and nutritious diet rich in fruits, vegetables, lean proteins, and whole grains. Avoid excessive caffeine, sugar, and processed foods, as they can contribute to stress and mood fluctuations.

Promoting Quality Sleep: Prioritize your loved one's sleep quality by establishing a regular sleep schedule and creating a conducive sleep environment. Ensure their bedroom is comfortable, quiet, and dark, and encourage relaxing bedtime routines to help them unwind.

Ensuring Proper Hydration: Keep your loved one well-hydrated by offering them water, herbal teas, or water infused with fruits throughout the day. Dehydration can exacerbate feelings of stress and fatigue, so ensuring an adequate fluid intake is important.

Fostering Social Connections: Encourage and help with social interactions for your loved one, whether it's with family members, friends, or support groups. Engaging in enjoyable activities and maintaining social connections can provide a sense of belonging and emotional support, helping to reduce stress.

Engaging in Meaningful Activities: Help your loved one pursue activities that bring them joy, relaxation, and a sense of purpose. This could include hobbies, creative projects, or reminiscence activities that tap into their interests and memories.

Seeking Professional Support: If your loved one's stress becomes overwhelming or difficult to manage, please seek the guidance of healthcare professionals specializing in dementia care. They can provide personalized strategies, coping mechanisms, and support tailored to your loved one's specific needs.

Integrating Stress Management into Your Loved One's Daily Routine:

Incorporating stress management techniques into your loved one's daily life need not be an overwhelming endeavor. Begin by selecting one or two strategies that resonate with them and gradually integrate them into their routine. Consistency is key; even small, consistent efforts can yield significant improvements in their physical health and overall well-being .

Chapter Summary:

Recognizing the profound impact of stress on your loved one's physical health is an important step toward promoting their holistic wellness. By proactively helping them manage stress through creating a calming environment, encouraging physical activity, providing a balanced diet, promoting quality sleep, ensuring proper hydration, fostering social connections, engaging in meaningful activities, and seeking professional support when needed, you can fortify their body against the harmful effects of chronic stress.

As you start this journey of stress management with your loved one, remember to be patient, compassionate, and adaptable. Celebrate the small victories along the way and remain committed to focusing on their physical and mental well-being.

By helping your loved one with dementia tame tension and embrace effective stress management strategies, you empower them to lead a more comfortable, fulfilling life, free from the burdens of chronic stress. Their physical health will benefit, and you'll see a renewed sense of resilience, vitality, and overall wellness in their daily life. Take the first step today and watch as the transformative power of stress management unfolds in your loved one's journey with dementia.

~

SUPPORTING YOUR LOVED ONE WITH DEMENTIA IN ACHIEVING PHYSICAL VITALITY: CRAFTING REALISTIC GOALS AND SUSTAINABLE ROUTINES

As a caregiver, supporting your loved one with dementia in their pursuit of physical vitality is a commitment to their overall well-being and quality of life. By helping them set achievable fitness goals and establish sustainable exercise routines tailored to their abilities, you can foster their physical health, improve their mood, and enhance their cognitive function. In this comprehensive guide, we will explore how you can help your loved one in crafting realistic fitness goals and developing routines that promote long-term adherence and success.

Crafting Achievable Fitness Goals for Your Loved One with Dementia:

The foundation of a successful fitness journey for your loved one lies in setting goals that align with their current abilities and interests. By carefully considering their starting point and defining clear, measurable goals, you can create a rewarding and fulfilling experience for them. Here's how to approach this important step:

Assess Their Starting Point: Begin by honestly evaluating your loved one's current fitness level, considering factors such as their exercise history, physical limitations, and overall health status. Understanding their baseline lets you tailor goals that are challenging yet attainable, ensuring a sense of progress and achievement along the way.

Define Clear, Measurable Objectives: Clarity is key when setting fitness goals for your loved one. Whether the aim is to walk a specific distance, perform a certain number of chair exercises, or simply incorporate more movement into their daily routine, make sure the goals are specific, measurable, and achievable. This approach provides a roadmap for success and lets you track their progress effectively.

Embrace Incremental Progress: Remember that fitness is a gradual process, especially for individuals with dementia. Break down larger goals into manageable, incremental steps that allow your loved one to experience a sense of accomplishment and maintain motivation throughout their journey. Celebrate the small victories along the way and focus on the progress they make, no matter how small.

Align Goals with Personal Interests: Choose activities that resonate with your loved one's interests and passions. When they genuinely enjoy their workouts, adherence becomes effortless. Whether it's dancing to their favorite music, engaging in gentle water exercises, or participating in a beloved sport adapted to their abilities, aligning their fitness goals with activities that bring them joy will transform exercise into a cherished part of their daily life.

Building a Sustainable Exercise Routine for Your Loved One with Dementia:

A well-structured exercise routine serves as the backbone of any successful fitness journey for your loved one. By crafting a program that is diverse, flexible, and tailored to their individual needs, you lay the foundation for long-term adherence and sustainable progress. Here's how to build a routine that stands the test of time:

Diversify Their Workouts: Incorporate a balanced mix of activities that target various parts of physical health, such as cardiovascular exercise, strength training, and flexibility work. This holistic approach not only prevents boredom but also ensures a well-rounded fitness experience. Aim to engage your loved one in activities that challenge their endurance, maintain their muscle strength, and improve their overall flexibility and mobility.

Find the Right Fit: Tailor the exercise routine to your loved one's abilities, preferences, and schedule. If they have limited mobility, consider incorporating chair exercises or gentle stretching routines. If they enjoy social interaction, explore group activities or classes designed for individuals with dementia. By finding a fit that aligns with their needs and preferences, you increase the likelihood of long-term adherence and enjoyment.

Prioritize Safety and Comfort: Ensure that the exercise environment is safe, secure, and comfortable for your loved one. Modify activities as needed to accommodate their physical limitations and provide any necessary support or assistance. Monitor their response to exercise and adjust the intensity or duration to prevent overexertion or discomfort.

Encourage Regular Movement: Incorporate physical activity into your loved one's daily routine, even if it's through small, manageable actions. Encourage them to take short walks, perform simple stretches, or engage in light household tasks that promote movement. Regular physical activity not only supports their fitness goals but also helps maintain their mobility and independence.

Provide Positive Reinforcement: Offer consistent encouragement and praise for your loved one's efforts and achievements. Celebrate their progress, no matter how small, and focus on the positive aspects of their fitness journey. Your support and positive reinforcement can be powerful motivators, helping them stay engaged and motivated.

Adapt and Adjust as Needed: Recognize that your loved one's fitness journey may evolve over time due to changes in their cognitive and physical abilities. Be open to adjusting their routine and goals as needed to ensure their safety, comfort, and continued enjoyment. Regularly assess their progress and make changes that align with their changing needs and preferences.

Seek Professional Guidance: Consult with healthcare professionals, such as physical therapists or occupational therapists, who specialize in working with individuals with dementia. They can provide valuable insights, recommend exercises, and offer guidance on adapting activities to your loved one's specific needs. Their knowledge can be invaluable in creating a safe and effective fitness plan.

Chapter Summary:

Supporting your loved one with dementia in their pursuit of physical vitality is a meaningful and rewarding endeavor. By helping them set achievable goals, build a sustainable routine, and maintain a positive mindset, you lay the foundation for improved physical health, enhanced cognitive function, and a better overall quality of life.

Approach your loved one's fitness journey with patience, compassion, and a willingness to adapt. Celebrate their victories, no matter how small, and view challenges as opportunities for growth and learning. Stay attuned to their needs, adjust your approach as necessary, and surround them with a supportive and encouraging environment.

Remember that the ultimate goal is not merely reaching a specific fitness milestone but fostering a sense of well-being, purpose, and enjoyment in your loved one's life. Trust in their abilities, find joy in the process, and let your commitment to their care guide them toward a life of enhanced physical vitality and fulfillment.

As you support your loved one in charting their path to physical vitality, celebrate the unique journey you share. Your dedication, love, and unwavering support will make a profound difference in their lives, helping them unlock their full potential and experience the many benefits of a physically active and engaged lifestyle.

$\sim$

SUPPORTING YOUR LOVED ONE WITH DEMENTIA IN NURTURING THE MIND-BODY SYMPHONY: UNLOCKING THE PATH TO HOLISTIC WELL-BEING

As a caregiver, supporting your loved one with dementia in their pursuit of holistic well-being involves nurturing the intricate connection between their physical and mental health. By helping them cultivate physical vigor, explore mindful practices, and harmonize their mind and body, you can guide them toward a more balanced, fulfilling existence. In this comprehensive guide, we will explore how you can help your loved one in unlocking the path to holistic well-being and promote their overall quality of life.

Cultivating Physical Vigor for Your Loved One with Dementia:

The foundation of holistic health for your loved one lies in nurturing their physical body with care and respect. By focusing on consistent physical activity, nourishing them with wholesome foods, and ensuring restorative sleep, you lay the groundwork for their optimal physical well-being. Here's how you can support them in elevating their physical health:

Encourage Regular Physical Activity: Engage your loved one in regular exercise appropriate for their abilities and interests. This can include gentle walks, chair exercises, or simple stretching routines. Regular physical activity not only supports their physical health but also releases endorphins, promoting a positive mood and emotional well-being.

Provide Nourishing Meals: Ensure that your loved one's diet includes wholesome, nutrient-dense foods that support their physical health. Incorporate a variety of fruits, vegetables, whole grains, lean proteins, and healthy fats into their meals. Help them to make healthy food choices and give them support during mealtimes.

Prioritize Restorative Sleep: Create a soothing bedtime routine for your loved one and ensure a comfortable sleep environment. Encourage them to maintain a consistent sleep schedule and provide any necessary assistance with their nighttime needs. Quality sleep is essential for their physical restoration, mental clarity, and emotional balance.

Exploring the Mind-Body Connection with Your Loved One with Dementia:

While physical health forms the foundation of well-being, nurturing your loved one's mental and emotional landscapes is equally important. By exploring and deepening their mind-body connection, you can help them tap into a powerful source of inner harmony and resilience. Here's how you can support them in cultivating this profound connection:

Encourage Mindful Practices: Introduce your loved one to simple mindfulness exercises, such as deep breathing or guided imagery. These practices can help reduce stress, anxiety, and agitation while promoting a sense of calm and inner peace. Engage in these practices together, creating a shared experience of mindfulness and connection.

Adapt Yoga for Their Abilities: Explore gentle yoga practices suitable for your loved one's physical abilities and cognitive level. Yoga combines purposeful movements, controlled breathing, and meditative focus, promoting a sense of unity between the mind and body. Help them to perform simple yoga postures or chair yoga exercises, focusing on their comfort and safety.

Incorporate Mindfulness into Daily Activities: Encourage your loved one to bring mindfulness into their daily life by focusing on the present moment during various activities. This can include savoring a meal, enjoying a calming sensory experience, or engaging in a favorite hobby with full attention. By incorporating mindfulness into their routine, you help them cultivate a greater sense of presence and well-being.

Harmonizing Mind and Body for Your Loved One with Dementia:

Supporting your loved one in their journey toward holistic well-being involves recognizing and honoring the symbiotic relationship between their mental and physical health. By integrating mindful practices and physical care into their daily routine, you create a solid foundation for their lasting vitality and happiness. Here's how you can help them harmonize their mind and body:

Create a Supportive Environment: Establish a calm and nurturing environment that promotes relaxation and reduces stress for your loved one. This can include organizing a clutter-free living space, incorporating soothing colors and textures, and providing a sense of safety and comfort. A supportive environment can have a positive impact on their overall well-being.

Encourage Self-Expression: Provide opportunities for your loved one to express themselves creatively, such as through art, music, or story-telling. These activities not only promote self-expression but also stimulate cognitive function and emotional well-being. Engage in these activities together, fostering a sense of connection and shared enjoyment.

Adapt to Their Unique Needs: Recognize that your loved one's journey toward holistic well-being is unique and may require adaptations based on their specific needs and abilities. Be patient, compassionate, and willing to adjust your approach as necessary. Celebrate their progress, no matter how small, and provide ongoing support and encouragement.

Collaborate with Healthcare Professionals: Work closely with healthcare professionals, such as doctors, occupational therapists, and mental health specialists, to create a comprehensive care plan that addresses your loved one's physical and mental well-being. Seek their guidance in implementing interventions and strategies that support your loved one's holistic health.

Chapter Summary:

Supporting your loved one with dementia in nurturing the mind-body symphony is a profound and meaningful endeavor. By helping them cultivate physical vigor, explore mindful practices, and harmonize their mind and body, you unlock the path to their holistic well-being and enhance their overall quality of life.

Approach this journey with patience, compassion, and a deep appreciation for the unique needs and experiences of your loved one. Celebrate the small victories, learn from challenges, and trust in the power of your love and support to guide them toward a more balanced and fulfilling existence.

Remember, the path to holistic well-being is not about perfection but about progress. Embrace each day as an opportunity to nurture your loved one's mind-body connection, fostering a sense of inner peace, resilience, and joy. Your unwavering dedication and support will create a profound impact on their life, helping them navigate the challenges of dementia with grace and dignity.

Cherish the moments of connection, the shared experiences of mindfulness, and the love that binds you. By supporting your loved one in nurturing their mind-body symphony, you not only enhance their well-being but also strengthen the bond you share.

Embrace the beauty of this journey, one mindful step at a time, and let the power of holistic well-being guide you and your loved one toward a life of greater harmony, resilience, and fulfillment.

∽

CARING FOR YOURSELF WHILE CARING FOR OTHERS: A GUIDE FOR CAREGIVERS

CARING for a loved one can be one of the most rewarding experiences, but it's not without its challenges. As a caregiver, you're giving your time, energy, and love to ensure your loved one's well-being. However, this selfless act can take a toll on you if you're not careful. Caregiver stress and burnout are common, affecting your ability to provide care and compromising your own health and happiness.

Recognizing the Signs

Caregiving can sometimes feel like you're navigating rough waters, with the waves of responsibility threatening to overwhelm you. Signs of caregiver stress may manifest differently:

- Physical exhaustion
- Emotional fatigue
- Irritability
- Sleep disturbances
- Changes in appetite
- Feelings of detachment or hopelessness

It's important to recognize these signs early on, as this is the first step toward regaining balance and preventing burnout.

Strategies for Self-Care

While caregiving is a selfless act, it's essential to focus on your own well-being. After all, you can't pour from an empty cup. Here are strategies to help you manage stress and avoid burnout:

- **Seek Support**: You need not go through this journey alone. Join caregiver support groups, either in-person or online, to share experiences and gain insights from others who understand what you're going through.
- **Delegate Responsibilities**: Don't be afraid to ask for help. Contact family members, friends, or professional services to share caregiving duties. Remember, asking for help is a sign of strength, not weakness.
- **Make Time for Yourself**: Dedicate time for activities that nourish your mind, body, and spirit. Whether it's reading, going for a walk, practicing meditation, or engaging in a hobby you enjoy, these moments of respite are important.
- **Stay Informed**: Knowledge is power. Learn as much as you can about your loved one's condition and the resources available to caregivers. This can help reduce uncertainties and make caregiving tasks feel more manageable.
- **Set Boundaries**: It's okay to say no sometimes. Establish clear boundaries on what you can and cannot do and communicate these boundaries with others to manage expectations and prevent resentment.
- **Practice Mindfulness**: Engage in mindfulness practices like meditation or yoga. These can help you stay centered, reduce stress, and enhance your emotional resilience.
- **Consult Professionals**: Don't hesitate to seek advice from healthcare providers, therapists, or counselors. Professional guidance can provide valuable coping strategies and emotional support.

The Path to Well-being

In the demanding role of a caregiver, it's easy to neglect your own needs. However, your well-being is the foundation on which effective caregiving rests. By embracing self-care and utilizing available resources, you can navigate the challenges of caregiving with strength and compassion.

Remember, caring for yourself is not just an act of self-preservation; it's an integral part of being a capable and loving caregiver. Empower yourself with the tools and support needed to maintain your health and spirit, ensuring you can continue to provide the care your loved one deserves.

∾

EMPOWERING YOURSELF: ESSENTIAL SELF-CARE FOR CAREGIVERS

CARING for a loved one is a noble and loving act that requires immense **Strength, Patience,** and **Resilience**. While it's a journey filled with rewarding moments, it also presents challenges that can test your limits. To sustain the care you provide, embracing self-care is not just important—it's essential. Here are strategies to help you nurture your well-being as you navigate the caregiving journey:

Establish Clear Boundaries: Setting boundaries is important for managing the demands placed on you. Understand your limits and communicate them clearly to your loved one and others involved in caregiving. This helps manage expectations and prevent feelings of resentment or overwhelm.

Seek and Accept Help: Remember, you're not an island, and asking for help is a sign of wisdom, not weakness. Whether it's soliciting family members to share caregiving duties or contacting professional services, getting support is vital. Delegating tasks lets you recharge and maintain your resilience.

Prioritize Time for Yourself: Integrate regular breaks into your schedule. Use this time to engage in activities that bring you joy and relaxation. Whether it's a hobby, exercise, or simply sitting quietly, these moments are essential for your mental and emotional health.

Nurture Your Health: Your physical well-being is the foundation of your ability to care for others. Focus on nutritious eating, regular physical activity, and adequate rest. Remember, taking care of your health enables you to be present for your loved one.

Embrace Mindfulness and Relaxation: Stress is an inevitable part of caregiving, but its impact can be mitigated. Practices such as meditation, yoga, or simply taking deep breaths can significantly lower stress levels and enhance your emotional equilibrium.

Connect with Support Networks: You're not alone in this journey. Connecting with others in similar situations can provide comfort, understanding, and valuable insights. Whether through support groups, online forums, or informal gatherings, these connections can be a source of strength and encouragement.

Seek Professional Support When Needed: If feelings of stress, anxiety, or depression become overwhelming, please seek professional help. Therapists and counselors can offer strategies to manage these emotions and support your well-being.

By adopting these self-care strategies, you can safeguard your health and well-being, enabling you to continue providing care with love and patience. Remember, caring for yourself is a testament to your commitment to your loved one. You're doing an incredible job, and it's okay—and necessary—to step back and care for yourself too.

～

CARING FOR YOURSELF: NAVIGATING CAREGIVER STRESS AND BURNOUT

As a dedicated caregiver, your primary focus is on providing compassionate care for your loved one. However, your own well-being is the foundation on which your caregiving ability rests. Caregiver stress and burnout can slowly creep in, gradually eroding your physical, emotional, and mental resilience. Acknowledging the signs of burnout and taking proactive steps to address them is key to maintaining your ability to provide the care your loved one needs.

Recognizing the Signs of Burnout

Being aware of the common indicators of caregiver burnout can help you take timely action to address the issue. Look out for:

- **Persistent Fatigue**: Feeling constantly tired, even after periods of rest, can signify physical and emotional exhaustion.
- **Increased Irritability**: Becoming easily frustrated or irritated by minor issues may be a sign of underlying stress.
- **Sense of Overwhelming**: Feeling that your caregiving duties have become insurmountable, leading to feelings of defeat or despair.

- **Sleep Disturbances**: Significant changes in your sleep patterns, such as difficulty sleeping or oversleeping, can be a red flag.
- **Emotional Distress**: Experiencing persistent anxiety, depression, or constant worrying can show emotional turmoil.
- **Self-neglect**: Prioritizing your loved one's needs for neglecting your own health and well-being is a concerning sign.

Recognizing these warning signs early on can help you take proactive steps to prevent further emotional and physical deterioration, letting you maintain your caregiving capacity.

Pathways to Well-being

To mitigate the risk of burnout and ensure you can continue providing compassionate care, consider these strategies:

- **Seek and Accept Support**: Utilize your network of friends, family, or community resources. Sharing caregiving responsibilities can alleviate stress and provide much-needed respite.
- **Embrace Self-Care**: Incorporate self-care practices into your daily routine, such as pursuing a hobby, engaging in exercise, or taking moments of quiet reflection. These activities can help replenish your energy and spirit.
- **Establish Boundaries**: Set realistic boundaries around your caregiving responsibilities to manage expectations and reduce feelings of being overwhelmed.
- **Focus on Health**: Maintain a healthy lifestyle by ensuring you're eating well, staying active, and getting adequate rest. Your physical health is the foundation for your caregiving abilities.
- **Seek Professional Guidance**: Don't hesitate to seek support from therapists or counselors if feelings of stress, anxiety, or depression persist. They can offer coping strategies tailored to your specific situation.

Caring for yourself is not an act of selfishness; it's a necessity. By recognizing the signs of burnout and taking proactive steps to address them, you can safeguard your well-being and ensure you can continue providing the best care for your loved one.

∼

FINDING BALANCE: NAVIGATING CAREGIVER STRESS WITH COMPASSION AND SUPPORT

CARING for a loved one is a journey marked by compassion and commitment, yet it's not without its challenges. The emotional and physical demands of caregiving can lead to stress and burnout, underscoring the critical importance of self-care for caregivers.

Here are empowering strategies to help you manage caregiver stress and maintain your well-being, ensuring you can continue to provide the best care for your loved one.

Building Your Support Circle

- **Engage with Support Networks**: Connect with friends, family, and caregiver support groups who understand your experiences. These connections offer emotional sustenance, practical advice, and a sense of community, helping to alleviate feelings of isolation.
- **Embrace Help**: Recognize that seeking help is a sign of strength, not weakness. Whether it's enlisting family members to share caregiving duties or hiring professional assistance, lightening your load can help prevent burnout.

Prioritizing Self-Care

- **Take Time for Yourself**: Regular breaks are essential. Dedicate time each day to activities that rejuvenate your spirit, whether it's a hobby, exercise, or simply enjoying a moment of solitude.
- **Mind Your Health**: Ensure you're eating nutritious meals, getting enough sleep, and staying physically active. Your physical health is the foundation for your ability to care for others.

Establishing Boundaries

- **Set Limits**: Clearly define what you can and cannot do. Setting boundaries helps manage expectations and respects your limits, ensuring you don't become overwhelmed.
- **Learn to Delegate**: Share responsibilities with others. Delegating tasks not only helps distribute the workload but also lets others contribute meaningfully to your loved one's care.

Organizational Strategies

- **Keep Organized**: Use planners, apps, or checklists to manage medical appointments, medication schedules, and important documents. Staying organized can significantly reduce stress and improve efficiency.

Seeking Professional Support

- **Consult Healthcare Professionals**: Regular check-ins with healthcare providers can offer guidance and support in managing your loved one's health and your own.
- **Consider Counseling**: A therapist or counselor can provide a safe space to explore your feelings, offering strategies to cope with stress and navigate the complexities of caregiving.

Remember, taking care of yourself isn't just beneficial for you—it's essential for the well-being of those you care for. By incorporating these strategies into your life, you can find balance and resilience on the caregiving journey. Let self-care and support light your path, ensuring you and your loved one thrive together.

~

THE POWER OF MINDFULNESS AND MEDITATION FOR CAREGIVERS

CARING for a loved one is a journey filled with love, sacrifice, and moments of deep connection. Yet, it's also a path that can be strewn with stress, exhaustion, and emotional turbulence. As caregivers, embracing self-care practices such as mindfulness and meditation can be transformative, offering a sanctuary of peace amidst the storm of caregiving responsibilities.

The Essence of Mindfulness and Meditation

Mindfulness and meditation are practices that call us back to the present moment, inviting us to experience life as it unfolds, without judgment or distraction. These practices teach us to observe our thoughts and emotions without getting entangled in them, fostering a state of calm awareness that can significantly alleviate the stress and emotional toll of caregiving.

Benefits for Caregivers

- **Stress Reduction**: Engaging in mindfulness and meditation can significantly lower stress levels, creating a sense of calm and tranquility even in challenging caregiving situations.

- **Enhanced Emotional Awareness**: These practices deepen our understanding of our emotional landscape, helping us recognize and manage our reactions and emotions more effectively.
- **Cultivated Resilience**: Regular mindfulness and meditation strengthen our emotional resilience, enabling us to navigate the complexities of caregiving with grace and adaptability.

Incorporating Mindfulness and Meditation into Daily Life

- **Start Small**: Begin with a few minutes of meditation each day. Focus on your breath or a simple mantra, gradually increasing the time as you become more comfortable with the practice.
- **Mindful Moments**: Integrate mindfulness into daily activities. Whether you're washing dishes, walking, or sitting with your loved one, practice being present, observing the sensations, thoughts, and emotions that arise.
- **Leverage Resources**: Explore guided meditations and mindfulness apps designed to support your practice. These can provide structure and variety, keeping your practice fresh and engaging.
- **Create a Routine**: Dedicate a specific time each day for mindfulness or meditation. This consistency helps cultivate a habit, making it easier to integrate into your life.
- **Be Compassionate with Yourself**: Approach your practice with kindness and patience. Mindfulness and meditation are skills that develop over time, and there will be days when it feels more challenging. Remember, the goal is not perfection but presence.

A Journey of Self-Care

For caregivers, mindfulness and meditation are not just practices but lifelines that can restore balance, peace, and well-being. As you navigate the caregiving journey, let these practices be your anchors, helping you to care for yourself with the same compassion and dedication you offer to your loved one. In cultivating your inner calm, you not only enhance your own well-being but also enrich the quality of care you provide, creating a ripple effect of peace and positivity.

❧

BALANCING CARE: NAVIGATING EXPECTATIONS AND SELF-CARE FOR CAREGIVERS

CARING for a loved one is a profound act of love and commitment. Yet, amidst the daily tasks and emotional support, it's easy for caregivers to overlook their own needs, leading to stress and burnout. Recognizing the fine balance between caregiving and self-care is essential. Taking care of yourself is essential for providing the best care. Let's explore how you can strike a healthy balance between caregiving and self-care.

Setting Realistic Expectations:

• **Recognize Limits**: We're all human, and there's only so much one person can do. Acknowledge that you have limitations, and don't beat yourself up for not doing it all. Accepting your boundaries will make caregiving more manageable.

• **Prioritize Tasks**: Not every task carries equal weight. Focus your energy on the most important responsibilities and let go of less important matters. This will help you manage your time and resources more efficiently.

• **Ask for Help**: There's no shame in needing help. Contact family members, friends, or professional services when you feel overwhelmed. Accepting help is a sign of strength, not weakness.

• **Communicate Clearly**: Being upfront about your needs and boundaries with others can prevent misunderstandings and unnecessary stress. Don't be afraid to voice your expectations to family members and the person you're caring for.

Caring for Yourself

• **Practice Self-Compassion**: Be kind to yourself. Remind yourself that you're doing the best you can in a challenging situation. Treat yourself with the same compassion you show your loved one.

• **Make Time for Self-Care**: Incorporate activities that rejuvenate your mind, body, and spirit into your daily routine. Whether it's reading, going for a walk, or practicing mindfulness, find what works for you and make it a priority.

• **Prioritize Healthy Habits**: Your physical well-being is the foundation for providing quality care. Eat nutritious foods, get enough sleep, and engage in regular physical activity to maintain your energy and resilience.

Adapting to Change

• **Expect the Unexpected**: Caregiving situations are often unpredictable. Remain open and flexible to new challenges, adjusting your strategies and expectations as needed.

• **Embrace Emotional Flexibility**: It's natural to experience a range of emotions throughout your caregiving journey. Allow yourself to feel and express your feelings and seek professional support if needed.

• **Celebrate Small Wins**: In the midst of caregiving's demands, it's easy to overlook the small victories. Celebrate the moments of connection, the tasks accomplished, and the challenges overcome.

Remember, caregiving is a journey filled with love, sacrifice, and resilience. By setting realistic expectations, embracing self-compassion, and maintaining flexibility, you can navigate this path with grace and strength. Caring for yourself is not just a necessity, but a critical part of providing the best care for your loved one.

DISCOVERING PURPOSE IN THE CAREGIVING PATH

CARING for a loved one is a profound journey filled with both challenges and cherished moments of connection. While demanding, this experience can be enriched by embracing its deeper meaning and purpose, which can serve as powerful sources of strength and resilience.

Finding Meaning in Caregiving

• **Appreciate the Value**: Take moments to reflect on the significance of your role. You're providing comfort, safety, and love, making a profound difference in your loved one's life. Recognizing the value in these actions can foster a deep sense of purpose.

• **Cherish the Small Moments**: Find joy in the everyday moments. A shared laugh, a remembered story, or a heartfelt connection can be deeply fulfilling. These instances highlight the unique bond caregiving can forge.

• **Embrace Personal Growth**: Caregiving can be a journey of personal development. Allow yourself to learn and grow from the experience, whether it's cultivating patience, empathy, or practical skills. This growth contributes to a sense of personal achievement and purpose.

Strategies for Managing Caregiver Stress

• **Prioritize Self-Care**: Self-care is not a luxury but a necessity. Ensure you're getting adequate rest, nutrition, and physical activity. Engaging in activities that bring you joy is essential for maintaining your well-being.

• **Build a Support Network**: You need not navigate caregiving alone. Connect with support groups, friends, family, or professionals who understand the caregiving journey. Sharing experiences and receiving support can lighten the emotional load.

• **Establish Boundaries**: Recognize your limits and communicate them clearly. Setting boundaries helps manage expectations and prevents resentment and burnout.

• **Seek Respite Care**: Utilize respite care services to take breaks when needed. Short-term care options can provide you with the time to recharge while ensuring your loved one is in safe hands.

• **Practice Mindfulness and Relaxation**: Incorporate mindfulness practices into your daily routine. Techniques like meditation, deep breathing, or yoga can reduce stress and enhance your emotional equilibrium.

Finding Balance

In caregiving, as in life, balance is key. While caregiving can be demanding, finding moments of joy, connection, and personal growth can infuse your journey with meaning and purpose. Remember, caring for yourself is integral to your ability to care for others. By adopting self-care strategies, building a support network, and embracing the unique opportunities for growth and connection caregiving presents, you can navigate this path with resilience and grace.

Caregiving is not just a role but a profound expression of love and dedication. In the midst of challenges, let the purpose and meaning you find guide you, providing strength and fulfillment on this rewarding journey.

FREQUENTLY ASKED QUESTIONS:

1. How can I motivate my loved one with dementia to participate in physical activities?

Answer: Start by choosing activities that align with their interests and abilities, making changes as needed to accommodate their current level of function. Incorporate elements of fun, such as music or incorporating their favorite pastime activities into the exercise. Also, keep activities short and simple, celebrating any form of participation to encourage a sense of accomplishment and motivation to engage in physical activities regularly.

2. What dietary considerations should I keep in mind to ensure proper nutrition for my loved one with dementia?

Answer: Focus on a balanced diet rich in fruits, vegetables, whole grains, lean proteins, and healthy fats to support overall health and cognitive function. Since individuals with dementia might experience changes in appetite or taste preferences, offer small, frequent meals and snacks that are nutrient dense. Pay attention to hydration, encouraging regular intake of fluids throughout the day. Consulting with a dietitian can provide personalized guidance tailored to their specific health needs and preferences.

3. How do I address sleep issues in someone with dementia to ensure they're getting enough rest?

Answer: Establish a consistent nighttime routine and a comfortable, quiet sleep environment. Limit caffeine and heavy meals before bedtime and encourage activities during the day to promote better sleep at night. Consider gentle, relaxing activities before bed, such as listening to soft music or reading, to help signal to their body that it's time to wind down. If sleep disturbances persist, consulting with a healthcare professional for further evaluation and management might be necessary.

4. My loved one often shows signs of stress and anxiety. How can I help alleviate these feelings?

Answer: Identify triggers of stress and try to reduce them. Create a calm, predictable environment and schedule. Use simple, reassuring communication and maintain a routine that includes activities they enjoy and find relaxing, such as walking in nature or engaging in a favorite hobby. Consider mindfulness or relaxation techniques that can be done together, like deep-breathing exercises or guided imagery, to promote calmness.

5. How can I ensure the safety of my loved one with dementia at home to prevent falls and injuries?

Answer: Conduct a thorough safety assessment of the home environment to identify and mitigate potential hazards. This may include installing grab bars in the bathroom, ensuring adequate lighting, removing tripping hazards, and using non-slip mats in slippery areas. Consider the use of wearable devices or home monitoring systems to alert caregivers to potential falls or emergencies. Regularly review and adjust safety measures as their mobility and cognitive abilities change.

By addressing these key aspects of care, caregivers can enhance the physical health and emotional well-being of their loved ones with dementia, creating a supportive and nurturing environment that caters to their evolving needs.

CASE STUDY:

MEET MARIA AND HER FATHER, Tom, who has been living with dementia for the past three years. Maria, a devoted daughter and primary caregiver, has been navigating the challenges of ensuring Tom maintains a nutritious diet and remains physically active, critical components in managing his condition and enhancing his quality of life.

Background: Tom, a 78-year-old retired schoolteacher with a love for gardening and a lifelong habit of walking daily, began showing signs of dementia, including memory loss, confusion, and occasional agitation. As his condition progressed, he started showing less interest in food and became more sedentary, spending much of his day sitting in front of the TV.

Challenges: Maria noticed the decline in her father's physical health and mood. He was losing weight, becoming weaker, and seemed more dispirited each day. She realized the need to focus on his diet and physical activity but was unsure where to start, given his changing preferences and abilities.

Strategies Implemented:

1. **Nutritious Diet:**

2. **Tailored Meal Planning:** Maria began to incorporate Tom's favorite foods into his diet, ensuring they were nutritious and catered to his needs. She introduced more fruits, vegetables, lean proteins, and whole grains, making meals colorful and appealing.

3. **Hydration:** She made sure Tom had a water bottle within reach throughout the day and offered him water-rich foods like cucumbers and watermelon to keep him hydrated.

4. **Dining Environment:** Maria created a calm and inviting dining atmosphere, playing soft music that Tom enjoyed during meals to make eating a more enjoyable experience.

5. **Regular Physical Activity:**

6. **Gardening:** Recognizing Tom's love for gardening, Maria encouraged him to spend time in the garden each day, helping him to plant new flowers and herbs, which provided both physical activity and a sense of accomplishment.

7. **Daily Walks:** Maria and Tom started going for short, gentle walks around the neighborhood, gradually increasing the distance as Tom's endurance improved. These walks became a cherished daily routine.

8. **Chair Exercises:** On days when going outside wasn't possible, Maria introduced Tom to simple chair exercises to keep him moving and improve his flexibility and strength.

Lessons Learned:

- **Personalization is Key:** Catering to Tom's preferences and abilities significantly increased his willingness to eat healthily and stay active.
- **Small Changes, Big Impact:** Incremental adjustments to Tom's diet and physical activity had noticeable effects on his physical health and mood.
- **Engagement Enhances Well-being:** Involving Tom in activities he enjoyed, like gardening, not only provided physical benefits but also improved his overall sense of well-being and engagement with life.

Outcome: Over several months, Maria observed positive changes in Tom's health and disposition. He became more engaged, his appetite improved, and he regained some of the weight he had lost. Their daily walks and gardening activities not only helped Tom stay physically active but also provided valuable bonding time, enriching their relationship.

Maria's dedication to adapting Tom's care to his needs and interests underscored the importance of personalized, compassionate care in enhancing the quality of life for individuals with dementia. Through patience, creativity, and commitment, caregivers can make a significant difference in the well-being of their loved ones.

∼

PART ELEVEN WRAP-UP:

1. **Personalize Meals:**
2. Incorporate the care recipient's favorite foods into their daily diet, ensuring these choices are nutritious and meet their dietary needs.
3. Experiment with colorful and varied food options to make meals visually appealing and nutritionally balanced.
4. **Enhance Hydration:**
5. Keep water easily accessible throughout the day to encourage regular hydration.
6. Offer water-rich foods as part of meals and snacks to increase fluid intake.
7. **Create a Pleasant Dining Atmosphere:**
8. Set up a calm and inviting eating area with minimal distractions.
9. Play soft music or sounds that the care recipient enjoys during meals to enhance their dining experience.
10. **Incorporate Physical Activities into Daily Routine:**

11. Identify activities the care recipient enjoys, such as gardening or walking, and incorporate these into their daily schedule.

12. Start with short sessions of physical activity and gradually increase duration as tolerated.

13. **Introduce Simple Exercise Routines:**

14. On days when outdoor activities are impossible, engage the care recipient in simple indoor exercises, such as chair exercises, to keep them physically active.

15. **Monitor Dietary and Physical Activity Adjustments:**

16. Keep a diary or log to track changes in the care recipient's diet, physical activity levels, and their effects on mood and health.

17. Adjust meal plans and activity levels based on observations and the care recipient's feedback.

18. **Seek Professional Guidance:**

19. Consult with healthcare professionals, such as dietitians or physical therapists, for personalized advice on nutrition and physical activities suited to the care recipient's health status and preferences.

20. **Foster Engagement and Independence:**

21. Encourage the care recipient's participation in choosing meals and engaging in physical activities, fostering a sense of independence and involvement.

22. **Celebrate Achievements:**

23. Acknowledge and celebrate small achievements and improvements in the care recipient's health, mood, and engagement levels.

24. **Focus on Caregiver Self-Care:**

25. Make sure you, as the caregiver, also take time for your own health and well-being, recognizing that effective caregiving requires looking after yourself as well.

∾

IN OUR NEXT PART...

IN OUR NEXT PART, we'll explore the essence of creating a robust support system—a cornerstone not just for navigating the intricacies of caregiving but for enhancing life's journey overall. Imagine crafting a sanctuary where empathy, understanding, and mutual support are the bricks and mortar holding the community together. This sanctuary isn't just a haven for those in need; it's a dynamic space where every member thrives on both giving and receiving support. We'll dig into practical steps to build this supportive ecosystem, emphasizing the transformative power of connecting with others who share similar paths. Whether through local groups, online communities, or one-on-one connections, the focus will be on cultivating relationships that offer strength and solace in times of need.

We'll highlight the importance of diversity within these networks—how different perspectives and experiences enrich our understanding and provide a more comprehensive support system. From recognizing when to seek help to offering your strength to others, this Part will serve as a guide to developing a support network that resonates with your personal journey. We'll also address common challenges in forming and maintaining these connections, offering strategies to overcome them. By fostering an environment of open communication, reciprocal support, and genuine connection, we can create a community that not only supports us through the caregiving journey but also enriches our entire life experience. Let's start this journey together, learning how to weave a tapestry of support that holds the power to transform lives.

~

PART TWELVE
CULTIVATING A NOURISHING CIRCLE OF SUPPORT

Building a supportive community is like planting a garden of resources and relationships; it requires patience, care, and nurturing to flourish. Whether you're a caregiver seeking solace, an individual craving connection, or anyone in between, cultivating a network of support is fundamental to navigating the complexities of life with resilience and strength. Here are actionable steps and insights on fostering a community that uplifts and sustains you:

∾

RECOGNIZE THE VALUE OF COMMUNITY:

Understand that a supportive community serves as a beacon of light during challenging times and a source of joy in moments of triumph. It provides a sense of belonging, enhances our resilience against stress, and enriches our emotional landscape.

Steps to Cultivate Your Support Network

• **Assess Your Social Landscape:** Begin by evaluating your current connections. Identify relationships that nourish your spirit and those that may require boundaries. Consider the roles different individuals play in your life and how they contribute to your sense of community.

• **Engage in Community Activities:** Actively participate in events, workshops, or classes that resonate with your interests. These settings offer fertile ground for sowing the seeds of new friendships and connections.

• **Leverage Social Media Mindfully:** Use online platforms to join groups or follow pages relevant to your interests and values. Digital communities can provide support and connection, especially when geographical constraints limit physical gatherings.

• **Volunteer Your Time and Skills:** Volunteering offers the dual benefit of contributing to a cause you care about while connecting with others who share your passion. This mutual interest can serve as a strong foundation for supportive relationships.

• **Start Your Own Support Group:** If existing groups don't meet your needs, consider creating your own space for shared experiences, whether it's a book club, a caregiver support group, or a fitness accountability circle.

• **Foster Open Communication:** Cultivate an environment of trust and openness within your community. Encourage members to share their experiences, challenges, and victories, fostering a culture of empathy and mutual support.

• **Practice Reciprocity:** A thriving community relies on give-and-take. Be willing to offer your support to others, whether through listening, advising, or helping with tasks. Reciprocity strengthens the bonds of community and ensures its longevity.

• **Celebrate Community Achievements:** Acknowledge and celebrate the milestones and achievements of your community members. Recognizing each other's successes reinforces the value of your collective support and encourages continued growth.

The Impact of a Supportive Community

A well-nurtured supportive community not only bolsters our emotional resilience but also promotes personal growth. It reminds us we are not alone in our journeys, providing a network of encouragement and understanding. In the garden of life, a supportive community is the sunlight that helps us grow, thrive, and blossom.

Remember, building a supportive community is an ongoing process that evolves with time. Be patient, stay open to new connections, and cherish the relationships that uplift you. In doing so, you'll find that the strength of your community becomes a powerful force in navigating life's ebbs and flows with grace and resilience.

≈

CRAFTING YOUR CIRCLE: HOW TO BUILD A STRONG SUPPORT NETWORK

A strong circle of support is an invaluable asset that can uplift you during life's challenges and celebrate your triumphs. Building a strong network takes intentionality and effort, but the rewards are immeasurable. Here's how you can craft a circle that provides strength and resilience:

Identify Your Needs: First, reflect on the areas where you need more support. Do you need someone to talk to, help with daily tasks, or a combination of both? Identifying your specific needs will guide you toward the right individuals or groups to include in your network.

Reach Out to Friends and Family: Your existing relationships can serve as the foundation of your support network. Open and honest communication is key to deepening these connections and letting loved ones know how they can best support you.

Join Community Groups or Clubs: Immerse yourself in local groups, clubs, or organizations that align with your interests or values. These settings provide fertile ground for meeting individuals who share your passions and can become valuable members of your support circle.

Volunteer in Your Community: Giving back through volunteering not only benefits others but also connects you with like-minded individuals. Working toward a shared goal can forge strong bonds and cultivate a sense of belonging.

Seek Professional Support: Sometimes, the support we need extends beyond what friends and family can provide. Please reach out to professionals, such as therapists, counselors, or support groups, to address specific challenges. Their knowledge and coping tools can be invaluable.

Be a Supportive Presence for Others: Remember, building a support network is a reciprocal process. Be there for others, listen without judgment, and offer a helping hand when you can. This fosters a culture of support and trust within your network.

Nurture Your Relationships: Like any meaningful relationship, your support network requires care and attention. Regularly check in with your circle, express your appreciation for their support, and please ask for help when you need it. Building and maintaining these relationships takes effort, but the rewards are immeasurable.

Remember, creating a supportive community isn't just about finding help; it's about building a space where you feel valued, heard, and empowered. By investing time and effort into these relationships and remaining open to both giving and receiving support, you'll develop a network that provides strength and resilience to face life's challenges with grace and determination.

∾

BUILDING A VILLAGE: FOSTERING COMMUNITY THROUGH GIVING AND RECEIVING

A SUPPORTIVE CIRCLE around you is essential to feeling secure, uplifted, and connected. It's about having individuals who celebrate your triumphs and offer a compassionate presence during challenging times. Here's how to weave a network that is both strong and nurturing:

Pinpoint What You Need: Start by identifying what type of support you're seeking. Do you need a motivating voice, assistance with daily tasks, advice, or simply someone who will listen without judgment? Knowing your specific needs will help you determine who to turn to.

Tap Into Your Existing Circle: You likely already have a network of friends, family, coworkers, or neighbors. Lean into these existing relationships. Often, people want to help but may not be aware that you're looking for support. Please reach out and express your needs.

Dive into Community Groups: If you have a hobby or a cause you're passionate about, look for community groups or clubs that share your interests. These settings are excellent for meeting people who might understand and relate to your experiences.

Give as Good as You Get: A strong community thrives on reciprocity. Be ready to offer your support to others as well. This way, you're building a culture of mutual aid where everyone feels valued and supported.

Open Up: True connections are formed through vulnerability and honesty. It's okay to share your feelings, worries, and dreams with people you trust. This openness can deepen your bonds and strengthen your support network.

Explore Support Groups: If you're dealing with specific challenges, support groups or workshops can be a lifeline. Sharing experiences with others in similar situations can provide comfort, practical advice, and a sense of community.

Go Digital: Don't overlook the power of the internet. There's a world of forums, social media groups, and online communities out there. Whether you're into gardening, gaming, or anything between, there's likely a virtual community waiting for you.

Building a support network doesn't happen overnight. But by embracing the spirit of community, opening yourself up to giving and receiving support, and consistently nurturing these connections, you'll find yourself surrounded by a group of people who offer strength, comfort, and joy as you navigate life's journey together.

∾

CRAFTING A CIRCLE OF TRUST: STRENGTHENING BONDS IN YOUR SUPPORT NETWORK

Creating a haven where everyone feels supported, understood, and valued is like cultivating a thriving community garden. It's about nurturing growth, fostering meaningful connections, and ensuring everyone has a place to blossom. Here's how you can cultivate this sacred space:

Understand Your Needs: Like selecting the right seeds for your garden, knowing what you're seeking in a support network is the important first step. Are you in need of emotional support, guidance, or a compassionate ear? Identifying your specific needs will help you seek companions who can provide the nourishment you require.

Gather with Those on Similar Paths: Seek groups or individuals who can relate to your experiences. This could be a local club, an online community, or a hobby group. Shared perspectives and values can sow the seeds of deep trust and understanding.

Keep the Lines of Communication Open: Trust flourishes in an environment of open communication. Share your thoughts and feelings honestly and lend an attentive ear to others. This two-way street of support and understanding can build strong, unbreakable bonds.

Embrace Diversity: A community thrives on the richness of diverse perspectives. Make sure everyone feels seen, heard, and valued. Celebrate the unique stories and backgrounds each individual offers – it's what makes your community vibrant and resilient.

Share and Care: A support network is as much about giving as it is about receiving. Share your knowledge, lend a helping hand, and please reach out when you need support. This give-and-take nurtures a strong, interconnected community.

Ensure a Safe Haven: Make sure your network is a place where everyone can share freely without fear of judgment or repercussions. Address any disagreements or discomforts with compassion and respect to maintain a safe, supportive environment for all.

By weaving these threads of trust, open communication, and mutual care, you create not just a support network, but a close-knit community where everyone can grow, share, and find solace. It's about cultivating a space where all are welcome, all are heard, and all are supported in their journey.

∼

CRAFTING YOUR SUPPORT ECOSYSTEM: A GUIDE TO DIVERSE NETWORKS

IN THE JOURNEY OF LIFE, having a robust support system isn't just beneficial; it's essential. Just as a garden thrives with a diverse array of plants, our well-being flourishes with a mix of support networks. Let's explore the types of networks that can enrich our lives:

Formal Organizations: Envision these as the structured trellises and frameworks in a garden, providing stability and guidance. Support groups, counseling centers, and community organizations offer professional and structured help. They are spaces where you can find specialized support, whether navigating health challenges, seeking educational guidance, or accessing community services. These organizations bring together individuals with shared experiences, offering a space for connection, understanding, and expert guidance.

Online Communities: Online communities are like sprawling vines that transcend borders, connecting people from all corners of the globe. Whether through forums, social media groups, or virtual meet-ups, these platforms allow for sharing experiences, advice, and support with a wide and varied audience. For those who may feel isolated in their physical surroundings, online communities can offer a sense of belonging and connection that's a click away.

Personal Relationships: The roots of our support network lie in personal relationships with friends, family, and mentors. These connections offer emotional nourishment, practical support, and the warmth of companionship. Cultivating these relationships requires time and care, but the depth of support and understanding they provide is unparalleled. They are our go-to people in times of joy and distress, offering a shoulder to lean on and a hand to hold.

Navigating life's ups and downs with a diverse support network enriches our journey, providing strength, comfort, and joy. By weaving together formal organizations, online communities, and personal relationships, we create a support ecosystem that nurtures our growth and resilience. Explore, connect, and nurture these connections, for they are the pillars on which we can lean and thrive.

Remember, just as a garden requires consistent tending and care, our support networks need nurturing and cultivation. By embracing the diverse sources of support available to us and tending to these connections, we create a rich and sustaining ecosystem that can uplift us through life's challenges and triumphs.

∼

NAVIGATING THE PATH TO SUPPORT: OVERCOMING OBSTACLES TOGETHER

CREATING a supportive community and reaching out for help can feel like navigating through a thick forest; it's easy to feel lost or overwhelmed by the underbrush of challenges and barriers. Yet, with determination and the right tools, you can clear a path to the support you need. Here's how:

Breaking Down Stigma's Walls: Mental health stigma can be a formidable barrier, casting shadows of judgment and misunderstanding. Education is our sunlight, dispelling these shadows and fostering an environment where seeking help is seen as a sign of strength, not weakness. Let's talk openly about mental health, sharing stories and facts that humanize and normalize these experiences.

Cultivating Trust Through Open Fields: A supportive community thrives on trust and openness, much like a field thrives under the open sky. Create spaces—whether physical or virtual—where everyone feels safe to share without fear of judgment. In these spaces, encourage honesty and vulnerability, laying the groundwork for deep, meaningful connections.

Professional Guidance as Our Compass: When the forest gets too dense, a professional guide can help us find our way. Therapists, counselors, and support groups are like compasses, pointing us toward paths we might not have seen on our own. They equip us with strategies and insights to navigate our challenges making the journey less daunting.

Setting Boundaries as Protective Clearings: Just as clearings in the forest offer respite and protection, setting personal boundaries safeguards our well-being. Recognize and communicate your limits, ensuring you have the space to breathe and grow. It's okay to step back and nurture yourself; self-care isn't selfish, it's essential.

Resilience as Our Root System: Deep roots let trees withstand storms; similarly, resilience helps us face life's challenges with strength. Develop resilience by embracing positive coping strategies like mindfulness, finding joy in hobbies, and surrounding yourself with positive influences. These roots will hold you steady, no matter the wind's strength.

Starting the journey to build a supportive community and seek help is courageous. Remember, every step forward, no matter how small, is progress. With patience, openness, and resilience, you can overcome barriers and find the support that enriches your life and fosters growth. Let's walk this path together, supporting each other every step of the way.

∾

FREQUENTLY ASKED QUESTIONS:

1. How can I start building my own supportive community when I feel isolated?

Answer: Begin by identifying areas where support could make a difference, such as emotional, practical, or informational support. Contact family and friends to express your needs and join local or online groups where you can share experiences and receive advice. Starting conversations, even if it's with one person, can be the first step toward breaking the cycle of isolation.

2. What strategies can I use to encourage active participation within my support group?

Answer: Foster an environment of open communication and mutual respect where everyone feels valued for their contributions. Regularly schedule activities or meetings that cater to the interests of the group members to keep engagement high. Acknowledge and celebrate the achievements of members to build a positive and supportive culture. Lastly, reach out to members who seem less engaged to understand their needs better and how the group can support them.

3. How can I find support groups relevant to my specific needs or situation?

Answer: Start by researching online for groups related to your specific needs or interests. Many organizations offer resources and directories for support groups. Social media platforms can also be a valuable tool for finding communities and forums. Additionally, healthcare professionals or local community centers may recommend support groups that cater to your specific circumstances.

4. How can I maintain my personal well-being while participating in a support community?

Answer: Set clear boundaries for yourself to avoid feeling overwhelmed by the needs of others. Practice self-care regularly and make time for activities that replenish your energy and bring you joy. Remember, being part of a support community means both giving and receiving support; expressing your own needs and seek help from the community when you need it.

5. What should I do if I don't feel like my current support group is the right fit for me?

Answer: It's important to feel connected and supported within your group. If you feel that the group is not meeting your needs, consider discussing your concerns with the group leader or members to explore possible changes. If the group still doesn't feel like the right fit, give yourself permission to explore other groups or communities that might align better with your needs and expectations. Remember, finding the right support group can take time, and it's okay to keep looking until you find a space where you feel comfortable and supported.

Building a supportive community is a dynamic and ongoing process. It requires patience, openness, and the willingness to both give and receive support. With these strategies in mind, you can create a network of support that enriches your life and the lives of those around you.

～

CASE STUDY: LINDA & RUTH

MEET LINDA, a 58-year-old caring for her 82-year-old mother, Ruth, who was diagnosed with early-stage Alzheimer's disease two years ago. Linda, an only child, felt overwhelmed with the caregiving responsibilities, juggling her job as a schoolteacher and her family life. However, over time, Linda discovered the immense value of building a supportive community around her and her mother. This case study explores how Linda navigated the complexities of caregiving by fostering a network of support and the lessons she learned along the way.

Background: Linda's mother, Ruth, was always independent, but as her Alzheimer's progressed, she required more assistance with daily activities. Linda struggled to keep up with her mother's needs, her job, and her own family. She felt isolated and stressed, unsure of where to turn for help.

The Turning Point: The turning point for Linda came when she went to a local Alzheimer's support group meeting. Here, she realized she was not alone in her journey. She met other caregivers who understood her challenges and offered practical advice and emotional support.

This experience encouraged Linda to actively seek and build a support network.

Building the Support Network: Linda took several steps to cultivate her support community:

Family and Friends:

Linda opened up to her close friends and family about her struggles, which she had hesitated to do. She was pleasantly surprised by their willingness to help. Her husband began accompanying Ruth on her morning walks, and her friends started dropping by to spend time with Ruth, offering Linda some respite.

Professional Services:

Recognizing she needed professional help; Linda hired a part-time home health aide specialized in Alzheimer's care. This not only ensured Ruth received professional care but also let Linda focus on her job and personal well-being.

Online Communities:

Linda joined several online forums for Alzheimer's caregivers. These platforms provided a space for Linda to ask questions, share her experiences, and learn from others across the globe. The tips and stories shared online became invaluable resources for Linda, helping her navigate her mother's condition with more confidence.

Local Support Groups:

The local Alzheimer's support group became a cornerstone of Linda's support network. The monthly meetings offered her a sense of community and belonging. She formed close friendships with several group members, and they often exchanged caregiving duties, providing each other with much-needed breaks.

Lessons Learned: Linda learned several important lessons through building and leaning on her support network:

- **The Power of Vulnerability:** By opening up about her challenges, Linda connected with others on a deeper level, fostering meaningful relationships and receiving the support she desperately needed.
- **Reciprocity in Support:** Linda found that giving support was as important as receiving it. Helping others in her support network gave her a sense of purpose and fulfillment.
- **Diversity in Support:** Linda realized that different types of support (emotional, practical, professional) were important to meet the varied challenges she faced. Diversifying her support network let her access the right help when needed.

Chapter Summary: Linda's journey highlights the transformative impact of building a supportive community for caregivers. Her proactive approach to seeking support, coupled with her willingness to offer help to others, not only improved her own quality of life but also enhanced the care provided to her mother. Linda's story serves as a powerful reminder of the strength found in community and the importance of fostering connections to navigate the caregiving journey with resilience and hope.

$\sim$

PART TWELVE WRAP-UP:
ACTION ITEMS FOR THE CAREGIVER:

BASED ON LINDA'S experience in building a supportive community for her caregiving journey, here are actionable steps for caregivers to consider:

1. **Open Up About Your Challenges:**
2. Share your caregiving experiences, challenges, and needs with family and friends. Let them know how they can help.
3. **Seek Professional Help:**
4. Consider hiring professional caregivers or home health aides specialized in caring for individuals with conditions similar to your loved one's. Research local agencies or services that offer the support you need.
5. **Join Online Support Forums:**
6. Find and participate in online communities and forums related to caregiving or your loved one's specific condition. Use these platforms to ask questions, share experiences, and learn from others in similar situations.
7. **Go to Local Support Group Meetings:**
8. Look for support groups in your area that cater to caregivers or specific conditions like Alzheimer's disease. Go to meetings

regularly to connect with others, exchange advice, and find emotional support.

9. **Use Respite Care Services:**
10. Investigate respite care options to give yourself a break. This could be through community services, volunteer organizations, or professional respite care providers.
11. **Cultivate Friendships with Fellow Caregivers:**
12. Build relationships with other caregivers you meet through support groups or online communities. Offer to exchange caregiving duties or simply provide a listening ear to each other.
13. **Explore Local Community Resources:**
14. Research local community centers, libraries, or nonprofit organizations that offer programs, activities, or services that could help you or your loved one.
15. **Educate Yourself and Others:**
16. Use resources available through support groups, healthcare providers, and reputable online sources to educate yourself about your loved one's condition. Share this knowledge with friends and family to improve their understanding and ability to help.
17. **Practice Self-Care:**
18. Make time for activities that rejuvenate you, whether it's exercising, reading, or pursuing a hobby. Recognize that taking care of yourself is essential to caring for someone else effectively.
19. **Communicate Needs Clearly:**
20. When asking for help, be specific about what you need, whether it's someone to watch your loved one for a few hours, help with household chores, or just someone to talk to.
21. **Be Open to Different Types of Support:**
22. Recognize that support can come in many forms (emotional, practical, informational) and from various sources. Be open to receiving help in ways you might not have considered.
23. **Document and Organize Resources:**

24. Keep a record of helpful contacts, services, and resources you come across. Organizing this information can make it easier to find the support you need when you need it.

These action items can help caregivers build a supportive network, manage caregiving responsibilities more effectively, and maintain their own well-being throughout the caregiving journey.

∾

IN OUR NEXT PART...

IN OUR NEXT PART, we're diving deep into the heart of caregiving - recognizing the undeniable importance of taking breaks for your well-being and the vitality of your care. It's about acknowledging that to give your best, you must feel your best. This isn't just about stepping away for a moment; it's about understanding the profound impact that rest and rejuvenation can have on your ability to provide compassion-ate, attentive care. We'll explore the essence of respite care, not as an optional luxury, but as an essential part of the caregiving process. This is about framing respite care in a new light, seeing it as an important support system that empowers you to continue your caregiving journey with renewed strength, patience, and love.

We'll guide you through the practicalities of integrating respite care into your life, from identifying the right respite care that aligns with your needs and those of your loved one to navigating the logistical parts of making it happen. We aim to give you the tools and insights necessary to make informed decisions about your respite care options, making sure you can take the breaks you need without worry.

It's about creating a balance that supports both you and your loved one, fostering a caregiving environment that is sustainable, nurturing, and filled with understanding. Join us as we explore how to embrace and implement respite care effectively, making sure you, the caregiver, have the support and time you need to thrive alongside your loved one.

~

PART THIRTEEN
TAKING A BREATHER: THE ESSENTIALS OF RESPITE CARE FOR CAREGIVERS

Taking care of someone you love is rewarding, but let's be honest, it can also be exhausting. Every caregiver needs a break now and then to catch their breath, focus on their own needs, and recharge their batteries. That's where respite care comes into play, offering a helping hand when you most need it.

Understanding Respite Care:

Imagine having someone reliable step into your shoes, taking care of your loved one while you take some time off. That's respite care for you. It's a temporary setup that gives you a chance to take a break, whether it's for a few hours to run errands or for a few days to go on a much-needed vacation.

Why Respite Care is a Game-Changer:

Constantly being in caregiver mode without a break can wear you down, leading to stress and burnout. That's not good for you or the person you're caring for. Respite care comes to the rescue by giving you some downtime. It's all about keeping you refreshed and ready to tackle your caregiving duties with renewed energy and patience.

Exploring Your Respite Care Options:

There's no one-size-fits-all regarding respite care. You've got options:

- **In-home care:** Someone comes over to your place to help out, giving you the freedom to step out or simply relax at home without worries.
- **Adult day programs:** These are great for your loved one to interact with others while you take care of your day-to-day tasks or relax.
- **Short-term residential stays:** Sometimes, a longer break is needed, and residential care facilities can offer temporary care for your loved one, giving you peace of mind.

Wrapping It Up:

Taking advantage of respite care is important for your well-being and ensures you can keep providing the best care for your loved one. Remember, taking time for yourself isn't selfish—it's necessary. So, please explore the respite care services available to you. It's all about finding the right balance that works for you and your loved one, ensuring you both stay happy and healthy.

～

EXPLORING YOUR BREAK OPTIONS: TYPES OF RESPITE CARE SERVICES

CARING for someone you love is a big job, and every now and then, you need a chance to step back and take a breather. That's where respite care comes in, offering you a well-deserved break while ensuring your loved one continues to receive the care they need. Let's dive into the different types of respite care services that can give you that moment of rest.

In-Home Respite Care:

Imagine someone stepping into your shoes, right in your own home, taking care of your loved one while you step out or simply take a nap in the next room. That's in-home respite care for you. Professionals or trained volunteers come to your place to provide the care needed, giving you the flexibility to manage your time without worrying about your loved one's well-being.

Adult Day Programs:

These programs are a win-win for everyone. Your loved one gets to enjoy a day filled with activities, socializing, and fun, while you get the time to handle other responsibilities or simply relax. It's a great way to

ensure your loved one is engaged and looked after, without you
needing to be there the whole time.

Short-Term Residential Stays:

Sometimes, a longer break is necessary, and that's where short-term
residential facilities come into play. Whether it's an assisted living
community or a nursing home, these places offer temporary care for
your loved one. It's a good option for when you need to recharge for
more than just a few hours, ensuring your loved one is in safe hands
while you take your break.

Caregivers must take care of themselves too, and respite care services
are there to help you do just that. Don't shy away from exploring these
options. Taking a break isn't a sign of weakness; it's a necessary step to
ensure you can continue providing the best care for your loved one
with renewed energy and patience.

~

RECHARGING YOUR BATTERIES: THE IMPORTANCE OF RESPITE CARE

LOOKING after a loved one is a task filled with love and dedication, yet it demands a lot from you, both body and soul. It's easy to get caught up in this cycle of care, often placing your own needs on the back burner. However, tapping into respite care services can be a game-changer, offering benefits not just for you, the caregiver, but also for the person you're caring for.

A Much-Needed Pause for Caregivers:

Respite care is that breath of fresh air for caregivers who've been deep in the trenches. It's a chance to step back, relax, and attend to your own needs, be it catching up on sleep, enjoying a hobby, or simply sitting in silence. This break can significantly reduce stress and prevent the all-too-common caregiver burnout, ensuring you're in the best shape to provide care.

New Experiences for Your Loved One:

While it's a break for you, it's also an opportunity for your loved one to interact with different people and enjoy many activities. This exposure can help break the monotony, offering them new experiences and the chance to form new bonds. It's a win-win situation where they get to enjoy a slice of life outside their routine while you recharge your batteries.

Strengthening Bonds:

Ironically, spending some time apart can actually bring you closer. Respite care makes sure when you're back, you're more patient, attentive, and genuinely present. This refreshed mindset can significantly enhance the quality of care you provide and strengthen your relationship with your loved one.

Looking After Your Health:

Regular use of respite care services lets you focus on your own health and well-being. It's an opportunity to go to medical appointments, engage in physical activity, or simply catch up on rest. Taking care of your health is not selfish; it's essential. A healthy caregiver is a more effective caregiver.

Respite care is an invaluable resource for caregivers, offering a necessary pause for rest and rejuvenation. It's about giving the best of you, not what's left of you. So, consider respite care not just as an option, but as an important part of your caregiving journey, ensuring both you and your loved one thrive.

∾

FINDING RELIEF: A GUIDE TO ACCESSING RESPITE CARE SERVICES

CARING for someone you love is a profound expression of commitment and affection. Yet, this journey can take a toll on your well-being. That's where respite care steps in, offering an important pause for caregivers to rejuvenate. But how do you tap into these services? Here's a simple guide to help you find the support you need.

Starting Points for Finding Respite Care:

- **Local Aging or Disability Agencies**: Your first port of call should be your local aging or disability services agency. They're the treasure trove of information on respite care options in your community and can guide you on how to get started.
- **Healthcare Professionals**: Your loved one's healthcare team can also be a valuable resource. Doctors, nurses, or social workers often connect with respite care services and can recommend options that cater specifically to your loved one's needs.
- **Online Platforms**: The internet is awash with resources to help you locate respite care. Websites like Caring.com or AgingCare.com not only list providers but also feature reviews

and ratings from other caregivers, giving you insights into their experiences.

- **Community Networks**: Don't overlook local community organizations, faith groups, and non-profits. These entities sometimes offer respite care services or can point you toward financial assistance programs to help cover costs.

Navigating Financial Support for Respite Care

- **Medicaid**: For eligible individuals, Medicaid can be a source of funding for respite care. Contact your local Medicaid office to explore eligibility and application procedures.
- **Veteran Affairs**: Veterans may have access to respite care help through the VA. These programs are designed to support veterans and their caregivers, covering respite care costs under certain conditions.
- **Insurance Plans**: Some private health insurance policies include respite care benefits. Contact your insurer to find out what's covered under your plan and the process for accessing these services.
- **Nonprofit Support**: Various nonprofit organizations offer grants or financial aid for respite care. Research could uncover organizations willing to help ease the financial burden of caregiving.

Remember, taking time for yourself isn't a luxury—it's a necessity. By exploring these avenues, you can access respite care services that let you recharge, ensuring you continue to provide loving care with renewed energy and dedication.

∾

BREAKING DOWN BARRIERS: MAKING RESPITE CARE WORK FOR YOU

Taking care of a loved one is a role filled with love and dedication, yet it's also one that demands much from us, physically and emotionally. Caregivers must remember the importance of their own well-being, and respite care services offer a valuable resource for this. This guide aims to shine a light on how to access these services while addressing the hurdles you might face.

Exploring Your Respite Care Options

- **In-Home Support**: Invite a professional caregiver into your home to care for your loved one, offering you a breather to attend to your needs.
- **Adult Day Programs**: These provide a nurturing environment for your loved one, filled with activities and social opportunities, giving you time to yourself.
- **Short-Term Residential Stays**: Temporary care in a facility ensures your loved one is well looked after, allowing you an extended period to recharge.

Tackling Common Hurdles to Accessing Respite Care

- **Feeling Guilty?**: It's natural to feel a twinge of guilt about taking time for yourself, but remember, recharging is essential to being the best caregiver you can be. It's not selfish; it's necessary.
- **Building Trust**: Entrusting your loved one's care to someone else can be daunting. Dedicate time to vet and get to know potential caregivers or facilities. This due diligence can ease your mind and build trust.
- **Worried About Costs?**: Yes, respite care can be expensive, but there are avenues for financial help. Look into Medicaid waivers, benefits for veterans, or grants from nonprofit organizations.
- **Finding Availability**: Especially in less populated areas, finding respite care can be challenging. Plan as far ahead as you can and lean on local networks for guidance and support.
- **Raising Awareness**: If you're unsure about what's available, you're not alone. Commit to learning more about the respite care services in your community. The more you know, the better equipped you'll be to take advantage of these resources.

Chapter Summary: Remember, caring for yourself isn't just a luxury—it's an integral part of being a caregiver. By leveraging respite care services, you're not only ensuring your loved one's needs are met but also taking essential steps to preserve your health and happiness. Facing the barriers to respite care head-on can empower you to find the support you need, enabling you to continue your caregiving journey with renewed energy and peace of mind.

∽

EMPOWERING CAREGIVERS: NAVIGATING SUPPORT AND RESPITE SERVICES

CAREGIVING, with its rewards and challenges, can be an intense journey, one that occasionally requires us to step back and recharge. Understanding when and how to take these necessary pauses is key to sustaining both our well-being and our ability to provide care. This is where respite care and support services become invaluable.

Diverse Respite Care Options

Respite care comes in several forms to fit different needs and situations:

- **In-Home Respite**: A professional caregiver steps into your home, taking over your duties and allowing you some time off. This option keeps your loved one in a familiar environment while you recharge.
- **Adult Day Programs**: These programs offer a safe and engaging space for your loved one to interact and stay active, granting you time to focus on other responsibilities or simply relax.
- **Residential Stays**: For a longer break, residential facilities

provide temporary care, ensuring your loved one is in good hands while you take an extended period to rest or travel.

Broadening the Support Network

Beyond respite care, a range of support services can help caregivers navigate their role more effectively:

- **Support Groups**: Joining a caregiver support group connects you with individuals in similar situations. These groups are a source of emotional support, advice, and a sense of belonging.
- **Counseling Services**: Professional counseling can aid caregivers in managing stress and emotional challenges. It's a confidential space to explore feelings and strategies for self-care.
- **Educational Workshops**: Learning sessions about caregiving techniques, effective communication, and self-care can enhance your caregiving skills and resilience.
- **Respite Vouchers**: Financial assistance through respite vouchers can make accessing respite care more feasible, reducing the worry about the cost of taking needed breaks.

Chapter Summary

For caregivers, finding a balance between the demands of caregiving and personal well-being is important. Leveraging respite care and support services is not just beneficial but necessary for maintaining this balance. These resources offer caregivers the support and breaks needed to continue their important work with renewed energy and perspective. Remember, focusing on your well-being ensures you can provide the best care for your loved one, making every step of this caregiving journey sustainable and fulfilling.

◇

MAXIMIZING RESPITE CARE: STRATEGIES FOR CAREGIVERS

CARING for a loved one is a deeply rewarding role, yet it's undeniable that it also comes with its own set of challenges. Recognizing when it's time to step back and recharge is essential not only for your well-being but also for the continued quality of care you provide. Respite care offers a temporary relief, letting caregivers take a well-deserved break. Here's how you can make the most out of respite care services:

Plan in Advance:

Before you find yourself overwhelmed, explore the respite care options in your community. Understanding what's available and having a plan can ease the process when you decide it's time for a break.

Communicate Clearly:

When arranging respite care, be upfront about your loved one's needs and routines. This makes sure the care they receive in your absence is consistent and tailored to their specific requirements.

Explore Additional Support:

Respite care is just one part of the support network available to caregivers. Look into counseling, joining support groups, or educational workshops designed to empower caregivers. These resources can provide valuable coping strategies and a sense of community.

Prioritize Your Well-being:

Use your time away from caregiving duties to focus on self-care. Whether it's indulging in a hobby, reconnecting with friends, or simply enjoying some quiet time, engage in activities that rejuvenate your spirit.

Fully Embrace Your Break:

It's natural to worry about your loved one while you're away, but it's important to trust the respite care you've arranged and allow yourself to relax and recharge. Remember, taking this time is beneficial not just for you but for your loved one too, as it ensures you can continue to provide the best care possible.

Using respite care effectively requires planning, communication, and a commitment to your own self-care. By making the most of these services, you can ensure a balanced approach to caregiving that benefits both you and your loved one. Remember, taking a break isn't a sign of weakness—it's an essential part of a sustainable caregiving journey.

FREQUENTLY ASKED QUESTIONS:

1. What is respite care, and why should I consider it?

Answer: Think of respite care as pressing the pause button on your caregiving duties. It's when someone else steps in to take care of your loved one for a while, giving you the chance to recharge, handle personal tasks, or relax. It's essential because constantly being on duty without a break can lead to stress and burnout. Taking a break helps you stay healthy and keeps your caregiving game strong.

2. What are my options for respite care?

Answer: You've got choices based on your needs and what's best for your loved one. In-home care is when a professional comes to your home to help out. Adult day programs provide a safe and engaging place for your loved one during the day. Short-term residential stays are available too, for when you need a longer break. Each option gives you the freedom to take care of yourself while knowing your loved one is in good hands.

3. How do I start using respite care? It seems overwhelming.

Answer: It's all about taking that first step. Start by checking out local resources or online to see what's available in your area. Talk to other caregivers for recommendations. Your loved one's healthcare provider can also guide you toward reliable respite care services. Remember, it's okay to start small with a few hours of respite care to see how it goes.

4. Can I afford respite care? I'm worried about the costs.

Answer: Costs vary, but there are ways to make respite care more affordable. Look into programs offered by local agencies or non-profits that may offer subsidized rates. Some insurance plans cover respite care, so it's worth checking with your provider. Also, consider community resources or family and friends who might volunteer their time to help out.

5. How can I trust someone else to care for my loved one?

Answer: Trust is a big deal, and it's natural to have concerns. Start by meeting potential respite care providers and ask plenty of questions about their experience and how they handle different situations. Have them spend time with your loved one while you're still around to see how they interact. Look for someone who communicates well and shows genuine care and understanding for your loved one's needs.

Remember, taking advantage of respite care is not a sign of weakness but a smart strategy for maintaining your well-being and ensuring you can continue providing the best care for your loved one.

～

CASE STUDY: SARAH & MICHAEL

Meet Sarah, a dedicated caregiver to her 75-year-old father, Michael, who has advanced Parkinson's disease. Sarah has been his primary caregiver for the last five years, navigating the challenges of his condition with love and patience. Recently, Sarah noticed her energy levels dwindling, her stress escalating, and her health suffering due to the continuous demands of caregiving. She loves her father deeply but realized that to continue caring for him effectively, she needed to take care of herself too.

Sarah's journey to finding balance began when she contacted her local caregiver support group for advice. Here, she learned about the critical importance of respite care—not just as a temporary relief but as an essential part of sustainable caregiving. She discovered various respite care options, including in-home care services, adult day programs, and short-term residential stays. After much consideration, Sarah started with in-home respite care for a few hours each week.

The first time Sarah left a caregiver with her father, she felt a mix of relief and guilt. However, she spent her time off reconnecting with old friends, catching up on sleep, and enjoying a leisurely walk in the park.

After returning home, she found her father content and well-cared-for, which alleviated her guilt and reinforced the value of taking breaks.

Over time, Sarah expanded her respite care plan to include an adult day program twice a week, which Michael grew to enjoy immensely. It offered him the chance to socialize, participate in activities suited to his abilities, and experience a change of scenery. Meanwhile, Sarah used this time to focus on her health, attending yoga classes and routine medical check-ups she had been postponing.

One of the most significant lessons Sarah learned was the importance of communicating her needs and setting clear boundaries. She realized that asking for help and taking time for herself did not make her a less dedicated caregiver; it made her a better one. Her relationship with her father strengthened, and she provided care with renewed patience and energy.

Sarah's case highlights the transformative impact of respite care on both caregivers and their loved ones. It underscores that taking breaks is not a sign of weakness but a strategic approach to maintaining the well-being of both the caregiver and the care recipient. Sarah's story teaches us that by embracing respite care, caregivers can find the balance needed to continue their caregiving journey with compassion, resilience, and love.

~

PART THIRTEEN WRAP-UP:
ACTION ITEMS FOR THE CAREGIVER:

1. **Research Respite Care Options**: Start by exploring various respite care services in your area, including in-home care, adult day programs, and short-term residential stays. Gather information on what each option offers and their costs.
2. **Join a Support Group**: Connect with local or online caregiver support groups. These groups can provide emotional support, practical advice, and insights into managing caregiving responsibilities more effectively.
3. **Assess Your Needs and Set Boundaries**: Take some time to reflect on your personal needs and the parts of caregiving that are most challenging for you. Based on this, set clear boundaries about what you can and cannot do.
4. **Communicate with Your Loved One**: Have an open and honest conversation with the person you're caring for about taking breaks for your well-being and how it ultimately helps both of you.
5. **Plan Your Respite Care**: Decide on the respite care that best suits your needs and start with a trial period to see how it works for you and your loved one. Adjust the plan as necessary based on your experiences.

6. **Schedule Regular Breaks**: Incorporate regular breaks into your caregiving routine. Whether it's a few hours a week or a longer period, schedule these breaks in advance.
7. **Use Respite Time Wisely**: Plan activities for your respite time that rejuvenate you, whether that's spending time with friends, engaging in a hobby, or simply resting.
8. **Monitor Your Loved One's Adjustment**: Keep an eye on how your loved one responds to the respite care arrangement. Ensure they feel safe and comfortable with the care they're receiving in your absence.
9. **Seek Financial Assistance if Needed**: Investigate if there are any financial assistance programs or insurance benefits available to help cover the costs of respite care.
10. **Reflect and Adjust**: After using respite care, take some time to reflect on its impact on your health and caregiving situation. Adjust your respite care plan as needed to ensure it continues to meet your needs.
11. **Prioritize Your Health**: Use the time freed up by respite care to focus on your own health. Schedule medical check-ups, exercise, and engage in activities that promote your physical and mental well-being.
12. **Cultivate a Culture of Openness**: Maintain open lines of communication with the respite care provider and your loved one. Share feedback and discuss any concerns or changes that may be needed to improve the experience for everyone involved.

IN OUR NEXT PART...

In our next Part, we dig into the essential realm of legal and financial planning, a critical part of securing peace of mind for both yourself and your loved ones. The journey of organizing your affairs may seem complex but it is an undeniable cornerstone of thoughtful preparation. We'll explore how to approach this task with clarity and purpose, ensuring your hard-earned assets are protected and your wishes are honored.

We'll start by unpacking the significance of drafting a comprehensive will, a step that lays the foundation for how your assets will be managed and distributed. Alongside this, we'll navigate the intricacies of setting up living wills and powers of attorney, documents that speak on your behalf when you're unable to do so. Our discussion will extend to the strategies for effective financial planning, including budgeting, saving for retirement, and ensuring adequate insurance coverage. By embracing these planning tools, you're not just preparing for the future; you're taking a proactive step toward a more secure and worry-free life for you and those you care about. Join us as we guide you through these critical considerations, offering the knowledge and insights you need to make informed decisions about your legal and financial well-being.

PART FOURTEEN
ESSENTIAL LEGAL AND FINANCIAL PLANNING FOR PEACE OF MIND

Preparing for the future is more than just a prudent step; it's an important part of ensuring your peace of mind and securing the well-being of your loved ones. Diving into the world of legal and financial planning might seem daunting, but it's necessary. Let's break down the essentials that you need to focus on:

Wills and Estate Planning:

Don't leave the distribution of your assets to chance. Drafting a will is the first step in making sure your estate is handled according to your wishes. Think about setting up trusts, deciding on guardians for any minors, and strategies for reducing taxes on your estate.

Living Will and Advance Directive:

These documents spell out your preferences for medical care if you're ever unable to voice your decisions. It's about making your healthcare wishes known ahead of time, ensuring they reflect your values.

Power of Attorney:

Appointing a power of attorney means choosing someone you trust to manage your financial or health matters if you're incapacitated. This person will step in to handle your affairs, making this decision one of the most significant in your planning process.

Financial Planning:

Creating a roadmap for your finances involves budgeting, saving, investing, and planning for retirement. It might be worth consulting with a financial advisor to tailor a plan that fits your unique goals and circumstances.

Insurance Needs:

Proper insurance coverage is your safety net against life's unpredictables. This includes health, life, disability, and property insurance. Regularly reviewing your coverage ensures it keeps pace with your changing needs.

Planning for Long-Term Care:

Considering the possibilities of long-term care, whether in a nursing facility or through home healthcare, is critical. Look into insurance or other financial strategies to cover these potential costs without burdening your loved ones.

Tax Considerations:

Every financial move you make has tax implications. Understanding how to navigate these can help you save significantly eventually. Professional advice can be invaluable here, making your financial plan as tax-efficient as possible.

Beneficiary Updates:

Life changes, and so might your list of beneficiaries. Regularly updating who you've designated on retirement accounts, insurance policies, and other critical documents ensures your assets go exactly where you intend.

Taking these steps now can significantly reduce stress and uncertainty for you and your family. Engaging with legal and financial experts can provide the guidance you need to navigate these waters smoothly. Planning today creates a foundation for a more secure tomorrow.

KEY LEGAL DOCUMENTS FOR FUTURE PLANNING: UNDERSTANDING THEIR IMPACT

Navigating the path to secure your future and the well-being of your loved ones involves understanding and preparing several key legal documents. These documents are essential tools in your planning arsenal, ensuring your wishes are honored and your assets are protected. Let's dig into their significance:

Wills: Laying the Foundation

A will is your voice after you pass away. It dictates how your assets should be distributed and can appoint guardians for minor children. Without a will, state laws take over, potentially leading to outcomes you wouldn't have chosen. It's the cornerstone of your estate planning, helping to avoid family disputes and ensuring your wishes are clear and legally binding.

Trusts: Beyond Simple Asset Distribution

Trusts offer a more nuanced approach to managing your assets, both during your lifetime and after. They can shield your estate from taxes, ensure privacy, and provide for loved ones who might need special arrangements, like minors or those with disabilities. Trusts bypass the public and often have long probate process, offering a smoother transition for your beneficiaries.

Power of Attorney: Ensuring Decision Continuity

The power of attorney allows someone you trust implicitly to decide on your behalf, should you become unable to do so. This encompasses:

- **Financial Power of Attorney**: This designee manages your financial affairs, ensuring bills are paid, and investments are handled according to your wishes.
- **Healthcare Power of Attorney**: This person makes healthcare decisions for you, guided by your preferences for treatment options or end-of-life care.

These documents are not just paperwork; they are expressions of your wishes and safeguards for your future. Working with a seasoned estate planning attorney is important in crafting these documents to reflect your desires accurately and legally. Regular reviews and updates are equally important, as life changes—such as births, marriages, or divorces—can affect your original plans.

By understanding and preparing these key legal documents, you're not just planning; you're securing peace of mind for yourself and your loved ones. It's a step toward making sure your legacy is preserved and protected, just as you envision.

~

SMART ESTATE PLANNING: SEAMLESS ASSET TRANSITIONS AND PEACE OF MIND

NAVIGATING the path of estate planning is like setting up a map for your loved ones, guiding them through what happens to your assets after you're gone. It's about making thoughtful decisions today to prevent unnecessary stress and financial burdens down the line. Here's how to approach estate planning with foresight and care:

Draft a Comprehensive Will:

Your will is the foundation of your estate plan. It outlines exactly who gets what, from your property to sentimental items. By naming an executor, you choose who will oversee the fulfillment of your wishes, ensuring your assets go to the right hands.

Use Trusts for More Than Just Asset Distribution:

Trusts offer a versatile way to manage your estate, providing benefits like avoiding the public eye during probate, cutting down on taxes, and setting up long-term provisions for minors or those with special needs. Trusts make sure your assets are managed and distributed according to your exact specifications.

Implement Powers of Attorney:

Life is unpredictable. Establishing a power of attorney for both health-care and finances ensures that if you're unable to make decisions, someone you trust will step in on your behalf. This covers everything from paying bills to making critical medical decisions, aligned with your wishes.

Healthcare Directives: Your Medical Wishes Respected:

A living will or healthcare directive speaks for you when you can't, outlining your desires for medical treatment. Appointing a healthcare proxy ensures someone is there to advocate for your wishes, providing clarity in difficult times.

Keep Beneficiary Designations Updated:

Life events like marriages, births, or divorces can change your intentions for your assets. Regularly review beneficiary designations on policies and accounts to ensure they reflect your current wishes.

Strategize for Taxes:

Estate taxes can take a significant chunk out of what you leave behind. Explore strategies to reduce this financial hit, such as gifting during your lifetime or setting up specific types of trusts, preserving more of your estate for your beneficiaries.

Regular Reviews: Keeping Your Plan Current

Life's constant changes mean your estate plan needs to evolve too. Regular reviews—at least every few years or after major life events—ensure your plan always matches your current situation and goals.

Professional Guidance is Key:

Estate planning can be complex, touching on intricate legal and financial areas. Enlist the help of professionals like estate planning attorneys and financial advisors to craft a plan that's both comprehensive and tailored to your unique circumstances.

Effective estate planning is about clarity, security, and peace of mind—for both you and your loved ones. By taking these steps, you're not just planning; you're protecting it, ensuring your wishes are honored and your legacy is preserved exactly as you envision.

～

RISKS OF SKIPPING FINANCIAL PLANNING: NAVIGATING WITHOUT A MAP

Not having a solid financial plan is like setting out on a journey without a map. It might not be immediately apparent, but the absence of a clear plan can lead to significant challenges and pitfalls down the road. Here's why it's important to have a financial roadmap:

Savings and Investment Challenges:

Without a financial plan, saving and investing become sporadic, lacking direction and purpose. Goals like retirement, education, or buying a home might seem out of reach as you miss out on compounded growth and the opportunity to build a substantial nest egg.

Budgeting Woes:

A plan is a budget's backbone. Without it, managing monthly expenses becomes a guessing game. This can lead to overspending, accumulating debt, and the constant stress of stretching each dollar. Consistently setting aside money for future needs becomes a challenge, affecting financial stability.

Insurance Gaps:

A solid financial plan includes protecting your assets and income through insurance. Without it, you're exposed to risks—health emergencies, property loss, or accidents can turn into financial catastrophes, wiping out savings or leading to debilitating debt.

Retirement Uncertainties:

One of the most significant risks of not planning is facing retirement unprepared. Without a dedicated strategy for retirement savings, you might find yourself unable to maintain your lifestyle or forced to rely on limited government support or family assistance in your golden years.

Estate Complications:

Ignoring financial planning often means neglecting estate planning. This oversight can leave your loved ones facing legal hurdles, confusion, and potential conflict over your assets and wishes after you're gone.

Missed Wealth-Building Opportunities:

A financial plan isn't just about saving; it's also about growing your wealth through informed investment choices and tax strategies. Without it, you might miss out on opportunities to increase your wealth, limiting your financial freedom and ability to achieve your dreams.

Skipping on financial planning is a gamble with your future security and well-being. It's never too late to start. By taking control and crafting a plan tailored to your goals, you can navigate life's journey with confidence, knowing you're prepared for whatever lies ahead.

~

INSURANCE: YOUR
FINANCIAL SAFETY NET

INSURANCE SERVES as a financial safety net, shielding you from the unpredictable storms of life. Whether it's a health emergency, a car accident, or a natural disaster, insurance steps in to mitigate the financial impact of these unforeseen events. Here's how insurance acts as a cornerstone of financial stability:

Transferring Risk:

At its core, insurance is about transferring the risk of financial loss from you to the insurance provider. By paying a premium, you're essentially handing over the financial risk of big, unexpected expenses to a company better equipped to handle them.

Asset Protection:

From your home to your car, your assets are investments worth protecting. Insurance covers the repair or replacement costs if they're damaged or lost, ensuring you need not drain your savings to restore your life back to normal.

Healthcare Costs:

Health insurance is more than just a policy; it's a lifeline. Covering everything from emergency surgeries to routine check-ups, it prevents medical bills from becoming financial burdens that can destabilize your finances.

Ensuring Business Continuity:

For business owners, insurance is pivotal in weathering unexpected setbacks. Be it property damage, legal liabilities, or business interruptions, the right insurance coverage helps keep the doors open and operations running, even in tough times.

Peace of Mind:

Perhaps the most significant role of insurance is the peace of mind it offers. Knowing you're covered in case of mishaps can relieve stress, allowing you to live, work, and enjoy life with less worry about "what ifs."

Insurance is not just a policy—it's a proactive strategy for protecting your financial future. By evaluating your needs and securing the right coverage, you're not just insuring your possessions; you're safeguarding your financial peace of mind and ensuring that, no matter what life throws your way, you have a reliable financial safety net ready to catch you.

~

KEEPING YOUR FINANCIAL HOUSE IN ORDER: THE VALUE OF PERIODIC REVIEWS

STAYING on top of your legal and financial plans isn't just about crossing items off your to-do list; it's about ensuring your peace of mind and securing your future. Life's constant changes and the ever-evolving legal and financial landscapes make regular reviews and updates of your plans not just beneficial but essential. Here's why:

Adapting to Life's Changes:

Life throws curveballs. From welcoming a new family member to career shifts or health changes, each significant life event can change your financial needs and goals. By sometimes reviewing your plans, you ensure they reflect your current situation and aspirations, keeping your path to financial security clear and customized.

Navigating Tax and Regulatory Shifts:

Tax laws and financial regulations are in a state of flux, with new amendments and policies introduced regularly. Keeping your legal and financial plans updated given these changes can safeguard you against unforeseen liabilities and capitalize on potential benefits, ensuring you're not leaving money on the table.

Safeguarding Your Assets:

Your asset protection strategies need to evolve alongside your asset portfolio. Regularly revisiting your plans can help identify new risks or exposure and adjust your protection measures. Whether it's tweaking your insurance coverage or restructuring your investment approach, staying proactive is key to asset preservation.

Monitoring Investment Performance:

The financial markets are dynamic, and the performance of your investments can shift. Regular reviews let you assess how your investments align with your risk tolerance and financial goals, making it possible to adjust your strategy proactively rather than reactively, ensuring your portfolio remains strong and growth-oriented.

Ensuring Peace of Mind:

Perhaps the most compelling reason to keep your legal and financial plans up-to-date is the peace of mind it brings. Knowing that you're prepared for the future and can handle whatever life throws your way can alleviate stress and leave you free to focus on the present.

Treating your legal and financial plans as living documents that require regular review and updates is important. Engaging with a financial advisor or attorney can help make sure your plans are not only current but also strategically aligned with your goals and life's changing circumstances. Remember, in the realm of personal finance, complacency can be costly, but diligence pays dividends.

～

EMPOWERING YOUR FUTURE: A GUIDE TO STARTING YOUR LEGAL AND FINANCIAL PLANNING

STARTING your legal and financial planning journey may seem daunting at first glance. Yet, with the right set of tools and guidance, you can lay a strong foundation for a secure future. Here's a roadmap to get you started:

Educational Resources:

Arm yourself with knowledge. Diving into many resources such as books, reputable online chapters, and webinars can illuminate the basics of estate planning, investing, and saving for retirement. Websites like Investopedia, NerdWallet, and the Financial Planning Association offer a wealth of information tailored to beginners.

Professional Guidance:

A journey like this often requires a navigator. Seeking advice from legal and financial professionals can give you customized strategies that align with your unique situation. For legal planning, including wills and trusts, a consultation with an estate planning attorney is invaluable. For financial planning, certified financial advisors can help craft a plan that matches your goals and risk tolerance.

Budgeting Tools:

A cornerstone of financial planning is a well-structured budget. Many apps and online tools, such as Mint or You Need A Budget (YNAB), offer intuitive platforms for tracking your spending and savings, helping you stay aligned with your financial goals.

Emergency Fund Essentials:

An emergency fund is your financial safety net. Aim to save a reserve of three to six months' worth of expenses, setting aside funds in a high-yield savings account where your money can grow but remains accessible.

Goal Setting:

Define what you're working toward. Whether it's homeownership, starting a business, or ensuring a comfortable retirement, setting clear, actionable goals gives your financial plan purpose and direction.

Will Preparation:

Don't overlook the importance of drafting a will. This document is fundamental in ensuring your assets are distributed according to your wishes. Online services like LegalZoom or Rocket Lawyer can offer a starting point, but consulting with a legal professional is recommended for complex estates.

Advanced Estate Planning:

For those with more intricate assets or concerns, digging into estate planning with a specialist can offer strategies for tax minimization, trusts, and more, ensuring your legacy is preserved exactly as you envision.

Stay Updated:

The financial and legal landscapes are ever-evolving. Subscribing to newsletters from trusted financial news sources and attending relevant seminars can keep you informed of the latest trends and laws affecting your planning efforts.

Legal and financial planning is not a one-time task but an ongoing process. By leveraging these resources and continually revisiting your plan, you can navigate your journey with confidence, knowing you're well-prepared for whatever lies ahead.

∾

FREQUENTLY ASKED QUESTIONS:

1. What's the first step in legal planning for the future, and why is it so important?

Answer: The first step is creating a will. It's important because it outlines how you want your assets distributed and ensures your wishes are followed. Without a will, state laws decide what happens to your assets, which might not align with your preferences. It's about clarifying your intentions and legally binding, so there's no confusion or conflict among your loved ones after you're gone.

2. I've heard a lot about Power of Attorney. What does it mean, and why do I need it?

Answer: A Power of Attorney (POA) is a document that allows you to appoint someone you trust to decide on your behalf if you're unable to do so. There are two main types: a Financial POA, which covers financial decisions, and a Healthcare POA, for medical decisions. Having a POA in place makes sure your affairs are managed according to your wishes, even if you're incapacitated. It's about entrusting someone with the authority to look after your well-being and assets, according to your guidelines.

3. Can you explain what living wills and advance directives are? How do they differ from a regular will?

Answer: Living wills and advance directives are documents that outline your preferences for medical treatment if you're unable to communicate them yourself. They can specify your wishes regarding life-support measures, resuscitation, and other medical interventions. Unlike a regular will, which deals with asset distribution after your death, living wills and advance directives focus on your healthcare preferences while you're still alive. They provide clarity and direction to healthcare providers and your family during difficult times.

4. How can I make sure my financial planning is solid? What should I focus on?

Answer: Solid financial planning starts with setting clear goals, budgeting, saving, and investing wisely. Focus on building an emergency fund, planning for retirement, and considering insurance needs to protect against unexpected life events. Consulting a financial advisor can provide personalized advice tailored to your situation, helping you navigate investments, tax strategies, and retirement planning to secure your financial future.

5. What's the best way to approach long-term care planning, and why is it important?

Answer: Long-term care planning involves preparing for potential healthcare needs and living arrangements as you age. It's important because it ensures you have a plan in place to manage healthcare costs, which can be significant, without burdening your family. Start by researching long-term care insurance options, understanding the benefits and limitations of each, and considering how they fit into your overall financial plan. Exploring these options early gives you the freedom to choose the care that best aligns with your wishes and financial situation.

Remember, legal and financial planning is not just about protecting assets; it's about ensuring peace of mind for you and your loved ones.

Taking proactive steps now can make a significant difference providing clarity, security, and a well-charted path forward.

❧

CASE STUDY: MARIA & TOM

LET'S talk about Maria and Tom, a couple who navigated the complex journey of legal and financial planning in their later years. Maria had been the primary caregiver for Tom, who was diagnosed with early-onset Alzheimer's at the age of 65. As Tom's condition progressed, Maria realized the importance of having a solid legal and financial plan in place, not only for Tom's care but also for their family's future.

At first, the thought of diving into wills, trusts, and financial planning seemed overwhelming to Maria. She felt out of her depth but knew it was important for ensuring Tom's well-being and securing their family's financial future. They started by drafting a will, a step that Maria found comforting. It gave her a sense of control, knowing that Tom's assets would be distributed according to their wishes.

Next, they explored living wills and advance directives. This was a difficult conversation, discussing scenarios in which Tom might not make his own medical decisions. However, once they made those decisions, Maria felt a weight lifted, knowing that Tom's healthcare preferences were documented.

Appointing a power of attorney was another critical step. Maria was chosen to manage Tom's financial matters and health decisions if he became incapacitated. This responsibility was daunting, but Maria felt honored to be trusted with Tom's care in such a real way.

Financial planning was an area where Maria sought professional help. They worked with a financial advisor to create a roadmap that included budgeting, saving, and investing strategies tailored to their goals and circumstances. This planning was pivotal in making sure they had the resources needed for Tom's long-term care, without compromising their financial security.

Insurance coverage was another area they had to revisit. Ensuring they had adequate health, life, and disability insurance became a priority, especially as they considered the potential costs associated with long-term care. They also made sure to regularly review and update their beneficiary designations, reflecting changes in their family dynamics.

One of the most significant lessons Maria learned through this process was the importance of regular reviews and updates to their legal and financial plans. Life was unpredictable, and as Tom's condition changed, so did their needs and priorities. Maria found peace of mind in knowing that their affairs were in order, letting her focus more on spending quality time with Tom.

This case study of Maria and Tom highlights the important role of legal and financial planning in caregiving. This process might seem daunting at first, but with the right support and resources, it can provide invaluable peace of mind and security for the future.

~

PART FOURTEEN WRAP-UP:
ACTION ITEMS FOR THE CAREGIVER:

HERE'S a list of action items for caregivers, inspired by Maria and Tom's journey, to ensure comprehensive legal and financial planning:

1. **Draft a Will**: Start by drafting a will to dictate how assets should be distributed. If unsure where to begin, seek legal advice to ensure all parts are covered.
2. **Set Up a Living Will and Advance Directive**: Clearly document healthcare preferences in case of incapacity to make decisions. This ensures healthcare wishes are known and can be honored.
3. **Appoint a Power of Attorney**: Choose a trusted individual to manage financial and healthcare matters if incapacitated. This decision is important, so consider it carefully.
4. **Consult with a Financial Advisor**: Create a financial plan that includes budgeting, saving, investing, and planning for retirement. Tailor the plan to fit unique goals and circumstances.
5. **Review Insurance Needs**: Ensure adequate coverage for health, life, disability, and property insurance. Regularly review policies to adjust coverage as needed.

6. **Plan for Long-Term Care**: Investigate options for long-term care, including insurance or financial strategies to cover potential costs without burdening loved ones.

7. **Understand Tax Considerations**: Every financial decision has tax implications. Seek professional advice to make the financial plan as tax-efficient as possible.

8. **Regularly Update Beneficiary Designations**: Life changes, such as births, marriages, or divorces, can affect plans. Regularly review and update beneficiary designations.

9. **Conduct Regular Reviews and Updates**: Life's unpredictable nature means plans need to evolve. Schedule regular reviews of legal and financial documents to ensure they match current situations and goals.

10. **Seek Support and Resources**: Don't navigate this process alone. Use resources, join support groups, and consider professional guidance to navigate the legal and financial planning process smoothly.

By following these action items, caregivers can create a strong foundation for their legal and financial planning, ensuring peace of mind and security for the future, much like Maria did for Tom.

~

IN OUR NEXT PART...

In our next Part, we will tackle a topic that's important yet often overlooked until it's urgently needed: respite care. Think of it as pressing pause, a chance for you, the caregiver, to catch your breath, recharge, and gather strength. We'll explore how integrating respite care into your routine isn't just beneficial; it's essential for maintaining your well-being and ensuring you can continue to provide the best care for your loved one with dementia. We'll guide you through understanding the different forms of respite care available, from in-home assistance to adult day care programs, and how to access these services. It's all about finding that important balance that lets you care for your loved one and yourself.

We'll dig into the financial parts of dementia care, a concern that weighs heavily on many caregivers' minds. Navigating the cost of care can be daunting, but we're here to show you that there are strategies and resources to help manage these expenses effectively. From crafting a dedicated dementia care budget to seeking financial assistance programs and maximizing insurance benefits, we'll give you practical steps to take. This journey might seem filled with challenges, but with the right information and support, you can find a path that eases the financial strain and lets you focus on what matters: providing love and care for your family member with dementia.

❧

PART FIFTEEN
STRATEGIES FOR NAVIGATING DEMENTIA CARE COSTS: A CAREGIVER'S FINANCIAL GUIDE

CRAFTING A DEMENTIA CARE BUDGET: TRACKING EXPENSES FOR FINANCIAL CLARITY

NAVIGATING the financial waters of dementia care requires foresight, planning, and knowledge of available resources. Here's a guide to help caregivers manage the costs associated with caring for a loved one with dementia, ensuring both financial stability and peace of mind.

Develop a Dedicated Budget: Crafting a budget that specifically addresses dementia care expenses is important. Include all potential costs such as medical treatments, prescriptions, in-home care, or residential care facilities. This targeted approach helps in assigning resources more effectively.

Meticulously Record Expenses: Keeping an accurate log of every expense tied to dementia care can unveil patterns and opportunities for savings. This comprehensive financial tracking is invaluable for both immediate and long-term planning.

Investigate Financial Assistance: Many avenues exist for financial support, ranging from government programs like Medicaid to nonprofit organizations offering aid to dementia patients. Dig into these options to alleviate the financial burden.

Engage with a Financial Professional: A financial advisor with experience in elder care can offer tailored advice, helping you strategize for both current and future dementia care needs. Their knowledge can guide critical decisions and financial changes.

Maximize Insurance Benefits: Ensure your current insurance plans, including health and long-term care insurance, optimally cover dementia-related costs. An in-depth review might reveal gaps in coverage or opportunities for more benefits.

Evaluate Care Alternatives: Alternatives like adult day care or part-time in-home care might offer more cost-effective solutions than full-time residential care. Assess the many care options to find a balance between quality care and manageable expenses.

Lean on Support Networks: The journey of caregiving is not one to walk alone. Engaging with support groups and counseling can provide not only emotional solace but also practical advice on handling the financial parts of dementia care.

Future-Proof Your Finances: Given the progressive nature of dementia, forward-thinking financial planning is essential. Setting up a trust or crafting a comprehensive financial roadmap can secure your loved one's care needs down the line.

While the financial strain of dementia care is undeniable, equipped with the right strategies and support, caregivers can navigate these challenges with greater ease and confidence. Remember, securing financial assistance and leveraging community resources can significantly ease the burden, letting you focus on providing compassionate care.

~

NAVIGATING FINANCIAL AID FOR DEMENTIA CARE

MANAGING the costs of dementia care can feel daunting. However, various strategies and resources can make this process smoother and more manageable. Here's how you can navigate the financial landscape of dementia care:

Research Government Benefits: Programs like Medicaid and Medicare might help with costs related to dementia care. Medicaid is especially useful for long-term care for those with limited finances.

Explore Grants and Scholarships: Look into financial aid from organizations focused on dementia care. The Alzheimer's Foundation of America and the Alzheimer's Association are good places to start.

Seek Charitable Organizations: Some charities offer financial support to families facing dementia. Organizations such as the National Alliance for Caregiving and the Family Caregiver Alliance can be valuable resources.

Create a Budget: Drafting a budget for dementia care expenses lets you track spending and manage costs effectively. A financial advisor can help to craft a detailed financial plan tailored to your needs.

Consider Long-Term Care Insurance: Check if your loved one's long-term care insurance covers dementia care. Understanding the policy's benefits can significantly reduce care-related expenses.

Use Respite Care Services: Respite care offers caregivers a necessary break, providing time to focus on personal and financial planning.

Look into Clinical Trials: Clinical trials may offer access to new treatments at low or no cost, potentially easing financial burdens.

Seek Mental Health Support: The financial stress of dementia care can affect your mental health. Consider consulting a therapist or joining a support group to navigate these challenges.

You're not navigating this journey alone. Support groups, healthcare professionals, and financial advisors for advice and support. By taking proactive steps to manage financial challenges, you can reduce stress and ensure quality care for your loved one.

~

STRATEGIZING FINANCIALLY FOR DEMENTIA CARE

CARING for a loved one with dementia involves not just emotional and physical dedication, but also financial planning. Here's a structured approach to manage the financial parts effectively:

Create a Budget: First, look closely at your finances. Lay out all your expenses against your income to see where your money goes each month. This clarity can highlight where you can reduce spending and reallocate funds toward care needs.

Research Financial Assistance Programs: Investigate support avenues like Medicaid, VA benefits, or long-term care insurance that might ease the financial burden of care. Local charities and community resources may also offer assistance or services at reduced costs.

Seek Professional Advice: Consulting with a financial planner or advisor with knowledge in elder care is invaluable. They can tailor a long-term financial plan to your unique situation, guiding you through estate planning, managing tax implications, and securing your retirement.

Consider Care Options: Evaluate various care settings – from in-home support to specialized memory care facilities. Understanding the costs and benefits of each can help you make an informed decision that aligns with your loved one's needs and your financial capacity.

Look for Cost-Saving Strategies: Actively seek ways to cut down on care expenses. This could mean negotiating rates with providers, choosing generic medications, or using senior discounts and subsidies.

Prioritize Self-Care: The financial stress of managing dementia care can take a toll. Lean on your support network, find solace in caregiver support groups, and engage in activities that rejuvenate your spirit and mind.

Explore Alternative Funding Sources: Brainstorm creative ways to boost your income – renting out space, selling items you no longer need, or considering part-time work. These strategies can provide a financial cushion for care expenses.

Navigating the cost of dementia care is a substantial challenge, but you're not in it alone. Draw on the knowledge of professionals and the strength of community resources to guide you through this journey, ensuring both you and your loved one are cared for.

$\sim$

NAVIGATING COST-EFFECTIVE DEMENTIA CARE OPTIONS

Facing the costs associated with dementia care can be daunting, yet there are strategies to manage these expenses effectively. Here's how you can ensure quality care without overwhelming financial pressure:

Explore Alternative Care Options: Traditional nursing homes or residential care facilities come with high costs. Look into adult day care centers or in-home care services as more affordable alternatives. These options can provide the care and stimulation for your loved one at a fraction of the cost.

Seek Financial Assistance: Various programs offer financial help for dementia care. Investigate Medicaid for potential coverage of long-term care needs. Also, many nonprofit organizations are dedicated to supporting dementia patients and their families with financial aid.

Create a Budget: Organizing a detailed budget for dementia-related expenses is important. This helps you track your spending and identify potential savings. A financial advisor with experience in caregiving situations can offer valuable assistance in crafting a budget that fits your needs.

Focus on Self-Care: The demands of caregiving can be intense. Remember to look after your own well-being by connecting with supportive friends or family and engaging in activities that replenish your energy. A well-cared-for caregiver is more effective and resilient.

Use Community Resources: Many communities provide support and services for dementia caregivers and patients. These might include educational workshops, respite care, or counseling, often at no cost. Leveraging these resources can provide more support and reduce out-of-pocket expenses.

Managing dementia care costs requires a blend of creativity, research, and support. By exploring alternative care solutions, seeking financial assistance, and using community resources, you can navigate this challenging time more smoothly while ensuring your loved one receives the care they deserve.

～

STRATEGIC FINANCIAL PLANNING FOR DEMENTIA CARE

ADDRESSING the costs of dementia care requires a thoughtful approach to financial management. Here are strategies to ease the financial burden and ensure your loved one receives the care they need:

Budget with Precision: Begin by closely examining your financial inflow and outflow. Crafting a detailed budget for dementia care helps identify potential savings and areas where funds can be reallocated.

Asset Optimization: Look into selling items that are no longer needed, like an extra vehicle or rarely used valuables. Downsizing your living situation or renting out part of your property can also provide a financial boost.

Consider a Reverse Mortgage: For homeowners, a reverse mortgage could be a good choice. This financial tool lets you access the equity in your home, turning it into usable funds for dementia care without selling your property.

Government Assistance Programs: Investigate government programs designed to help with long-term care costs. Medicaid, for example, may cover certain dementia care services for those who qualify.

Professional Financial Guidance: Engaging with a financial advisor with expertise in elder care can be invaluable. They can help navigate the complexities of long-term financial planning for dementia care, offering tailored advice and strategies.

Community Support: Many communities offer resources and support for dementia caregivers, including financial assistance programs, respite care, and support groups. Leveraging these resources can provide both emotional and financial relief.

Prioritize Your Well-being: The financial and emotional weight of dementia care can be immense. It's essential to care for your own health and well-being, seeking support from your network and professional counselors as needed.

By using these strategies, you can navigate the financial challenges of dementia care ensuring both you and your loved one are supported through this journey.

∽

NAVIGATING FINANCIAL STRAIN WITH DEMENTIA CARE: A GUIDE TO SUPPORT AND SELF-CARE

MANAGING the financial demands of dementia care can be overwhelming. However, there are strategies and support systems available to help ease this burden. Here's a roadmap to finding balance and support:

Budget Creation: First, lay out a detailed budget that captures all dementia-related expenses. This could range from medical treatments and medications to caregiving services. A clear financial picture is the first step toward effective management.

Financial Assistance Exploration: Many programs offer financial support to those caring for loved ones with dementia. Investigate options like Medicaid, Medicare, and other disability benefits. Each program has its eligibility criteria and benefits, so it's worth exploring what might be available to you.

Future Financial Planning: Consulting with a financial planner who understands the intricacies of dementia care can be beneficial. They can guide you in preparing for both current and future financial needs, ensuring a stable plan is in place.

Support System Engagement: The emotional toll of caregiving, compounded by financial stress, can be significant. Contacting family, friends, or joining support groups can provide a much-needed outlet and source of comfort and advice.

Self-Care Prioritization: Amidst the challenges, don't forget to take care of yourself. Engaging in activities that rejuvenate your spirit and relax your mind is important. Whether it's through exercise, hobbies, or simply taking a quiet moment for yourself, self-care is key.

Community Resource Utilization: Many communities offer resources geared toward supporting caregivers of individuals with dementia. These can range from informational sessions to financial aid. Local organizations or religious groups often have programs designed to help caregivers.

In navigating the financial aspects of dementia care, remember that resources and support networks are available to help you through this journey. By seeking assistance, engaging with your community, and taking care of your own well-being, you can manage the challenges that come with dementia care more effectively.

∼

USING RESPITE CARE SERVICES: A KEY TO SUSTAINABLE DEMENTIA CAREGIVING

CARING for a loved one with dementia is a journey filled with love, challenges, and significant responsibilities. Amidst these responsibilities, it's vital for caregivers to remember their own well-being. Here's how incorporating respite care services can be a game-changer:

Respite Care Services: These services are a lifeline for caregivers. They provide temporary care for your loved one, letting you rest and recharge. Whether it's for a few hours or for a couple of days, respite care can prevent caregiver burnout and ensure you're at your best for your loved one.

Financial Assistance for Care: The cost of dementia care can be daunting, but financial assistance programs are available to help. Investigate programs like Medicaid and Veterans Affairs benefits, which may cover costs of respite care. Local Alzheimer's associations and nonprofit organizations also often have resources or grants available specifically for dementia care.

Effective Budgeting: A dedicated budget for dementia care expenses allows for clearer financial management and planning. Tracking all costs related to care can help identify where financial assistance is needed most. Financial planners specializing in elder care can offer invaluable advice, helping you navigate through financial planning and potential cost-saving strategies.

Community Support: Leverage the power of community resources. Many communities have senior centers, support groups, and Alzheimer's associations that provide not just emotional support but also practical resources and information on managing dementia care, including affordable respite care options.

Alternative Care Options: Exploring different care settings, like adult day care programs or assisted living facilities, might offer more sustainable financial and care solutions. These settings not only cater to the unique needs of individuals with dementia but also provide regular respite for caregivers.

Remember, focusing on your health and well-being is not an act of self-ishness; it's a necessity. By incorporating respite care into your care-giving plan, you ensure you have the energy, patience, and strength to provide the compassionate care your loved one deserves. Please reach out for support and use the resources available to you as a caregiver.

∿

FREQUENTLY ASKED QUESTIONS:

1. How do I start planning for the costs of dementia care?

Answer: Start by creating a dedicated budget for dementia-related expenses. List out all potential costs, including medical treatments, caregiving supplies, in-home care, or residential care fees. This will help you understand the financial commitment involved and plan. It's also wise to meticulously record all expenses related to care to identify areas where financial changes can be made.

2. Are there any financial assistance programs available for dementia care?

Answer: Yes, there are several options you might explore. Government programs like Medicaid can provide support for those who qualify, covering parts of long-term care. Additionally, various nonprofit organizations offer financial aid and resources specifically for individuals with dementia and their caregivers. Research and contact these organizations to understand the eligibility criteria and application process.

3. When should I consider professional financial advice for managing dementia care costs?

Answer: It's beneficial to engage with a financial professional, especially one experienced in elder care, early. They can offer personalized advice on managing current expenses and planning for future needs. A professional can guide you through estate planning, insurance options, and potential tax implications, ensuring a well-rounded approach to financial management in dementia care.

4. How can I make sure my insurance plans are optimized for dementia care?

Answer: Review your current health and long-term care insurance policies to understand what parts of dementia care are covered. You might need to adjust your plans or consider more coverage based on your loved one's specific needs. Consulting with an insurance professional can provide clarity on the benefits and limitations of your policies, helping to maximize the support you receive.

5. What cost-effective care options are available for someone with dementia?

Answer: Look into alternative care settings that might offer more affordable solutions without compromising the quality of care. Adult day care programs, for example, provide care and social interaction for your loved one during the day, which can be less expensive than full-time residential care. In-home care services, where you can control the hours and level of care provided, can also be a flexible and potentially more affordable option. Always assess the many care options available to find the best fit for your budget and your loved one's needs.

Navigating the financial parts of dementia care is undoubtedly challenging, but remember, you're not alone. There are resources, support networks, and professionals ready to help you. Trying to understand and manage these costs effectively can provide peace of mind for you and your loved one.

CASE STUDY: MARY'S JOURNEY WITH RESPITE CARE AND FINANCIAL PLANNING

MEET MARY, a 68-year-old retired teacher who became a full-time caregiver for her husband, John, diagnosed with early-stage dementia two years ago. Mary's story is one of love, dedication, and learning the hard way about the necessity of self-care and financial planning in the caregiving journey.

The Challenge:

Mary devoted her days and nights to caring for John, ensuring his comfort and safety. While she managed the emotional and physical demands of caregiving with grace, the financial strain of dementia care and the lack of personal time took a toll on her well-being. Mary felt exhausted, isolated, and worried about their future finances.

The Turning Point:

The turning point came when Mary went to a local Alzheimer's support group meeting, where she heard about respite care. She learned that respite care could give her the break she desperately needed, offering temporary care for John and allowing her some time to herself. Mary also realized the importance of a solid financial plan to manage the costs of dementia care. She decided it was time to make changes.

Action Taken:

1. **Respite Care**: Mary explored various respite care options and started with in-home care services for a few hours each week. This break allowed her to reconnect with friends, go to her own medical appointments, and simply rest.
2. **Financial Planning**: Mary met with a financial advisor specializing in elder care. Together, they crafted a detailed budget for John's care, investigated potential government benefits like Medicaid, and reviewed their insurance policies to ensure maximum coverage for dementia-related expenses.
3. **Community and Support**: Mary continued to go to the Alzheimer's support group, finding comfort and practical advice from others in similar situations. She learned about more resources and financial aid programs for families affected by dementia.

Lessons Learned:

- **The Importance of Respite**: Mary learned that taking regular breaks was not a luxury but a necessity for her health and the quality of care she could provide for John. Respite care became an integral part of their care plan.
- **Financial Planning is Crucial**: By addressing their financial situation head-on, Mary alleviated much of the stress associated with the costs of dementia care. She learned to navigate the complex landscape of care funding, insurance, and government assistance.
- **Community Support is Invaluable**: The support group gave Mary not just emotional support but also practical advice and resources. She found that sharing experiences with others in similar situations made her feel less alone and more empowered.

- **Self-Care is Essential**: Mary recognized that caring for herself was as important as caring for John. By incorporating self-care into her routine, she was better equipped to handle the challenges of caregiving.

Mary's journey highlights the challenges and solutions in navigating dementia care, emphasizing the need for respite, financial planning, and community support. Her experience serves as a reminder to other caregivers of the importance of taking care of themselves while they care for their loved ones.

PART FIFTEEN WRAP-UP:
ACTION ITEMS FOR THE CAREGIVER:

1. **Explore Respite Care Options**: Research and identify respite care services in your area, such as in-home care, adult day care programs, or temporary residential care facilities. Determine which option best suits your needs and schedule regular breaks to recharge.
2. **Schedule a Financial Planning Session**: Arrange a meeting with a financial advisor with experience in elder care. Prepare to discuss your current financial situation, explore funding options for dementia care, and develop a comprehensive financial plan.
3. **Investigate Government and Community Assistance**: Look into eligibility for government programs like Medicaid or Veterans Affairs benefits that can help cover the costs of dementia care. Additionally, explore local nonprofit organizations and charities that offer financial aid or services at reduced costs.
4. **Review Insurance Policies**: Thoroughly review your existing health and long-term care insurance policies to understand what dementia-related expenses are covered. Consider

adjusting your coverage if necessary to ensure ideal benefits for dementia care.

5. **Join a Support Group**: Find a local or online support group for caregivers of individuals with dementia. Participation in these groups can provide emotional support, practical advice, and information on resources and coping strategies.

6. **Create a Care Budget**: Develop a detailed budget specifically for dementia care expenses. Include all potential costs such as medical treatments, caregiving supplies, in-home care services, or residential care fees. Regularly update this budget to reflect any changes in care needs or financial situation.

7. **Document All Care Expenses**: Start meticulously recording every expense related to dementia care. This will help in identifying spending patterns, managing the budget more effectively, and preparing for potential tax deductions or reimbursements.

8. **Focus on Personal Well-being**: Schedule time for self-care activities that rejuvenate your spirit and health. Whether it's exercise, hobbies, or simply taking a walk, ensure you set aside time for activities that help you relax and de-stress.

9. **Educate Yourself on Dementia Care**: Seek educational resources, workshops, or seminars that focus on dementia care. Gaining a deeper understanding of the condition and care strategies can improve your caregiving approach and confidence.

10. **Plan for Long-Term Care Needs**: Consider the future care needs of your loved one with dementia. Start exploring long-term care options and make preliminary plans for transitions that may become necessary as the condition progresses.

By following these action items, caregivers can better manage the demands of caring for a loved one with dementia, ensuring both their own well-being and the best care for their loved one.

∾

IN OUR NEXT PART...

In our next Part, we'll dig into the transformative power of technology in dementia care, highlighting how it can significantly ease the caregiving burden while enhancing the safety and well-being of individuals with dementia. As caregivers, embracing technology may seem overwhelming at first, but understanding its potential to streamline care, improve safety, and foster communication can change the caregiving landscape for the better. We'll explore various technological tools, from simple apps that help manage daily tasks and medication reminders to more advanced systems that track health and activity, ensuring peace of mind for both caregivers and their loved ones. This exploration will not only introduce you to the range of options available but also guide you on how to select and implement these technologies effectively in your care strategies.

We'll discuss the importance of staying informed and adaptable as technology evolves. The rapid pace of innovation in healthcare technology promises even more support and resources for those navigating the challenges of dementia care. By keeping abreast of new tools and platforms, caregivers can continue to provide compassionate, effective care, ensuring their loved ones remain safe, engaged, and supported. Our guide will give practical advice on leveraging technology to its fullest potential, empowering you and your loved one to face the journey of dementia with confidence and hope. Join us as we explore how technology is reshaping dementia care, offering solutions that make a significant difference in the lives of those affected by this condition.

~

PART SIXTEEN
ENHANCING DEMENTIA CARE THROUGH TECHNOLOGY: SIMPLIFYING CAREGIVING AND IMPROVING SAFETY AND WELL-BEING

EMBRACING TECHNOLOGY: TRANSFORMING DEMENTIA CARE FOR THE BETTER

NAVIGATING the journey of dementia care presents unique challenges and responsibilities for caregivers. This path requires constant vigilance, empathy, and innovation. Thankfully, the rise of technology in healthcare has ushered in a new era of support for both caregivers and those living with dementia. Let's dig into how technology can significantly ease the caregiving burden and enhance the safety, comfort, and well-being of individuals with dementia.

Technology's Impact on Dementia Care:

Integrating technology into dementia care has been nothing short of transformative. It offers tools that help with monitoring safety, ensuring consistent medication management, and simplifying daily care routines. This technological evolution means caregivers can now access many resources designed to make their roles more manageable and to provide enriched care experiences.

Key Benefits and Tools:

- **Enhanced Safety and Monitoring**: Devices and apps designed for real-time location tracking and activity tracking can provide peace of mind by ensuring the safety of individuals with dementia. Wearables and home tracking systems can alert caregivers to potential issues, such as wandering or falls, allowing for prompt response.

- **Medication Management**: Automated medication dispensers and reminder apps help make sure individuals with dementia take their medications correctly and on time, reducing the risk of missed doses or overdosing.
- **Improved Communication**: Technology helps with better communication between individuals with dementia, their caregivers, and healthcare providers. Digital platforms and social apps can help maintain social connections, reducing feelings of isolation.
- **Cognitive Assistance**: Apps and games designed to support cognitive function can offer engaging ways for individuals with dementia to stimulate their minds, potentially slowing the progression of cognitive decline.
- **Care Coordination**: Digital tools and platforms let caregivers efficiently organize and manage care tasks, appointments, and health records, streamlining the caregiving process.

Implementing Technological Solutions:

Embracing technology in dementia care begins with identifying the specific needs and challenges faced by the individual with dementia. From there, caregivers can explore and select appropriate technological tools that address these needs. Choose user-friendly solutions that seamlessly integrate into daily routines, making sure they enhance, rather than complicate, the caregiving experience.

Chapter Summary:

The role of technology in dementia care is invaluable, offering innovative solutions that improve the quality of life for individuals with dementia and their caregivers. By leveraging these technological advancements, caregivers can provide more effective, compassionate care, ensuring their loved ones remain safe, engaged, and supported throughout their dementia journey. As we continue to explore and develop new technologies, the future of dementia care looks increasingly hopeful, promising even greater support and empowerment for those navigating this challenging path.

~

NAVIGATING DEMENTIA CARE WITH TECHNOLOGY: A GUIDE TO ESSENTIAL TOOLS

IN DEMENTIA CARE, technology stands as a beacon of hope, offering innovative solutions that can significantly enhance the safety, independence, and quality of life of those affected by dementia. For caregivers, navigating the many technological options available can be daunting. Here's an overview of different types of technology that have proven invaluable in dementia care:

Monitoring Devices: A cornerstone in dementia care, monitoring devices offer caregivers insights into the daily activities and health of their loved ones. From wearable devices that track sleep patterns and physical activity to advanced systems that monitor vital signs, these tools help to detect early signs of health changes or emergencies.

GPS Trackers: Wandering is a common issue in dementia care. GPS trackers, whether as wearable devices or embedded in everyday items like shoes or bracelets, empower caregivers to quickly locate their loved ones if they wander off, providing peace of mind and enhancing safety.

Reminder Apps: Staying on top of medication schedules, appointments, and daily routines can be challenging for individuals with dementia. Reminder apps serve as a digital aide-memoire, issuing notifications for medications, appointments, and even encouraging hydration and movement throughout the day.

Electronic Memory Aids: Memory loss can be one of the most challenging parts of dementia, both for the individual and their loved ones. Electronic memory aids, such as digital photo frames that display cherished memories or voice-activated devices that offer reminders of important personal information, can help support cognitive functions and foster a sense of connection to their life's narrative.

Assistive Communication Devices: As dementia progresses, verbal communication may become difficult. Assistive communication devices range from simple tools like picture boards that help express needs or preferences to sophisticated speech-generating devices that enable more complex communication, thus preserving the dignity and autonomy of the individual with dementia.

Embracing technology in dementia care not only aids in managing the condition's daily challenges but also opens up new avenues for interaction and engagement. By integrating these tools into care routines, caregivers can enhance the well-being of their loved ones while also alleviating burdens associated with caregiving responsibilities. As technology continues to evolve, so too will the opportunities to improve the lives of those living with dementia and their caregivers.

~

TRANSFORMING DEMENTIA CARE THROUGH TECHNOLOGY: REAL-WORLD SUCCESS STORIES

IN THE JOURNEY of dementia care, technology has emerged as a key ally, offering innovative solutions that profoundly affect the lives of those living with dementia and their caregivers. Here are a few case studies illustrating how technology has made a real difference:

Enhancing Safety with Monitoring Systems: For caregivers, one of the top concerns is ensuring the safety of their loved ones, especially those prone to wandering. A family in California implemented a comprehensive monitoring system equipped with GPS tracking and motion sensors in their home. This system provided peace of mind by alerting them anytime their loved one tried to leave the house unattended. Additionally, the system tracked the individual's medication intake, sleep patterns, and activity levels, enabling the family to tailor care and interventions more effectively.

Bridging Communication Gaps with Apps: Communication challenges can significantly affect the quality of life for individuals with dementia. In a care facility in Florida, caregivers introduced a specialized communication app designed for those with cognitive impairments. The app featured easy to understand interfaces, visual prompts, and the ability to send personalized messages. This innovation let residents express their needs more clearly, participate in social activities, and maintain connections with their families, significantly reducing frustration and enhancing their sense of independence.

Therapeutic Experiences through Virtual Reality: Virtual reality (VR) offers a unique opportunity for cognitive stimulation and emotional engagement. A memory care center in Oregon incorporated VR therapy into their care program, giving residents immersive experiences tailored to their interests and life histories. Through VR, individuals could revisit cherished places, engage in favorite pastimes, or relax in calming environments. This approach not only stimulated cognitive function but also evoked positive emotions and memories, contributing to an improved sense of well-being among the residents.

Chapter Summary: These case studies underscore the transformative potential of technology in dementia care. By leveraging tools like monitoring systems, communication apps, and virtual reality, caregivers can address some of the most pressing challenges of dementia care. These technological solutions not only enhance safety and help with communication but also provide meaningful therapeutic experiences that enrich the lives of individuals with dementia. As technology continues to advance, its role in dementia care promises even more innovative and impactful ways to support those affected by this condition and their caregivers.

~

NAVIGATING THE COMPLEXITIES OF TECHNOLOGY IN DEMENTIA CARE:

INCORPORATING technology into dementia care presents a host of advantages, making daily caregiving tasks more manageable and enhancing the quality of life for individuals with dementia. From medication reminders to GPS tracking for safety, technology opens new avenues for care and engagement. It offers platforms for social interaction and activities tailored to stimulate cognitive functions, keeping individuals connected and mentally active.

However, integrating technology in dementia care is not without its challenges and concerns, which justify careful consideration:

Privacy and Dignity Concerns: The use of monitoring devices and tracking technology raises significant privacy issues. It's important to balance ensuring safety and respecting the individual's privacy and dignity. Transparent communication about the use and purpose of these technologies is key to addressing privacy concerns.

Financial Barriers: The cost associated with implementing technological solutions in dementia care can be prohibitive for many families. High-tech devices and systems often come with a hefty price tag, making them inaccessible to those with limited financial resources.

Finding cost-effective solutions and exploring financial assistance programs becomes essential to broaden access to these technologies.

Usability Challenges: Technology designed without considering the specific needs of individuals with dementia may prove more frustrating than helpful. The cognitive and physical challenges associated with dementia require user-friendly, accessible technology. Simplified interfaces and intuitive design are critical to ensuring the effectiveness of tech-based interventions.

Training and Support: For technology to be successfully adopted in dementia care, both caregivers and individuals with dementia may require training and ongoing support. Making sure caregivers are comfortable and proficient in using technological tools is crucial for the technology to be a valuable asset rather than a source of frustration.

Ethical Considerations: The ethical implications of using technology in dementia care, such as autonomy and consent, must be carefully navigated. Engaging in open discussions with the individual with dementia and their family members about technology can help address these ethical concerns.

Chapter Summary:

While technology holds promise for transforming dementia care, navigating the associated challenges and concerns is essential for its successful implementation. By focusing on privacy, addressing financial and usability barriers, providing adequate training, and considering ethical implications, technology can serve as a powerful tool to support individuals with dementia and their caregivers, enhancing safety, engagement, and overall well-being.

∾

SELECTING AND IMPLEMENTING TECHNOLOGY IN DEMENTIA CARE: A PRACTICAL GUIDE

IN THE JOURNEY of dementia care, technology stands as a beacon of support, offering tools that can significantly ease the caregiving process while enhancing the safety and well-being of those with dementia. Here's a guide to navigating the selection and implementation of technology solutions effectively:

Assess Needs and Preferences: Begin by understanding the specific needs and challenges faced by your loved one with dementia. Consider factors such as their level of cognitive function, mobility, and preferences when selecting technology solutions.

Safety First: Safety tracking systems, including motion sensors, door alarms, and GPS trackers, can be lifesavers for caregivers. These systems provide peace of mind by alerting caregivers to potential safety issues and helping track the location of their loved one if they wander.

Simplify Medication Management: Medication management apps are invaluable in ensuring timely medication adherence. Look for apps that offer customizable reminders, track medication intake, and alert caregivers about missed doses or refill needs.

Engage and Stimulate: Seek apps and programs designed to engage individuals with dementia cognitively. From memory games to music therapy apps, these tools can provide enjoyable ways to stimulate cognitive functions and maintain engagement with the world.

Help with Communication: In the era of digital connectivity, tools like video calling apps and simplified messaging platforms can help maintain social connections and combat loneliness. Consider devices and apps that are user-friendly and cater to the cognitive abilities of your loved one.

Monitor Health Remotely: Wearable health trackers and telehealth platforms can offer insights into the health status of your loved one, allowing for early detection of potential issues. These devices can monitor vital signs, sleep patterns, and physical activity levels, providing valuable data to caregivers and healthcare providers.

Support for Caregivers: Don't overlook the value of online caregiver support platforms. These communities offer a space to connect with others in similar situations, share experiences, and access a wealth of information and resources related to dementia care.

Emergency Preparedness: A personal emergency response system (PERS) can be a critical safety net, enabling your loved one to easily call for help in case of a fall or emergency. Choose a device comfortable to wear and easy to use.

Implementing Technology Solutions:

- **Start Small:** Introduce new technology gradually to avoid overwhelming your loved one. Begin with the most pressing need and build from there.
- **Educate and Train:** Teach your loved one how to use the technology, if possible. Patience and repetition are key.
- **Evaluate and Adjust:** Regularly assess the effectiveness of the technological solutions in place. Be ready to make changes based on your loved one's evolving needs and the effectiveness of the tools.

By thoughtfully selecting and implementing technology solutions, caregivers can not only improve the safety and quality of life for individuals with dementia but also find greater support and ease in their caregiving roles. Remember, the goal is to enhance care and connection, making the journey easier for both you and your loved one.

~

HARNESSING TECHNOLOGY: EMPOWERING CAREGIVERS AND INDIVIDUALS WITH DEMENTIA

IN DEMENTIA CARE, technology emerges as a pivotal ally, offering innovative tools that promise to enhance quality of life, foster connectivity, and bolster safety for individuals navigating the complexities of dementia. The key to unlocking the full potential of these technological innovations lies in effective education for both caregivers and those with dementia. Here's why it's important:

Elevating Quality of Life: Technology holds the power to sustain the independence of individuals with dementia, connecting them to their passions and preserving cherished memories. Educating caregivers on the best use of these tools can significantly enrich the lives of those they support.

Strengthening Communication: From video chats to reminder systems, technology bridges the gap between caregivers and individuals with dementia. Mastery of these tools can transform communication, dispel isolation, and deepen bonds.

Ensuring Safety: The digital realm offers a suite of tools, including GPS tracking and home monitoring, designed to safeguard those with dementia. Knowledgeable use of these technologies enables caregivers to swiftly manage emergencies and avert potential hazards.

Stimulating Cognition: Brain-training applications and memory games stand as testaments to technology's potential in cognitive engagement. When caregivers are versed in integrating these tools into daily routines, they can play an important role in sustaining mental acuity and slowing the disease's progression.

Supporting Caregivers: Beyond aiding those with dementia, technology also serves as a pillar for caregivers, streamlining task management and fostering community connections. Learning to navigate these resources can alleviate the caregiving burden, promoting organization and emotional well-being.

The journey toward effectively using technology in dementia care is twofold, requiring both the willingness to embrace digital solutions and the commitment to educate all involved parties. As caregivers and individuals with dementia become proficient in these tools, they unlock new possibilities for enhancing care, fostering independence, and maintaining dignity throughout the dementia journey.

∾

EMERGING TECHNOLOGIES: SHAPING THE FUTURE OF DEMENTIA CARE

THE LANDSCAPE of dementia care is on the cusp of transformation, driven by rapid advancements in technology. From artificial intelligence to wearable gadgets, the potential for these innovations to redefine care is immense. Here's a glimpse into the future:

Artificial Intelligence (AI): AI stands at the forefront of change, offering breakthroughs in early detection and tailored treatment strategies. By analyzing patterns in vast datasets, such as health records or sensor data, AI could predict disease progression and optimize care plans.

Virtual Reality (VR): VR technology offers a gateway to worlds that can stimulate cognition and evoke cherished memories for those with dementia. Beyond cognitive benefits, VR provides serene escapes, helping to soothe the distress that often goes along with dementia.

Internet of Things (IoT): IoT devices extend the reach of caregivers, offering real-time insights into the well-being of individuals with dementia. From monitoring vital signs to ensuring home safety, IoT connects the dots to support seamless care.

Robotics: In the realm of companionship and care, robotics emerges as a promising ally. Robots, equipped with empathetic AI, can offer social interaction, perform routine tasks, and even remind patients about medications, enriching the care experience.

Telemedicine: The rise of telemedicine breaks down geographical barriers, making specialist care accessible from home. This innovation is valuable for dementia patients, reducing the stress of hospital visits and enabling continuous, personalized care.

Personalized Medicine: The era of one-size-fits-all treatment is giving way to personalized approaches, thanks to strides in genetics and biomarker research. This precision medicine could tailor treatments to individual profiles, enhancing efficacy and patient outcomes.

Gamification: By transforming cognitive exercises into engaging games, technology can motivate and captivate the minds of those with dementia. These digital platforms not only entertain but also work to sharpen cognitive functions, offering a fun twist on traditional therapies.

Wearable Devices: The simple act of wearing a device could unlock a wealth of health insights. Tracking everything from heart rate to sleep patterns, wearable tech provides a continuous health snapshot, aiding in the holistic management of dementia.

As we navigate the path forward, these technological advancements promise not only to enhance the quality of care for individuals with dementia but also to empower caregivers with tools that make their roles more manageable and fulfilling. In this journey toward innovation, the potential to transform lives shines brightly, heralding a future where dementia care is not just about managing symptoms but enhancing life's quality at every stage.

~

FREQUENTLY ASKED QUESTIONS:

1. What types of technology can help me keep my loved one with dementia safe at home?

Answer: Safety is a top priority in dementia care. Technologies like GPS trackers can help monitor your loved one's location, especially useful if they usually wander. Additionally, home tracking systems equipped with motion sensors and cameras can alert you to any unusual activity, ensuring their safety within the home. These tools offer peace of mind by keeping you informed of your loved one's well-being in real-time.

2. How can technology help with medication management for someone with dementia?

Answer: Managing medications can be challenging. Automated medication dispensers and reminder apps are invaluable tools in this part. They can alert your loved one when it's time to take their medication and ensure the correct dosage is dispensed, reducing the risk of missed or incorrect doses. This helps maintain their medication regimen accurately and safely.

3. Are there any technological solutions to help with the communication difficulties my loved one is experiencing?

Answer: Yes, technology can play a significant role in enhancing communication. Apps designed for simplified messaging and video calling can help maintain social connections, reducing feelings of isolation. For more advanced communication needs, speech-generating devices and apps that convert text to speech or use pictorial interfaces can help with interaction, helping your loved one express their needs and feelings more effectively.

4. Can technology help improve the cognitive abilities of my loved one with dementia?

Answer: Absolutely. There are many apps and games designed specifically to support cognitive functions, offering exercises that stimulate memory, attention, and problem-solving skills. Engaging with these activities can be both enjoyable and beneficial for your loved one, potentially slowing cognitive decline and enhancing their quality of life.

5. I'm overwhelmed with caregiving tasks. How can technology ease this burden?

Answer: Caregiving comes with a heavy load of responsibilities. Digital tools and platforms can help streamline care management, letting you organize health records, appointments, and daily care tasks efficiently. Online support communities can also provide emotional support and practical advice, helping you feel less alone in your caregiving journey. Leveraging technology not only improves care for your loved one but can also significantly reduce your stress and workload.

Integrating technology into dementia care offers many benefits, enhancing safety, communication, and overall well-being. By exploring and adopting appropriate technological solutions, you can provide compassionate and effective care for your loved one while also taking care of your own needs.

~

CASE STUDY: GEORGE AND THE POWER OF TECHNOLOGY IN DEMENTIA CARE

GEORGE, a 72-year-old man with early-stage dementia, lives with his daughter, Emily, who has taken on the role of his primary caregiver. Emily, balancing her job and family commitments alongside caring for George, found herself overwhelmed by the demands of ensuring her father's safety and well-being. However, their story changed when Emily leveraged technology to enhance George's care.

Integrating Technology into Dementia Care

Emily began by introducing a simple GPS tracking device in George's watch, addressing her primary concern—George's occasional wandering. This device let Emily monitor George's location through her smartphone, giving her peace of mind when she was at work. The GPS tracker proved invaluable one afternoon when George took an unscheduled walk to the park. Thanks to the tracker, Emily was able to quickly locate and safely bring George back home.

Next, Emily implemented an automated medication dispenser to manage George's medications, ensuring he took the correct doses at the right times. The dispenser was programmed to alert George with a beep and a visual signal, making it easier for him to maintain his medication regimen independently. This not only helped in reducing medication-related errors but also fostered a sense of independence in George, who took pride in managing his medications.

Enhancing Communication and Cognitive Engagement:

To tackle the challenges of communication and social isolation, Emily introduced George to a tablet with user-friendly apps designed for seniors with cognitive impairments. The tablet became a tool for George to video chat with family members, play cognitive games, and enjoy music from his youth, which visibly lifted his spirits and engaged his mind.

Lessons Learned:

From Emily's experience, several key lessons emerged:

1. Start Small and Simple: Introduce technology gradually, focusing on the most pressing needs first. This approach prevents overwhelm and allows for smoother adaptation for the individual with dementia.

2. Involve the Person with Dementia: Whenever possible, involve your loved one. This inclusion can enhance their cooperation and make the use of technology a positive experience.

3. Customize Solutions: Tailor technological tools to fit the specific needs and preferences of your loved one. Personalization increases the likelihood of acceptance and effectiveness.

4. Seek Support and Training: Seek support and training on using these technologies. Many communities and online platforms offer resources for caregivers.

5. Monitor and Adjust: Continuously monitor the effectiveness of the technology in meeting your care goals and be ready to make changes as needed.

Chapter Summary:

Through Emily's journey, we see the transformative impact technology can have in managing dementia care. By strategically incorporating technological tools, caregivers can enhance the safety, independence, and quality of life for their loved ones with dementia, while also easing their own caregiving burden. Emily's story is a testament to the power of technology in reshaping dementia care, offering hope and practical solutions for caregivers navigating this challenging journey.

∼

PART SIXTEEN WRAP-UP:

Action Items for the Caregiver:

1.   **Research and Select Appropriate Technology Tools**: Begin by researching technology tools that address the specific needs of your loved one with dementia. Focus on devices for safety monitoring, medication management, and cognitive engagement.

2.   **Introduce GPS Tracking Device**: Invest in a GPS tracking device suitable for the individual with dementia, such as a wearable watch or bracelet. This tool will help monitor their location and ensure their safety during wandering episodes.

3.   **Set Up an Automated Medication Dispenser**: Acquire an automated medication dispenser to manage the medication regimen accurately. Look for a dispenser with auditory and visual alerts to remind your loved one when it's time to take their medication.

4.   **Explore Tablets and Senior-Friendly Apps**: Select a user-friendly tablet and download apps designed for seniors with cognitive impairments. Choose applications that help with video chatting with family, cognitive games, and music or activities that your loved one enjoys.

5.   **Educate Yourself and Your Loved One**: Learn how to use the technology effectively. If possible, involve your loved one in this learning process to increase their comfort and engagement with the new tools.

6.   **Monitor and Adjust as Needed**: Regularly assess how well the technological solutions are working. Be ready to make changes based on your loved one's response and any changes in their condition.

7.   **Seek Community Support**: Look for community resources or online forums where you can learn from other caregivers' experiences with technology in dementia care. Sharing insights and challenges can be valuable.

8.   **Focus on Privacy and Dignity**: Always consider the privacy and dignity of your loved one when implementing monitoring technologies. Discuss the purpose and use of these tools to maintain trust.

9.   **Explore Financial Assistance for Technology**: Investigate if there are any financial assistance programs or subsidies available that can help cover the cost of necessary technology tools for dementia care.

10. **Implement a Backup Plan**: Despite the best technological aids, always have a non-technological backup plan in place for emergencies. Ensure there is a clear procedure for what to do in case of technology failure or other unforeseen issues.

11. **Practice Patience and Compassion**: Remember that adapting to new technologies can be challenging for individuals with dementia. Approach the implementation process with patience, compassion, and a willingness to go at your loved one's pace.

∼

IN OUR NEXT PART...

IN OUR NEXT PART, we will dive into the ins and outs of navigating the transition to long-term care facilities, a pivotal moment that many families face with trepidation and uncertainty. We'll break down the process into understandable pieces, guiding you through recognizing when it's time for this significant change, what to expect, and how to prepare both yourself and your loved one for the move. It's about making informed decisions, understanding the benefits of professional care environments, and ensuring a smooth transition that focuses on the well-being and comfort of your family member. We'll also tackle the emotional parts of this transition, offering strategies to cope with the feelings of guilt, loss, and change that often go along with this decision.

We'll explore the practicalities of selecting the right long-term care facility. This includes understanding the different types of care available, what to look for during visits, questions to ask, and how to evaluate if a facility aligns with your loved one's needs and preferences. Financial planning, a part that can feel overwhelming, will be demystified, giving you a roadmap to navigate the costs associated with long-term care. By the end of this Part, you'll feel empowered with the knowledge and tools needed to make the best decision for your loved one, ensuring they receive the care, respect, and quality of life they deserve during their time in a long-term care facility.

∽

PART SEVENTEEN
NAVIGATING THE TRANSITION TO LONG-TERM CARE FACILITIES

Deciding on a move to a long-term care facility for a loved one is a decision fraught with emotion and concern. Recognizing the need for this transition is the first step toward ensuring the safety and well-being of your family member. Here are key signs that might show it's time to consider professional care:

Health Deterioration: When health issues become more complex and demand constant medical attention, long-term care facilities can provide the comprehensive support that might be beyond what family caregivers can offer.

Increasing Safety Risks: Challenges with mobility, frequent falls, or struggles with daily self-care can signal that the home environment might no longer be the safest option. Facilities are designed to reduce these risks and offer support.

Caregiver Stress: If the physical and emotional toll on the caregiver becomes overwhelming, it might be time to explore long-term care options. This move can ensure the well-being of both the caregiver and the person receiving care.

Social Withdrawal: Loneliness and isolation can negatively affect health. Long-term care facilities offer community and social engagements that can enrich your loved one's life.

Financial Planning: While concerns about cost are valid, in some scenarios, the resources and care provided by facilities can be more cost-effective than extensive in-home care, especially when considering the level of care and amenities offered.

Acknowledging these signs and considering a move to a long-term care facility is a step toward focusing on the health and happiness of your loved one. Involve them in the conversation as much as their condition allows, and to research and visit potential facilities to find the best fit for their needs and preferences.

∼

UNDERSTANDING LONG-TERM CARE CHOICES

Choosing the right long-term care option is an important step for families navigating the journey of aging or managing chronic conditions. Here's a closer look at the many long-term care facilities available, to help make an informed decision that aligns with the individual's needs and preferences:

Nursing Homes: These facilities are equipped to offer comprehensive 24-hour medical care and assistance with daily activities. They cater to individuals who require constant medical attention and support due to severe health conditions.

Assisted Living Facilities: For those who need help with daily tasks but wish to maintain a level of independence, assisted living offers a balanced solution. Residents live in their own rooms or apartments and have access to communal dining and social activities, with staff available to help with personal care.

Memory Care Units: Specialized care units for individuals with Alzheimer's disease or dementia. These secure environments are designed to manage the unique challenges of memory loss, offering structured activities and therapies to support cognitive function.

Continuing Care Retirement Communities (CCRCs): CCRCs provide a spectrum of care from independent living to skilled nursing, all within the same community. This option is ideal for those seeking a stable environment that can adapt to their changing needs.

Hospice Care Facilities: Focused on providing compassionate end-of-life care, hospice facilities support individuals with terminal illnesses. The goal is to ensure comfort and dignity in the final stages of life, with emotional support extended to family members.

In-Home Care: This option lets individuals receive personalized care and assistance in the familiar setting of their own home. Services can range from help with daily activities to skilled nursing care, depending on the individual's requirements.

Each long-term care option offers unique benefits tailored to different levels of need, lifestyle preferences, and health conditions. Weigh these options carefully, considering factors like the quality of care, cost, and the individual's personal comfort and happiness. Consulting with healthcare professionals and visiting potential facilities can provide valuable insights to aid in this significant decision.

∾

NAVIGATING THE
EMOTIONAL JOURNEY TO
LONG-TERM CARE:

MOVING into a long-term care facility marks a significant shift in life's journey, often bringing a mix of emotions for the person moving and their family. This step involves adapting to a new living environment and lifestyle, which can stir feelings of uncertainty, loss, and even relief. Understanding and addressing these emotions is key to a smoother transition.

Feeling a Sense of Loss: One of the most profound impacts is the sense of loss experienced by many. This isn't just about moving from one home to another; it's about what that home represents—autonomy, memories, and a significant part of one's identity. Adjusting to this change requires time and emotional support to grieve and accept the new phase of life.

Combating Loneliness and Isolation: Leaving behind a community and stepping into an unfamiliar setting can spark feelings of loneliness. Even in a facility surrounded by others, the sense of being uprooted can be isolating. It's important for individuals and their families to actively engage in building new connections within the facility to foster a sense of belonging and community.

Dealing with Fear and Anxiety: The unknown aspects of life in a long-term care facility can trigger fear and anxiety. Worries about the quality of care, adapting to new routines, and the stigma sometimes associated with such facilities can weigh heavily on someone's mind. Addressing these fears openly with staff, family, and through counseling can help mitigate these concerns.

Finding Relief and Reassurance: For some, the move to a long-term care facility comes as a relief. It offers reassurance they will receive the care and support they need, which might have been a source of worry when living independently. This sense of security can significantly ease the emotional burden of the transition.

The emotional journey of transitioning to long-term care is deeply personal and can encompass a wide range of feelings. It's important for both the individual and their support network to acknowledge these emotions, seek support systems, and try to make the new environment feel like home. Engaging with the community, personalizing the living space, and maintaining open lines of communication with caregivers and family can all contribute to a more positive transition experience.

Ultimately, navigating this emotional landscape with empathy, patience, and understanding can help transform the experience into one of growth and new beginnings.

∾

NAVIGATING FINANCIAL PLANNING FOR LONG-TERM CARE:

UNDERSTANDING AND PREPARING for the financial aspects of long-term care is important. As you or a loved one approach this stage, here are key steps to consider to ensure financial readiness:

Assess Personal Finances: Begin with a thorough review of personal savings, investments, and any other financial resources. This includes looking at retirement accounts, personal savings, and any assets that could be used for care expenses.

Explore Long-Term Care Insurance: Investigate long-term care insurance options. This insurance is specifically designed to cover costs rarely handled by regular health insurance, such as daily living assistance. It's important to understand the terms, coverage limits, and the best time to buy a policy.

Understand Government Assistance: Familiarize yourself with government programs like Medicaid and benefits from Veterans Affairs, which can provide significant support for long-term care expenses. Each program has its own eligibility criteria, so it's important to determine if you or your loved one qualifies.

Discuss Family Contributions: Openly discuss potential financial support with family members. Discuss expectations, abilities, and limitations regarding financial assistance.

Budget and Financial Planning: Develop a detailed budget that accounts for current financial status and expects future long-term care expenses. This can help in identifying how much needs to be saved or set aside for these costs.

Seek Professional Advice: Consulting with a financial advisor or planner with experience in elder care can be invaluable. They can offer personalized advice on managing assets, planning for long-term care expenses, and making sure your financial plan aligns with your care needs.

By taking these steps, you can create a more secure financial foundation for long-term care. Planning ahead allows for greater choice and control over the care received, ultimately leading to better outcomes for individuals and their families.

~

DECIDING ON PROFESSIONAL CARE: FACTORS TO CONSIDER

DECIDING to transition to professional care is a significant decision that impacts both the individual requiring care and their loved ones. Here are essential factors to consider, helping ensure the choice aligns with the best interests and well-being of everyone involved.

Healthcare Needs: Assess the level and type of healthcare required. Professional care facilities are equipped to offer specialized attention, catering to complex health conditions that may be challenging to manage at home.

Safety Concerns: Safety is paramount. If there's a risk of falls or if the individual has medical conditions that require constant supervision, a professional care setting can give a safer environment round-the-clock support.

Social Opportunities: Loneliness and isolation can affect one's health. Professional care settings offer social activities and opportunities to interact with others, enriching the individual's social life.

Impact on Caregivers: Caring for a loved one can be rewarding but also physically and emotionally taxing. Transitioning to a professional setting can alleviate the strain on caregivers, letting them focus on their health and well-being too.

Financial Planning: Understand the costs associated with professional care and explore how they fit into your financial plan. Consider all potential funding sources, including private insurance, government assistance, and personal savings.

Quality of Life: Evaluate how a move to professional care might enhance the individual's quality of life. Factors like access to various amenities, engaging activities, and the overall environment of the facility are important.

Caregiver Burnout: Recognize the signs of caregiver burnout. If caregiving is becoming unsustainable, transitioning to a facility can ensure the individual continues to receive high-quality care while giving the caregiver necessary respite.

Health and Wellness: Consider the comprehensive benefits a professional care setting can offer, including nutritional meals, fitness programs, and regular health monitoring, contributing to overall health and wellness.

Personal Preferences: Above all, respect the wishes and preferences of the person needing care. Engage in open and honest discussions to understand their feelings and concerns about moving to professional care.

By thoughtfully considering these factors, you can navigate this complex decision-making process making sure the move to professional care is in the best interest of all involved.

～

NAVIGATING THE TRANSITION TO LONG-TERM CARE: ADDRESSING CONCERNS AND FEARS

THE MOVE to a long-term care facility is a significant change that can evoke a range of emotions, concerns, and fears in individuals and their families. Understanding and addressing these feelings is essential to help with a smoother transition and ensure the comfort and well-being of everyone involved.

Concerns About Independence: Fear of losing one's independence is a common concern. Highlight how the facility supports residents in maintaining their autonomy. Encourage active participation in care planning and daily activities to foster a sense of control and empowerment.

Adjusting to a New Environment: The thought of leaving behind a familiar home can be daunting. To ease this transition, encourage personalizing the new living space with cherished items and mementos. Familiarizing oneself with the facility and its staff before moving can also make the new environment feel more welcoming.

Worries About Social Isolation: Concerns about loneliness or feeling isolated are understandable. Encourage engagement in the facility's social activities and events to foster connections with peers. Forming new friendships and bonds can significantly enhance the sense of belonging and community.

Quality of Care: The quality of care is a legitimate concern for many. Encourage open dialogue with the care team to express care preferences and needs. It's important for individuals to feel heard and to know that they can voice concerns or requests.

Financial Stress: The financial implications of long-term care can be overwhelming. Explore all financial options, including insurance, Medicaid, and other assistance programs, to alleviate concerns. Consulting a financial advisor or social worker can provide clarity and assistance in navigating these financial challenges.

Addressing these concerns requires empathy, patience, and open communication. Listen to and validate the individual's feelings, providing reassurance and support throughout the transition process. By proactively discussing and addressing these fears, you can help ease the emotional burden and move to long-term care a more positive experience for everyone involved.

∿

SMOOTH SAILING THROUGH TRANSITION: PRACTICAL TIPS AND STRATEGIES

STARTING ANY TRANSITION, whether it's moving into a long-term care facility, changing careers, or adapting to any new phase in life, requires careful planning and support. Here are several practical tips and strategies to help make your transition process smooth:

Plan Ahead: Before diving into the transition, outline your goals and the steps needed to achieve them. A detailed plan can guide your actions and make the process more manageable.

Stay Organized: Keeping everything organized can significantly ease the transition process. Maintain a list of important tasks, deadlines, and contacts to ensure you have everything you need at your fingertips.

Time Management: Allocate specific periods for transition-related tasks to make the most of your time. Breaking down tasks into smaller, more manageable chunks can also prevent feelings of overwhelm.

Seek Support: Don't go through the transition alone. Lean on family, friends, or professionals for support. Sharing your experiences and challenges can provide relief and potentially offer new solutions.

Embrace Positivity: Keep a positive outlook on the changes ahead. Viewing the transition as an opportunity for growth and new experiences can make the process more rewarding.

Focus on Self-Care: It's easy to neglect your own needs during a period of change. Remember to take care of your physical and emotional well-being by getting enough rest, eating well, and engaging in activities you enjoy.

Be Adaptable: Transitions rarely go exactly as planned. Be ready to adapt your plans based on new information or changes in circumstances to continue effectively.

Reflect on the Experience: Once you're settled into the new situation, take time to reflect on the transition process. Consider what went well and what could have been done differently for future reference.

By using these strategies, you can navigate transitions more smoothly and confidently. Remember, transitions are a natural part of life, and with the right approach, they can lead to personal growth and new opportunities.

~

FREQUENTLY ASKED QUESTIONS:

1. How do I know it's the right time to move my loved one to a long-term care facility?

Answer: The decision to move a loved one to long-term care is deeply personal and can be challenging. Signs it might be time include increasing difficulty in managing their health and safety at home, frequent medical needs that exceed your caregiving capabilities, and noticeable decline in their quality of life. Consider your well-being, as caregiver burnout can affect the level of care you're able to provide.

2. What should I look for in a long-term care facility?

Answer: Look for a facility that meets your loved one's specific health care needs, particularly one with experience in handling dementia if applicable. Consider the staff-to-patient ratio, the availability of medical and emergency services, and the cleanliness and safety of the environment. It's also essential to assess the facility's activities and programs designed to enhance residents' quality of life. Visiting the facility, talking to staff, and connecting with other families can provide valuable insights.

3. How can we make the transition easier for our loved one?

Answer: Making the transition smooth involves preparing your loved one emotionally, which might include discussing the move in advance, focusing on the positive aspects, and involving them in the decision-making process as much as their condition allows. Personalizing their new space with familiar items from home can also help make the new environment feel more comfortable and less intimidating.

4. How can I stay involved in my loved one's care after the move?

Answer: Stay actively involved by visiting regularly, participating in care planning meetings, and maintaining open communication with the facility's staff about your loved one's condition and care. Most facilities welcome family involvement and can provide updates and reports on your loved one's progress. Building a good relationship with caregivers and staff can make sure your loved one receives the best care.

5. What are ways to manage the costs associated with long-term care?

Answer: Managing the costs involves exploring all available funding sources, including private insurance, Medicaid, veterans' benefits, and other assistance programs. It's also wise to consult with a financial planner or eldercare attorney who can offer advice on protecting assets and planning for long-term care expenses. Some families also consider personal resources, such as savings, retirement accounts, or even selling or renting property, to finance care.

Transitioning a loved one to long-term care is a significant step that requires careful consideration and planning. By addressing these questions and seeking support from professionals and caregiver communities, you can navigate this challenging process with greater confidence and peace of mind, ensuring the best outcome for your loved one.

CASE STUDY: MARTHA AND HER MOTHER'S JOURNEY TO LONG-TERM CARE

MARTHA, a 55-year-old high school teacher, had been caring for her 82-year-old mother, Ellen, who was diagnosed with Alzheimer's disease five years ago. At first, Martha managed well supported by home health aides. However, as her mother's condition progressed, the challenges and responsibilities intensified beyond Martha's capacity.

Recognizing the Need for Change

Ellen's health deteriorated, requiring constant medical attention that Martha struggled to provide. Frequent falls became a concern, signaling that their home might no longer be the safest environment for Ellen. Martha, juggling her job and caregiving, felt the toll on her physical and emotional well-being, leading to caregiver burnout. She noticed her mother's increasing isolation, missing the social interactions that once brought her joy.

The Decision-Making Process

After months of contemplation and discussions with her family, Martha recognized it was time to consider a long-term care facility for Ellen. The decision was fraught with guilt and uncertainty, but Martha knew it was in her mother's best interest. They started researching and visiting facilities, focusing on those offering specialized memory care units.

Martha involved Ellen in the decision-making process, ensuring her mother's preferences and needs were respected. They evaluated each facility's medical care capabilities, safety measures, and social activities. Financial planning was a significant concern, but Martha discovered that the cost of in-facility care was offset by the comprehensive services provided, making it a cost-effective solution in their situation.

Lessons Learned

Through this journey, Martha learned the importance of acknowledging when professional care is needed. She realized that transitioning to a long-term care facility was not a failure on her part, but a decision made out of love and concern for her mother's well-being. Martha found peace in knowing her mother was in a safe environment, receiving medical attention, and engaging in social activities.

Engaging with support groups for caregivers, Martha shared her experiences, learning she was not alone in her feelings of guilt and overwhelm. These connections gave her emotional solace and practical advice on navigating the transition.

Chapter Summary

Ellen's move to a long-term care facility marked a new chapter for both mother and daughter. Martha saw improvements in her mother's quality of life, thanks to the specialized care and social engagements the facility provided. Martha could return to her teaching job full-time, relieved from the constant worry about her mother's safety and health. The transition taught Martha the value of self-care and the importance of seeking support, letting her be a better daughter and caregiver from a place of strength and peace.

PART SEVENTEEN WRAP-UP:
ACTION ITEMS FOR THE CAREGIVER:

1. **Assess the Individual's Current Needs:**
2. Evaluate the loved one's health condition, safety risks, and daily living needs to determine the level of care required.
3. **Research Long-Term Care Facilities:**
4. Look into facilities with a good reputation that specialize in the care needed, such as memory care units for dementia patients.
5. **Involve Your Loved One in the Decision:**
6. Engage the person requiring care in conversations about the transition as much as their condition allows, respecting their preferences and concerns.
7. **Visit Potential Facilities:**
8. Schedule visits to potential care facilities to assess the environment, staff, and the services provided. Consider both the quality of care and the opportunity for social engagement.
9. **Consult Healthcare Professionals:**
10. Talk to healthcare providers about the best care setting for your loved one based on their medical and personal needs.
11. **Financial Planning:**
12. Review personal finances, insurance coverage, and

government assistance programs like Medicaid to understand how to fund the cost of care.

13. Consider consulting a financial advisor for guidance on managing long-term care expenses.

14. **Prepare for the Emotional Journey:**

15. Acknowledge and address your feelings about the transition. Seek support from friends, family, or caregiver support groups to navigate the emotional parts of this decision.

16. **Plan the Move:**

17. Once a facility is chosen, plan the move by deciding what personal items to bring to make the new space feel like home and scheduling the moving day.

18. **Stay Involved:**

19. After the move, remain actively involved in your loved one's care. Regular visits and participation in care planning meetings can make sure their needs are being met.

20. **Take Care of Yourself:**

21. Recognize the importance of self-care. Use the respite from caregiving duties to recharge and address your health and well-being.

22. **Build a New Routine:**

23. Establish a new routine that includes visiting your loved one, engaging in your own interests, and connecting with others who understand your experience.

24. **Monitor and Evaluate the Care Received:**

25. Regularly assess the quality of care and your loved one's satisfaction with the facility. Be ready to advocate for changes or improvements as needed.

By following these action items, caregivers can navigate the transition to long-term care more smoothly, making sure their loved ones receive the care they need while also taking care of their own well-being.

❧

IN OUR NEXT PART...

In our next Part, "Embracing the Sunset: Compassionate Approaches to End-of-Life Care," we'll explore the delicate art of providing support during the most profound moments of life. Understanding how to navigate this sensitive time is important, not just for the well-being of those on their final journey, but also for the peace of mind of their loved ones and caregivers. We'll dig into the importance of creating a nurturing environment that respects the dignity and wishes of the individual, offering strategies for pain management, emotional support, and the celebration of life's legacy. This Part aims to guide caregivers through the process of making end-of-life care a meaningful and comforting experience, emphasizing the power of empathy, respect, and love in facing life's final chapter.

We will provide practical advice on helping with heart-to-heart conversations about end-of-life wishes, understanding the options for care, and managing the complexities of grief and loss. By fostering a deeper understanding of the emotional and spiritual needs of those nearing the end of their journey, caregivers can learn how to offer solace and support in ways that honor the individual's life and preferences. We'll also touch on the benefits of involving professional care teams, including hospice and palliative care professionals, to ensure comprehensive support that aligns with the patient's needs and values.

Through compassionate care and thoughtful preparation, caregivers can help create a peaceful transition, making sure the final days are filled with dignity, comfort, and love.

~

PART EIGHTEEN
EMBRACING THE SUNSET: COMPASSIONATE APPROACHES TO END-OF-LIFE CARE

PLANNING FOR PEACE: A GUIDE TO COMPASSIONATE END-OF-LIFE PREPARATION

WHEN WE TALK about the final chapters of life, it's important to approach them with kindness, understanding, and open hearts. Preparing for and navigating end-of-life care is not just about medical decisions; it's about honoring the wishes and dignity of those nearing life's end and ensuring their journey is filled with love and respect.

Central to end-of-life care is the power of open communication. It's important to discuss the desires and preferences someone has for their final days. This includes discussions on medical treatments, pain management preferences, emotional and spiritual needs, and even the smaller, personal touches they wish to include in their care.

Such conversations should ideally involve not just the individual but also their loved ones and healthcare providers. It's a collaborative effort that ensures everyone understands and respects the individual's wishes, providing a supportive network that upholds these decisions with compassion and dedication.

A key focus is ensuring the highest possible quality of life. This often involves working closely with healthcare teams to create a care plan that aligns with the person's values and desires, possibly incorporating palliative care or hospice services designed to offer comfort and reduce suffering.

Addressing the emotional and spiritual aspects of end-of-life care is equally important. Creating space for meaningful reflection, connection, and the completion of any unfinished business can significantly affect the individual's and their family's peace of mind. Whether through cherished rituals, sharing memories, or simply spending quiet moments together, these practices can offer solace and a sense of closure.

Ultimately, the journey through end-of-life care is deeply personal and unique to each individual. By fostering open dialogue, honoring personal wishes, and focusing on comfort and quality of life, we can support those at life's end to navigate this path with dignity, respect, and love. It's a collective effort that not only honors the individual but enriches the lives of all involved, leaving a lasting legacy of compassion and understanding.

~

UNDERSTANDING YOUR OPTIONS: NAVIGATING END-OF-LIFE CARE

WHEN WE TALK about caring for someone nearing the end of their life, it's all about ensuring they're comfortable and supported. Let's break down the main options available, so you can make informed choices about care that aligns with your loved one's wishes and needs.

Hospice Care: Hospice care is all about comfort. It's for individuals in the final stages of a terminal illness, where the focus shifts from trying to cure the illness to easing symptoms and providing emotional and spiritual support. This care can be provided at home, in a hospice center, or even in some nursing homes and hospitals. It's a comprehensive approach that includes pain management, help with daily activities, and counseling for both the patient and their family, continuing with grief support after the loved one has passed.

Palliative Care: Palliative care takes a broad approach, aimed at improving life quality for anyone with a serious illness, not just those at the end of life. It can be provided alongside treatments meant to cure. This care addresses pain, symptoms, and the emotional and spiritual needs of the patient, involving a team of specialists working together to support both the patient and their family.

Advance Care Planning: This is about making your wishes known before you reach a point where you can't communicate them yourself. It involves choosing someone to decide on your behalf (a healthcare proxy), putting your healthcare wishes in writing (through a living will), and conversing with family and healthcare providers about what's important to you. Advance care planning ensures your preferences for care are understood and respected.

Exploring these options can help make sure care at the end of life is in line with the patient's wishes, offering peace of mind to everyone involved. It's important to have open discussions with healthcare providers and family members to make sure these wishes are known and can be followed when the time comes.

～

FINDING PEACE IN LIFE'S FINAL CHAPTER

TALKING about preparing for the end of life brings up a lot of emotions —fear, sadness, maybe even anger. It's natural to feel all these things, and it's okay to let yourself feel them. If you find them overwhelming, talking to friends, family, or even a counselor can help.

This time can also be deeply spiritual. It's a chance to look back on your life, to connect with what you believe in, and maybe find some peace in those beliefs. It's a time for making amends, for forgiving and asking for forgiveness, and for reflecting on what your life has meant. Simple practices like meditation, prayer, or being in nature can offer comfort.

On a practical level, there's a lot to think about too. Making a will, figuring out your healthcare wishes, and talking about these plans with your family can ease a lot of worry. It means you can spend your energy on more important things—like finding peace and acceptance.

Finding that peace is really about embracing every part of life, including its end. It's about being grateful for the moments you've had, staying present, and letting go of the things you can't control. Surround yourself with love, do things that make you happy, and try to create meaningful moments.

Everyone's journey toward acceptance and peace at the end of life is unique. There's no right way to feel or to grieve. What's most important is giving yourself grace and space to navigate this journey in your own way, supported by love and compassion from those around you.

～

GUIDING YOUR LOVED ONE THROUGH THEIR FINAL CHAPTER

Helping a loved one navigate the end-of-life journey is profound and heartfelt work. It's about lending emotional support and practical help when they need it most. Here are ways you can stand by them:

Just Be There: Sometimes, your presence is the most comforting support you can offer. Listen, share a quiet space, or simply hold their hand.

Acknowledge Their Feelings: It's important to let your loved one express their emotions without judgment. Let them know it's okay to feel scared, angry, or peaceful—whatever they're going through.

Honor Their Choices: Always respect the decisions your loved one makes about their care. It's their journey and feeling in control can bring them comfort.

Help Out with the Day-to-Day: Lend a hand with the daily chores, be it cooking, cleaning, or running errands. Such tasks can seem monumental to someone dealing with end-of-life care.

Manage the Care: Offer to keep track of appointments and medications. Being the point of communication between healthcare providers and other family members can relieve a lot of stress.

Make Their Space Comforting: Creating a calm and soothing environment can significantly affect your loved one's well-being. It could be as simple as playing their favorite music or arranging a bouquet of flowers by their bedside.

Encourage Them to Indulge a Little: Encourage self-care that brings them joy, whether that's a favorite snack or a gentle massage.

Take Care of Yourself: Supporting someone at the end of life is emotionally taxing. Ensure you're also getting the support you need, so you don't burn out.

Share and Create Memories: Spend time reminiscing about the good times. Putting together a memory book or a collection of photos can be a beautiful way to connect and remember.

Be Patient and Compassionate: Everyone's journey with grief and acceptance is unique. Offer your patience and understanding as you both navigate this time together.

Supporting your loved one through the end of their journey is a testament to your love and devotion. It's about being there, in whatever way they need, and ensuring their final chapter is peaceful and meaningful.

~

EMBRACING THE JOURNEY: UNDERSTANDING DEATH AND DYING

IT'S normal to feel uneasy when thinking about death and dying. It's a journey into the unknown, and uncertainty can be frightening. Let's talk about some of the common fears and misconceptions around this subject and how we can find comfort in understanding them better.

Fear of the Unknown: Wondering what happens after we pass is a big question many of us grapple with. Whether or not there's an afterlife, or simply nothing at all, can weigh heavily on our minds. It's okay not to have all the answers. Many find peace by embracing the mystery and finding comfort in the natural cycle of life.

Worrying About Pain: The thought of a painful end is daunting. However, modern medicine and palliative care have made great strides in making sure people can remain comfortable. Teams specializing in end-of-life care focus on easing pain and providing a peaceful transition.

Fear of Being Alone: facing death alone can be scary. But remember, you're surrounded by people who care—family, friends, healthcare workers, and maybe spiritual guides. Making your end-of-life wishes known early ensures those around you know how to support you best.

Misconceptions About Death: Some believe that talking about death might hasten its arrival or that it's a subject best left untouched. In reality, open conversations about death are healthy. They help us accept our mortality and make important decisions about our final wishes.

If these fears are on your mind, know that it's all right to seek support. Whether it's talking with a counselor, exploring spiritual beliefs, or simply having heartfelt conversations with loved ones, support is available. Practices like meditation or engaging in meaningful activities can also offer solace.

Addressing fears and misconceptions about death isn't easy, but it's an important part of coming to terms with our mortality. By confronting these fears, we can find a sense of peace and readiness for when the time comes. Death is a part of life's natural cycle, and understanding it better can help us live our lives more fully and with gratitude.

~

COLLABORATING WITH HEALTHCARE TEAMS FOR COMPASSIONATE END-OF-LIFE CARE

As someone nears the end of their life, the support and expertise of healthcare professionals become invaluable. This team, which may include doctors, nurses, social workers, and chaplains, plays a critical role in ensuring comfort, dignity, and care during these final stages. Here's how you can work effectively with them to support your loved one:

Keep Communication Open: Being open and honest with the care team is key. Share your loved one's wishes, any symptoms they're experiencing, and your family's concerns or preferences about their care. This helps in creating a care plan that aligns with your loved one's needs and values.

Understand Everyone's Role: Each healthcare professional brings a unique set of skills to end-of-life care. Doctors and nurses manage physical symptoms, social workers provide emotional support and help navigate healthcare systems, while chaplains offer spiritual care. Knowing who to turn to for different needs can make the process smoother.

Make Decisions Together: End-of-life care involves many difficult decisions, from pain management strategies to whether to use life-sustaining treatments. Engage in shared decision-making with the healthcare team, considering the pros and cons of each option given your loved one's wishes.

Honor Cultural Values: People's end-of-life preferences are often deeply influenced by their cultural, spiritual, or religious beliefs. Ensure the healthcare team is aware of these preferences so that care can be tailored to respect them.

Advocate for Family Support: While the primary focus is on your loved one, it's also a challenging time for family and friends. Work with the healthcare team to address the emotional and practical needs of everyone involved, ensuring support is available for coping with grief and loss.

Ensure Seamless Care: Good communication among healthcare professionals is important for providing consistent care. Advocate for regular updates and meetings between team members to discuss care strategies, symptom management, and any changes in your loved one's condition.

Discuss Advance Care Planning: If possible, encourage conversations about advance care planning early on. Understanding your loved one's wishes regarding end-of-life care helps guide the healthcare team in making decisions that reflect those wishes when the time comes.

Navigating end-of-life care is a profound journey, and a compassionate, coordinated approach from the healthcare team can make all the difference. By fostering a collaborative relationship with these professionals, you can help ensure your loved one's final days are comfortable and meaningful.

$\sim$

CREATING A SANCTUARY: COMFORT AND PEACE IN THE FINAL JOURNEY

ENSURING comfort and peace for someone in their final days is a deeply loving act. Here are ways to create a serene environment that supports their physical and emotional well-being:

Managing Pain Effectively:

- Collaborate closely with healthcare professionals to tailor a pain management plan that addresses the unique needs of your loved one. This might include medications, gentle physical therapies, or alternative approaches like acupuncture.
- Adjust the room to promote relaxation. Consider soft lighting, soothing music, and ensuring the bedding is cozy.
- Encourage your loved one to share their feelings about pain and discomfort openly, so changes can be made to improve their comfort.

Fostering Emotional Well-being:

- Being there to listen and provide emotional support is invaluable. Let them share their thoughts, fears, and desires freely, and acknowledge their feelings.

- If they find comfort in spiritual or religious practices, make space for these activities. This might bring them peace and solace.
- Help them reminisce, sharing joyful memories, and connecting deeply with family and friends can offer great comfort and a sense of closure.

Ensuring Comfort:

- Attend to their basic needs with gentle care, ensuring they are clean, nourished, and hydrated.
- Maintain a tidy and calm space, personalized with items that mean a lot to them, making the environment feel safe and familiar.
- Allow them autonomy, letting them make choices about their care and surroundings.

Encouraging Visits from Loved Ones:

- Invite close friends and family to spend quality time, offering their presence and love.
- Educate visitors on how to best support their loved one ensuring their interactions are comforting and not overwhelming.

Considering Hospice Care:

- If not already involved, bringing in hospice care can provide specialized support for pain management, emotional comfort, and more, helping to create a peaceful environment.

Creating this sanctuary for your loved one is about more than physical comfort; it's about honoring their life, supporting their journey, and surrounding them with love as they approach the end of their path.

∾

FREQUENTLY ASKED QUESTIONS:

1. How can I start a conversation about end-of-life wishes with my loved one?

Answer: Starting this conversation is one of the most caring actions you can take. Begin by choosing a quiet, comfortable moment, and express your desire to honor their wishes regarding end-of-life care. Emphasize the importance of knowing their preferences for medical treatments, comfort measures, and even their thoughts on hospice care. This dialogue should be approached with sensitivity, letting them share as much as they feel comfortable.

2. What are the key components of compassionate end-of-life care?

Answer: Compassionate end-of-life care focuses on comfort, dignity, and respect for the individual's wishes. Key components include pain management, emotional and spiritual support, assistance with daily activities, and providing a peaceful environment. It also involves supporting family members through the process and after the loss, emphasizing the importance of creating meaningful moments and memories in the final days.

3. How can we ensure our loved one's pain is well-managed?

Answer: Work closely with healthcare providers to develop a comprehensive pain management plan tailored to your loved one's needs. This may include medications, non-pharmacological methods like massage or relaxation techniques, and regular assessments to adjust the plan as needed. Communication is important; encourage your loved one to express their comfort level and any changes in pain.

4. What should we consider when deciding between hospice and palliative care?

Answer: The choice between hospice and palliative care depends on the individual's stage of illness and the goals for their care. Palliative care can be provided at any stage of a serious illness, focusing on relieving symptoms and improving quality of life. Hospice care is specifically designed for the final months of life, emphasizing comfort and support for both the individual and their family. Discussing options with healthcare providers can help determine which approach aligns best with your loved one's needs and preferences.

5. How can I support my loved one in finding peace and fulfillment in their final days?

Answer: Supporting your loved one in finding peace involves listening to their fears, hopes, and desires without judgment. Help with conversations that let them reflect on their life, acknowledge their legacy, and express any unresolved issues or wishes. Create an environment that reflects their personality and comforts, incorporating favorite music, scents, or keepsakes. Encourage visits from friends and family to share memories and love, and consider spiritual or religious support if it aligns with their beliefs.

Navigating end-of-life care is a profound responsibility that requires compassion, communication, and respect for the individual's wishes. By seeking guidance from healthcare professionals and providing a supportive and loving presence, caregivers can help ensure their loved one's final journey is peaceful and meaningful.

$\sim$

CASE STUDY: GRACE'S JOURNEY TO PEACEFUL END-OF-LIFE CARE

GRACE, a vibrant 78-year-old with a love for gardening and poetry, had been living with advanced heart disease. As her condition progressed, her family faced the difficult realization it was time to focus on quality of life and comfort. Her daughter, Emily, became her primary caregiver.

At first, Emily tried to manage everything on her own, from medication schedules to aiding with daily tasks. However, as Grace's health declined, the physical and emotional toll on Emily intensified. It was during a challenging night, after Grace had a minor fall, that Emily recognized they needed more support.

Opening the Conversation: Emily sat down with Grace one quiet afternoon, amidst her beloved garden, to talk about her wishes for the end of her life. It was a tough conversation, filled with tears but also laughter as they reminisced about cherished memories. Grace expressed her desire not to pursue aggressive treatments that would only prolong her suffering. She wished for comfort, to be surrounded by her family and friends, and to enjoy her days without the burden of hospital visits.

Seeking Professional Support: Understanding Grace's wishes, Emily contacted a local hospice care organization. A nurse, specializing in end-of-life care, visited them at home to discuss what hospice care involved and how it could support Grace's desire for comfort and dignity. They formulated a care plan that included pain management, emotional support for both Grace and her family, and assistance with daily care needs.

Creating a Sanctuary: Emily transformed Grace's room into a peaceful sanctuary, bringing in fresh flowers from the garden and setting up a small speaker to play Grace's favorite classical music. Friends and family were encouraged to visit, share stories, and offer their love and support. Hospice provided a volunteer who specialized in legacy projects, helping Grace to compile her poems into a small book as a gift to her family.

Lessons Learned: From this journey, Emily learned the importance of open communication about end-of-life wishes and the value of seeking support. She realized that hospice care was not about giving up but about honoring her mother's wishes for a dignified and peaceful end of life. Emily saw firsthand the difference in her mother's quality of life with proper pain management and the comfort of being at home surrounded by love.

The experience also highlighted the need for self-care. Joining a support group for caregivers, Emily found a space to share her feelings, learn from others' experiences, and navigate her grief. It reminded her she wasn't alone on this journey.

Chapter Summary: Grace's final weeks were filled with love, comfort, and peace. The hospice team's support enabled Emily to be a daughter again, rather than a caregiver, letting her cherish the precious moments with her mother. Grace passed away peacefully, surrounded by her family, leaving behind a legacy of love and memories cherished by all who knew her. Through this experience, Emily learned the profound impact of compassionate care and the importance of honoring the wishes of loved ones at the end of life.

PART EIGHTEEN WRAP-UP:

1. **Start Conversations About End-of-Life Wishes**: Start open, honest discussions with your loved one about their preferences for end-of-life care, including medical interventions, pain management, and personal touches they would like in their care plan.
2. **Research Hospice and Palliative Care Options**: Look into local hospice and palliative care services. Understand what they offer, how they align with your loved one's wishes, and what steps are needed to enroll.
3. **Create a Comfortable Environment**: Transform the living space of your loved one into a peaceful sanctuary. Include personal items that bring them joy, such as photos, favorite books, or music.
4. **Arrange for Professional Support**: Contact a hospice care organization to discuss a care plan tailored to your loved one's needs. Ensure it includes pain management, emotional support, and assistance with daily activities.

5. **Plan for Visitors**: Coordinate visits from friends and family. Create a schedule that allows your loved one to enjoy the company without becoming overwhelmed.

6. **Engage in Legacy Projects**: Help your loved one with projects that let them leave a legacy, such as compiling a collection of their writings, recipes, or creating a photo album.

7. **Educate Yourself on Medication Management**: Work with healthcare providers to understand your loved one's medication schedule, especially for pain management. Learn how to administer medications and recognize signs of discomfort or pain.

8. **Focus on Self-Care**: Look after your own well-being. Join support groups, seek counseling and ensure you have time for rest and relaxation.

9. **Document Important Information**: Keep a record of all essential documents, care plans, and healthcare provider information in an easily accessible place.

10. **Discuss and Plan Financial Aspects**: Understand the costs associated with hospice and palliative care. Explore coverage options through insurance, Medicaid, or Medicare, and discuss how family members can contribute.

11. **Familiarize Yourself with Grief Resources**: Research grief support services for yourself and your family to use both before and after your loved one passes.

12. **Celebrate Life**: Encourage the sharing of happy memories, stories, and the celebration of your loved one's life with friends and family, creating positive moments together.

By following these action items, caregivers can make sure their loved ones receive compassionate, respectful care in their final days, aligning with their wishes and providing comfort for both the individual and their family.

~

IN OUR NEXT PART...

In our next Part, "The Heart of Caregiving: Balancing Love, Duty, and Personal Growth," we dig into the complexities and nuances of the caregiving role, unraveling the layers of emotions, responsibilities, and unexpected joys that define this journey. Caregiving, often seen as a duty, is much more than that—it's an act of love and compassion that can profoundly shape both the giver and receiver. We'll explore the delicate balance between caring for a loved one and maintaining one's own well-being, emphasizing the importance of self-care, setting boundaries, and finding moments of joy amidst the challenges. This Part aims to guide caregivers through the emotional landscape of their role, offering strategies to manage stress, foster personal growth, and deepen the connection with their loved ones. Through personal stories, expert insights, and practical advice, we hope to illuminate the path for caregivers, showing them how to navigate the complexities of their role with grace, resilience, and love.

∾

PART NINETEEN: THE HEART OF CAREGIVING: BALANCING LOVE, DUTY, AND PERSONAL GROWTH

EXPLORING THE CHALLENGES AND REWARDS OF CAREGIVING:

STARTING the journey of caregiving can profoundly shape one's life, weaving together a tapestry of emotional highs and lows. It's a path that demands much, both physically and emotionally, yet it's also rich with opportunities for personal growth and deep fulfillment.

At the heart of caregiving lie the emotional challenges that can sometimes feel overwhelming. It's natural to grapple with feelings of sadness, guilt, and worry as you navigate the complexities of caring for someone dear. These feelings can weigh heavily, making days seem longer and more taxing. The physical demands of caregiving, from managing medications to helping with daily activities, can leave little room for self-care, leading to exhaustion and stress.

Beyond the physical and emotional toll, caregiving can sometimes feel like a solitary road, marked by moments of isolation and the profound sorrow of seeing a loved one in distress. Test the spirit, yet they are also the crucible within which profound growth and fulfillment can occur.

Despite its challenges, caregiving can strengthen bonds, building a deeper, more meaningful connection with the loved one in your care. It's in these moments of tenderness and care that a profound sense of purpose emerges, illuminating the true value of your role. The gratitude and love that flow from these interactions can transform the caregiving experience, offering moments of joy and satisfaction amidst the hardships.

Caregiving also offers a unique lens through which to view life, nurturing a deeper appreciation for the small, everyday moments and fostering a sense of compassion and empathy that extends beyond the immediate circle of care. The resilience developed through this journey is a testament to the human spirit's capacity to adapt and find strength even in the most challenging circumstances.

In embracing the caregiving journey, with its ups and downs, it's important to seek support and allow oneself moments of rest and reflection. Finding balance can help in navigating the journey with grace, making sure both you and your loved one are cared for.

The caregiving journey, with all its intricacies, is a profound journey of love and sacrifice. This path, while challenging, can lead to immense personal growth and a deeper understanding of the bonds that tie us to one another. In the act of caregiving, we find not just the essence of our humanity but also the capacity for immense love and compassion.

~

REFLECTING ON PERSONAL GROWTH:

FROM RUTH:

Reflecting on the journey of caregiving, I recall a formative period when I stepped into the role of caregiver for my grandfather, who was battling a prolonged illness. This was a chapter of my life filled with challenges, but it was also a time that profoundly shaped my character and outlook on life.

At first, I found myself overwhelmed by the responsibilities and the emotional toll of seeing a loved one in pain. My days were a mix of medication schedules, doctor's appointments, and moments of trying to offer comfort and companionship. During this period, I discovered an inner strength I didn't know I had. The resilience required to face each day, to adapt to new challenges, and to continue providing care, taught me a lot about my own capabilities and limits.

One particular moment stands out vividly in my memory. It was a quiet evening, and I was helping my grandfather get ready for bed—a routine we had perfected. As I helped him settle in, he took my hand, looked me in the eyes, and thanked me for being there for him. It was a simple gesture, but it conveyed so much love and gratitude. Then I truly understood the impact of my role as a caregiver—not just in the practical sense, but on an emotional and spiritual level as well.

This journey with my grandfather deepened my empathy and compassion, not only for him but for others experiencing similar struggles. I learned to listen more intently, to offer support without words, and to value the quiet moments of connection that occur even in hardship.

Caregiving reshaped my understanding of love and sacrifice. It taught me that love is not just a feeling but an action—a series of small, daily acts of kindness and care that can significantly affect someone's life.

Looking back, my experience as a caregiver was one of the most challenging yet rewarding chapters of my life. It pushed me to grow in ways I hadn't expected, fostering resilience, empathy, and a deeper appreciation for the bonds we share with our loved ones. Through this experience, I came to understand that while caregiving can be demanding, it also offers the unique opportunity to see the strength of the human spirit and the capacity for love and compassion that lives in each of us.

∼

DISCOVERING PURPOSE AND FULFILLMENT ON THE CAREGIVING JOURNEY:

CAREGIVING TRANSFORMS LIVES, not just for those receiving care but also for the caregivers themselves. This role comes with its own set of challenges, yet it holds the potential to profoundly affect one's sense of purpose and meaning in life. For many, stepping into the role of a caregiver leads to a profound reassessment of what matters, shifting priorities and reshaping values in significant ways.

At the heart of caregiving is the act of giving oneself to the well-being of another, which inherently brings a deep sense of fulfillment and purpose. It's in these moments—whether they're spent in quiet companionship, managing daily care tasks, or navigating medical appointments—that caregivers often discover a strong sense of accomplishment and pride. This sense of purpose is rooted in the positive impact caregivers have on the lives of those they care for, creating a bond that's both unique and deeply meaningful.

Caregiving invites a powerful introspection, urging caregivers to ponder over life's big questions and reevaluate what's genuinely important. Many caregivers develop a new appreciation for the fragility of life, the strength found in vulnerability, and the unparalleled value of time spent with loved ones. This shift in perspective often leads to a reordering of life's priorities, placing a greater emphasis on relationships, compassion, and empathy over material success or societal accolades.

This journey also fosters the growth of admirable traits such as patience, resilience, and understanding. Caregivers learn the art of patience through the slow progression of care, resilience through the ups and downs of their loved one's health, and empathy by putting themselves in the shoes of those they're caring for. These traits not only enhance the caregiver's character but also enrich their interactions with the world around them.

Caregiving can illuminate a path to gratitude, making one thankful for the moments of health, joy, and togetherness. This role, despite its demands, can offer a clearer perspective on life's true gifts, instilling a sense of gratitude for the present moment.

Caregiving is more than just a set of tasks; this journey can significantly change one's sense of purpose and meaning in life. It encourages a reevaluation of what's significant, fostering a life enriched with compassion, understanding, and a deep sense of fulfillment. Through the act of caring for another, caregivers often find themselves, discovering profound purpose and meaning.

$$\sim$$

GROWING THROUGH CAREGIVING: FINDING STRENGTH AND PURPOSE

TAKING care of someone can feel overwhelming at times, but believe it or not, this journey can be one of the most rewarding experiences of your life. Instead of seeing it just as a heavy responsibility, try to view it as a unique chance for personal growth and discovery.

Why See Caregiving as a Chance for Growth?

·   **Build Patience and Empathy**: Being there for someone in need teaches us to slow down, listen, and empathize with others. It's about stepping into their shoes and seeing the world from their perspective.

·   **Discover Inner Strengths**: Facing caregiving challenges head-on can reveal strengths you might not have known you had. It's about finding resilience in tough times and learning to navigate situations with grace.

·   **Deepen Connections**: This journey can strengthen the bonds between you and your loved one. It's an opportunity to share moments, big and small, and cherish them deeply.

·   **Learn Gratitude**: Caregiving helps us appreciate the small victories and the everyday moments. It teaches us to be grateful for our health, our relationships, and the time we have with our loved ones.

· **Find Fulfillment**: There's a profound sense of fulfillment that comes from making a difference in someone's life. It's about giving love and support and knowing it matters.

Sure, caregiving has its tough days, but it's also filled with moments of love, laughter, and learning. If you approach it with an open heart and a willingness to grow, you'll find the journey can be enriching.

So, let's embrace caregiving not just as a duty, but as an opportunity to grow, to love more deeply, and to find new meaning in our lives. Remember, you're not just giving care; you're growing, learning, and connecting on a deeply human level.

∼

SELF-CARE AND RESILIENCE FOR CAREGIVERS: NURTURING YOURSELF WHILE NURTURING OTHERS

LOOKING after someone in need is a big job that can take a lot out of you. To keep going without burning out, it's super important to look after yourself, know where your limits are, and build up your strength, both inside and out. Here's how you can do just that:

Make Time for You: You've got to see self-care as something that's as important as any appointment. Find time for things that make you happy and relaxed. It could be anything from getting lost in a good book, meditating, hitting the gym, to laughing with friends. Looking after your mind and body is key.

Draw the Line: It's okay to say no. Setting limits with the person you're caring for and others around you means you won't feel swamped. Sometimes, you might need to ask for help or take a breather, and that's okay. Boundaries help you keep your energy levels up and stress levels down.

Lean on Others: Don't do it all on your own. Joining a support group, chatting with a counselor, or venting to friends and family who get it can make a huge difference. Sharing your journey can give you a boost and some handy tips on handling the tricky parts.

Be Kind to Yourself: Remember, nobody's perfect. Go easy on yourself and understand that it's fine not to have all the answers or to feel over-whelmed sometimes. Treating yourself with kindness, especially when things don't go as planned, can help you bounce back quicker.

Stay Healthy: Eating right, staying active, getting enough sleep, and keeping those not-so-great habits in check are all part of taking care of yourself. When you're healthy, you've got more energy to give to the person you're caring for.

Do What You Love: Make sure you're still doing things that light you up. Whether it's a hobby, listening to your favorite tunes, enjoying nature, or getting creative, these refill your tank and keep you feeling like you.

Stay Present: Practices like deep breathing, meditation, or yoga can help you keep your cool and stay focused, especially on tough days. These tools can help you manage stress and keep your strength up when you need it most.

Taking care of yourself isn't selfish; it's essential. By making yourself a priority, setting clear boundaries, and building up your resilience, you're not just helping yourself; you're making sure you're there for your loved one in the best way possible.

~

BUILDING YOUR CAREGIVING VILLAGE: THE POWER OF SUPPORT NETWORKS

TAKING care of someone is a big deal, and let's be honest, it can get tough. That's why having a group of people you can rely on—family, friends, support groups, or doctors—is like having a secret super-power. It's not just about having someone to talk to when things get hard (though that's super important). It's about all the kinds of help they can give you.

A Shoulder to Lean On: Sometimes, you need to vent, cry, or share a laugh with someone who gets it. Having people who can be there for you emotionally is a big deal. It's comforting to know you're not alone.

An Extra Pair of Hands: Whether it's helping with the day-to-day stuff, like cooking or cleaning, or the big things, like doctor's appointments, having folks who can chip in is a lifesaver. It means you're not carrying the load all by yourself.

Wisdom and Tips: There's a lot to know about taking care of someone, especially if they're dealing with health issues. Support groups and healthcare pros can share all sorts of useful info and advice that can make things easier for you and your loved one.

Time for You: You can't pour from an empty cup, right? When you have people to back you up, you can find time to recharge your batteries. Whether it's hitting the gym, reading a book, or taking a nap, taking care of yourself is super important.

Meeting Fellow Caregivers: There's something special about connecting with others in the same boat. They know exactly what you're going through, and they might have some great advice or a listening ear when you need it.

Creating your support network—your caregiving village—isn't just a good idea; it's essential. It makes the tough times a little easier and reminds you you need not do everything on your own. So, reach out, ask for help, and remember, it's okay to lean on others.

~

CAREGIVING: STORIES OF LOVE, RESILIENCE, AND TRANSFORMATION

BEING a caregiver is more than just a role; it's a journey filled with love, challenges, and incredible moments that leave a lasting impact on both the caregiver and the person receiving care. These stories showcase just how powerful and transformative caregiving can be.

· Then there's *Lily*, who cared for her aging grandmother with dementia. Through the confusion and memory loss, Lily remained her grandmother's anchor, finding ways to connect with her even on the toughest days. Lily would play her grandmother's favorite songs, sparking moments of clarity and joy that were precious to them both. This experience taught Lily the true meaning of patience and the power of small moments to bring light in darkness.

These stories illuminate the profound sense of fulfillment and satisfaction that comes from caregiving. Beyond the challenges lie opportunities for growth, deeper connections, and an enriched understanding of what it means to care for another. Caregiving is a testament to the strength of the human spirit and the incredible impact we can have on each other's lives.

FREQUENTLY ASKED QUESTIONS:

1. How can I handle the emotional stress of caregiving without feeling overwhelmed?

Answer: Handling emotional stress begins with acknowledging your feelings - it's okay to feel overwhelmed, sad, or frustrated. These emotions are a normal part of caregiving. Find healthy outlets for your stress, like talking to a friend, journaling, or engaging in a hobby you love. Remember, seeking support from caregiver support groups or a counselor can provide relief and practical strategies for managing stress. Taking time for yourself isn't selfish; it's necessary to recharge and provide the best care for your loved one.

2. How do I balance caregiving duties with my personal life and work?

Answer: Balancing caregiving with personal life and work requires setting clear boundaries and focusing on tasks. Communicate openly with your employer about your caregiving situation; you may be surprised at the flexibility or support they can offer. Lean on your support network for help with caregiving duties, and don't shy away from using respite care services when you need a break. Remember, maintaining your own health and well-being is important to being a effective caregiver.

3. What are some ways to maintain a strong connection with my loved one as I care for them?

Answer: Maintaining a strong connection involves engaging in activities you both enjoy and can share. Whether it's reminiscing over old photos, listening to their favorite music, or enjoying nature, these moments can strengthen your bond. Be present and listen actively when they share their thoughts or emotions, showing empathy and understanding. Tailoring activities to their abilities and interests ensures they feel valued and respected.

4. How can caregiving lead to personal growth?

Answer: Caregiving can lead to personal growth by teaching you resilience, empathy, and the importance of human connection. It challenges you to develop new skills, from medical knowledge to emotional intelligence. This journey often brings a deeper appreciation for life, the strength found in vulnerability, and the value of each moment. Many caregivers find that through the challenges, they discover their own strength, develop a greater sense of purpose, and learn the true meaning of unconditional love.

5. How do I deal with the guilt of feeling burdened by caregiving?

Answer: Dealing with guilt starts by recognizing that feeling burdened is a natural response to the demands of caregiving, not a sign of failure or lack of love. Allow yourself to acknowledge these feelings without judgment. Share your feelings with trusted friends, family, or a support group who can offer perspective and understanding. Remember, taking breaks and seeking help when needed doesn't make you less of a caregiver—it makes you a more effective and compassionate one. Practicing self-compassion and setting realistic expectations for yourself are key to managing feelings of guilt.

Navigating caregiving is a profound journey that tests limits but also offers unparalleled opportunities for love, connection, and personal growth. Remember, you're not alone—seek support, take care of yourself, and embrace the journey with compassion and grace.

～

CASE STUDY: MARIA'S JOURNEY THROUGH CAREGIVING

MARIA, a 52-year-old mother of two, stepped into the role of caregiver when her mother, Elena, was diagnosed with early-stage Alzheimer's disease. The diagnosis came as a shock to the family, but Maria, being the closest in proximity and emotionally to Elena, naturally assumed the role of her primary caregiver.

At first, Maria found the caregiving role manageable. Elena's symptoms were mild, and she enjoyed the added time spent with her mother. However, as Elena's condition progressed, the demands of caregiving went up significantly. Maria juggled her job, her children's needs, and her mother's care. The emotional toll of watching her mother's decline, combined with the physical demands of caregiving, began to weigh heavily on Maria.

Challenges Faced:

1. **Emotional Stress:** Maria struggled with feelings of sadness and guilt. She mourned the loss of her mother's former self and felt guilty when she experienced frustration or anger over her caregiving responsibilities.

2.   **Physical Exhaustion:** As Elena's needs became more complex, Maria's physical exhaustion escalated. She had difficulty finding time for herself, leading to burnout.

3.   **Isolation:** Maria felt isolated from her friends and broader family. Her world narrowed to her caregiving responsibilities, leaving little room for social interactions.

4.   **Finding Balance:** Maria struggled to balance her role as a caregiver with her responsibilities as a mother, employee, and individual with her own needs.

Turning Points:

1.   **Seeking Support:** Maria joined a local support group for caregivers of Alzheimer's patients. Here, she found a community of people who understood her struggles and could offer practical advice and emotional support.

2.   **Setting Boundaries:** Maria learned the importance of setting boundaries for herself. She started to say no to more responsibilities and asked for help from her siblings and children in caring for Elena.

3.   **Self-Care:** Maria realized that taking care of herself was not selfish but essential. She began to carve out time for activities that rejuvenated her, such as weekly yoga classes and reading.

4.   **Focusing on Quality Time:** Maria shifted her focus from the tasks of caregiving to the quality of time spent with her mother. They enjoyed simple pleasures together, like looking through old photo albums and walking in the park.

Lessons Learned:

1.   **The Importance of Support:** Maria learned that seeking support, both emotionally and practically, was important in managing the stresses of caregiving. Support groups and family became invaluable resources.

2.   **Self-Care is Essential:** Maria discovered that caring for herself let

her be a better caregiver to her mother. Self-care was not a luxury but a necessity.

3.   **Finding Joy in the Journey:** Despite its challenges, caregiving brought Maria closer to her mother. They shared moments of joy and connection that Maria cherished.

4.   **Strength and Resilience:** Maria found strength she didn't know she had. She developed resilience in the face of adversity, learning to adapt and find solutions to new challenges.

Maria's journey through caregiving was marked by challenges, growth, and profound personal development. It taught her the importance of compassion, both for herself and for her mother, and highlighted the strength of human connection in the face of life's most challenging moments.

∽

PART NINETEEN WRAP-UP:

1. **Join a Support Group:** Seek local or online support groups for caregivers. These groups can offer emotional support, practical advice, and a sense of community with others who understand your journey.

2. **Set Clear Boundaries:** Determine what you can realistically handle and communicate your limits to family and friends. It's okay to say no to more responsibilities to prevent burnout.

3. **Schedule Regular Self-Care:** Make self-care a priority by scheduling time for activities that rejuvenate you. This could be exercise, hobbies, relaxation techniques, or simply quiet time alone.

4. **Ask for Help:** Don't hesitate to ask for help from family members, friends, or professional services. Delegate tasks when possible to lighten your load.

5. **Educate Yourself:** Learn as much as you can about your loved one's condition. Understanding the disease can help you anticipate needs and changes in their care.

6. **Implement Memory Care Activities:** Engage your loved one in activities that stimulate their mind and memories, such as looking through photo albums, listening to their favorite music, or simple puzzles.

7. **Focus on Quality Time:** Focus on spending quality time with your loved one. Cherish the moments of connection and joy, even in the midst of caregiving tasks.

8. **Plan for the Future:** Begin planning for future care needs, including financial planning, legal considerations, and potential long-term care options.

9. **Maintain Social Connections:** Make an effort to stay connected with friends and maintain social activities outside of caregiving to prevent isolation.

10. **Practice Mindfulness:** Incorporate mindfulness or meditation practices into your routine to manage stress and stay present.

11. **Document Important Information:** Keep a detailed record of medical information, medication schedules, doctor's appointments, and daily care routines for your loved one.

12. **Celebrate Small Victories:** Acknowledge and celebrate the small victories and positive moments in your caregiving journey to maintain a positive outlook.

These action items can help caregivers manage the challenges of their role while also finding fulfillment and maintaining their well-being.

～

IN OUR NEXT PART...

In our next Part, we dig into the rich tapestry of caregiving, exploring both its challenges and rewards through the lens of personal stories and experiences. This journey is not a solitary one; it's a shared path that many walk with courage, love, and resilience. Each story is a beacon of light, offering insights and understanding, and forging connections that transcend the boundaries of our individual journeys. As we venture into these narratives, we find solace in the shared struggles and triumphs, drawing strength from the knowledge that we are part of a larger community of caregivers. These stories serve as a reminder of the profound impact of caregiving on both the giver and the receiver, highlighting the deep, often unspoken bond that caregiving nurtures. Through these narratives, we aim to create a space of empathy, support, and understanding, inviting you to see your reflection in the stories of others and to recognize the universal themes of love, sacrifice, and growth that define the caregiving experience.

As we prepare to turn the page to this new chapter, remember that your story, too, is an invaluable part of this collective journey. Sharing your own experiences can be a powerful act of healing and connection, offering comfort to those who may feel isolated in their roles. This Part is not just about listening; it's an invitation to engage, to share, and to find your voice within the chorus of caregivers who have navigated the complexities of this path. It's a call to embrace the vulnerability that comes with sharing and to find strength in the solidarity of shared experiences. Let these stories inspire you to reflect on your own journey, to find meaning in the challenges, and to celebrate the profound connections that caregiving fosters. Together, let's explore the heart of caregiving, discovering the beauty and transformation that lie within the act of caring for another.

~

PART TWENTY - CONNECTING THROUGH STORIES: FINDING SOLACE AND STRENGTH TOGETHER

As WE WRAP up our journey together, let's reflect on the incredible power of sharing our personal stories and experiences. Through these stories, we find common ground, understanding, and a deep sense of connection with one another. Each narrative, with its unique challenges, triumphs, and insights, serves as a bridge, bringing us closer and reminding us of our shared humanity.

The act of sharing our stories is not just about recounting events; it's about opening our hearts and letting others see the world through our eyes. It's about vulnerability, courage, and the profound impact of knowing someone else has walked a path similar to ours. These stories offer comfort, inspire change, and foster a sense of community that transcends the pages of this book.

I invite you, the reader, to see this not as an end but as a beginning. A beginning of more conversations, more sharing, and more connections. Whether it's with friends, family, or strangers who share similar experiences, let your story be heard. You never know who might find hope, inspiration, or a sense of belonging through your words.

In the tapestry of life, each thread is significant, each color vibrant, and each pattern unique. Together, our stories weave a rich fabric of human experience that is both diverse and unified. As you move forward, carry with you the stories you've read here, and please add your own to the ever-growing quilt of human connection.

Thank you for sharing this journey. May you find strength in your story and in the stories of others, and may you continue to build connections that illuminate the shared paths of our lives.

～

NEW PERSPECTIVES
THROUGH SHARED STORIES

Diving into the stories of others opens up a world where we see life through a different lens, offering us new perspectives and insights we might have overlooked. It's like stepping into someone else's shoes, even if just for a moment, and viewing the world from where they stand. This journey of sharing and listening to personal tales is not just about understanding others; it's a gateway to discovering uncharted parts of our own selves and the world.

Each story shared is a beacon, illuminating paths we've never walked and experiences we've never lived. It challenges our preconceived notions, questions our biases, and enriches our understanding of what it means to be human. These narratives, in their raw and unfiltered form, have the power to reshape our worldview, making us more empathetic, more compassionate, and more connected to the tapestry of human experience.

In the stories of others, we find lessons we didn't know we needed, comfort in shared struggles, and joy in collective triumphs. They remind us that our own experiences, while unique, are part of a larger, interconnected narrative. This realization fosters a sense of belonging and solidarity, knowing that our personal journeys contribute to the rich mosaic of human life.

As you reflect on the stories you've encountered, consider how they've shifted your perspective or opened your mind to new ideas. Embrace this newfound understanding as a tool for growth and connection, letting it guide you in your interactions and your journey through life.

Let's carry forward the curiosity and openness that these stories have sparked in us, remaining ever receptive to the lessons and insights they offer. In doing so, we not only enrich our own lives but also contribute to a world that values understanding, empathy, and the unbreakable bonds of our shared humanity.

~

SHARING YOUR STORY: A GUIDE TO AUTHENTIC, IMPACTFUL STORYTELLING

Sharing your personal story is a powerful way to connect with others, offering insights and fostering understanding. But doing so in an authentic, impactful, and privacy-respecting manner is important. Here are tips to help you share your experiences effectively:

Know Your Why: Before sharing, ask yourself why you want to share your story. Understanding your motivation—whether it's to heal, educate, connect, or inspire—can guide how and what you share.

Set Your Boundaries: It's okay not to share everything. Decide in advance which parts of your story you're comfortable sharing and which parts you'd rather keep private. Your comfort matters most.

Stay True to Yourself: Your story is uniquely yours. Share it in a way that feels true to who you are, using your voice and style. Authenticity resonates more than perfection.

Respect Others' Privacy: If your story involves others, think about their privacy. Change names or details if necessary to protect their identities, and consider asking for their permission if their part in your story is significant.

Focus on the Takeaway: While the specifics of your story are important, the underlying message or lesson sticks with people. Highlight the insights or growth that came from your experiences.

Be a Good Listener: Storytelling is a two-way street. Be open to hearing and valuing the stories of others. This reciprocal exchange can deepen connections and mutual understanding.

Practice Empathy: Remember, everyone's story is different. Approach both sharing and listening with empathy, recognizing the courage it takes to open up and the value of diverse experiences.

By following these tips, you can share your story in a way that honors your experiences and respects your audience. Whether in a one-on-one conversation, in a group setting, or through written or digital formats, your story has the power to inspire, connect, and heal. Remember, every story shared is a gift to those who hear it.

~

BUILDING COMMUNITY
THROUGH STORIES:

SHARING our personal stories isn't just about opening up—it's about building bridges. It's about finding those threads that tie us all together, weaving a tapestry of experiences that highlight our shared humanity. This exchange of narratives is important for creating a community that thrives on empathy, understanding, and mutual support.

There's incredible power in realizing, "Hey, I've been there too," or "I know exactly how that feels." It breaks down the walls we often put up, thinking our struggles are ours alone to bear. Suddenly, you're not just a person with a story; you're part of a larger narrative, a community that gets it, that's been through it too, and that's there to support you.

Encouraging each other to share and connect over these stories is like laying down steppingstones across a river. It helps us cross difficult waters, knowing there's a hand to hold on the other side. This sense of belonging, of being part of something bigger, can be healing and empowering.

So, I urge you to reach out, to share your journey, and to listen to those around you. You might find that giving your story, you receive so much more—a community that stands with you, that laughs and cries with you, and that helps you see you're never alone.

In this ever-connected world, let's use our stories to bring us closer, to create a space where everyone feels understood and accepted. Let's remind each other of the strength found in shared experiences and the comfort in collective empathy. Your story matters, and it has the power to bring us together.

~

EMBRACING VULNERABILITY: THE PATH TO CONNECTION AND GROWTH

It is important to recognize the power of vulnerability in fostering genuine connections with others and experiencing transformative personal growth. By allowing ourselves to be open and authentic with others, we create space for deeper relationships and a sense of belonging fulfilling. Embracing vulnerability enables us to showcase our true selves and find acceptance and support. So, let us embrace vulnerability, open up to others, and see the immense impact it can have on our lives.

~

CONCLUSION: JOURNEY'S REFLECTION - THE HEART OF CAREGIVING

As we draw this guide to a close, it's essential to step back and reflect on the journey we've traversed together. The path of caregiving, woven with challenges, rewards, personal growth, and profound connections, is a testament to the strength and resilience of the human spirit.

Caregiving, in its essence, is an act of love and selflessness. It's a role that demands much from us—patience, empathy, and sacrifice—but also offers in return immeasurable rewards. The deep connections forged in the crucible of care, the personal growth sparked by the challenges faced, and the satisfaction found in making a real difference in someone's life are treasures that enrich our lives beyond measure.

As caregivers, we embark on a journey that transforms us. We learn the true meaning of resilience as we navigate the emotional highs and lows, finding strength we never knew we had. We discover the power of empathy, letting us connect with our loved ones in ways that transcend words and touch the essence of our being. And through the act of giving, we receive—lessons in love, insights into the human condition, and moments of profound joy and gratitude.

Let this guide be a reminder that you are not alone on this journey. Across the world, countless individuals share this path with you, each with their own stories of struggle, hope, and triumph. By reaching out, sharing experiences, and supporting one another, we build a community of caregivers bound by a common purpose and a shared understanding.

As we conclude, I encourage you to carry forward the lessons learned, and the insights gained. Embrace the role of caregiver with an open heart and a resilient spirit. Allow yourself to be vulnerable, to seek support when needed, and to celebrate the small victories along the way. Remember, the act of caregiving is not just about providing care; it's about nurturing the soul, both yours and your loved ones.

May you find strength knowing that your efforts make a world of difference. May you find comfort in the connections forged on this journey. And may you find fulfillment in the love shared and the lives touched.

Thank you for embracing the call to care. Your journey is a beacon of hope and a testament to the boundless capacity for love and compassion that lives within each of us. Let's move forward with courage, knowing that in the heart of caregiving lies the essence of our shared humanity.

~

ABOUT THE AUTHOR

With a rich career spanning over four decades in psychiatric and mental health nursing, Rae brings a wealth of compassionate insights and profound wisdom to both his writing and speaking engagements.

As a distinguished member of Toastmasters International for over 30 years, Rae has honed his communication skills and self-confidence, enabling him to impart valuable personal development insights. His unique style combines conversational ease with direct engagement, making his books and presentations not only informative but also deeply relatable.

Rae's approach is marked by a blend of wry humor and sage advice, drawing from a lifetime of experiences in nursing and a commitment to continuous personal growth. Although retired from his nursing career, he continues to thrive in his roles as a writer, speaker, and mentor, empowering others to realize their full potential.

Beyond his professional pursuits, he has been productive as a do-it-yourselfer in renovating three older homes, one being a heritage home. As a legal boarding home, it had the reputation of being a brothel and illicit drug distribution center at a point in time. He also worked with building contractors to create three new homes and doing all the interior decorating and exterior landscaping himself with the help of his wife Sandra.

Rae is an avid gardener, cultivating a lush array of flowers, shrubs, and vegetables.

Residing in the picturesque Kelowna, British Columbia, Rae shares his life with his wife Sandra, a fellow retired nurse, their son Jeffrey, daughter-in-law Jennifer, and the joy of his life, granddaughter Maybelle. His journey is a testament to the power of lifelong learning and the pursuit of excellence in every endeavor.

~

ALSO BY RAE A. STONEHOUSE

VISIT HTTPS://LIVEFOREXCELLENCE.STORE/ for a selection of personal/professional self-development books by Rae A. Stonehouse.

If you have found this book to be helpful, please leave us a warm review wherever you purchased it.

www.ingramcontent.com/pod-product-compliance
Lightning Source LLC
Chambersburg PA
CBHW062129040426
42335CB00039B/1813